STUDY GUIDE & LABORATORY MANUAL

PHYSICAL EXAMINATION & HEALTH ASSESSMENT

9TH EDITION

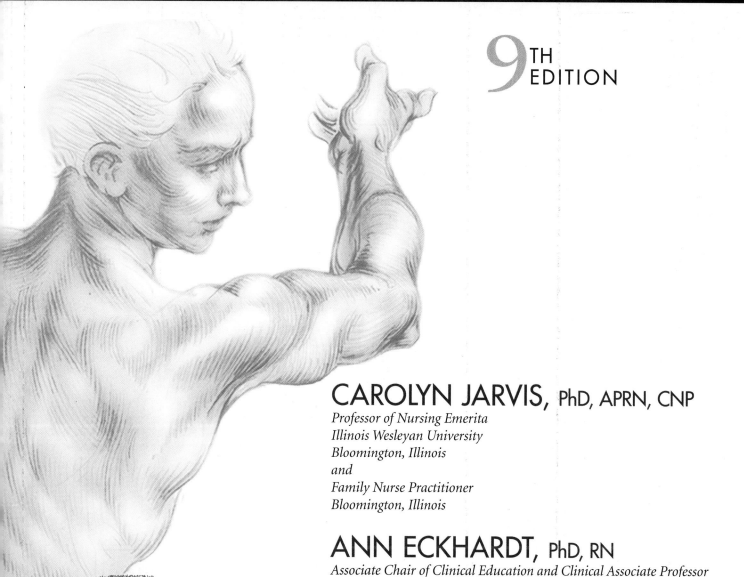

CAROLYN JARVIS, PhD, APRN, CNP
Professor of Nursing Emerita
Illinois Wesleyan University
Bloomington, Illinois
and
Family Nurse Practitioner
Bloomington, Illinois

ANN ECKHARDT, PhD, RN
Associate Chair of Clinical Education and Clinical Associate Professor
College of Nursing and Health Innovation
University of Texas at Arlington
Arlington, Texas

Elsevier
3251 Riverport Lane
St. Louis, Missouri 63043

Content Strategist: Heather Bays-Petrovic
Content Development Manager: Danielle M. Frazier
Publishing Services Manager: Deepthi Unni
Project Manager: Thoufiq Mohammed
Design Direction: Brian Salisbury

Printed in the United States of America

Last digit is the print number: 9 8 7 6 5 4 3 2 1

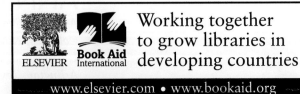

Contributors

Lydia Bertschi, DNP, APRN, ACNP-BC
Assistant Professor
Illinois Wesleyan University
Bloomington, Illinois
Chapter 19, Thorax and Lungs, Chapter 20, Heart and Neck Vessels, Chapter 21 Peripheral Vascular System, Chapter 22, Abdomen

Amanda Kemp, MSN, RN
Simulation Coordinator
School of Nursing
Illinois Wesleyan University
Bloomington, Illinois
Chapter 33, Next-Generation NCLEX® (NGN) Examination–Style Unfolding Case Studies

Pat Thomas, CMY, FAMI
East Troy, Wisconsin
Original Illustrations

Preface

This *Study Guide & Laboratory Manual* is intended to accompany the textbook *Physical Examination & Health Assessment*, 9th edition. You, the student, will use it in two places: in your own study area and in the skills laboratory.

As a *Study Guide*, this workbook highlights and reinforces the content from the text. Each chapter corresponds to a chapter in the textbook and contains activities and questions in varying formats to promote your mastery of content from the text. Fill out the lab manual chapter and answer the questions before coming to the skills laboratory. This will reinforce your lectures, expose any areas in which you have questions for your clinical instructor, and prime you for the skills laboratory/clinical experience.

Once in the skills laboratory, use the *Laboratory Manual* as a direct clinical tool. Each chapter contains assessment forms on perforated, tear-out pages. Usually you will work in pairs and perform the regional physical examinations on each other under the tutelage of your instructor. As you perform the examination on your peer, you can fill out the regional write-up and turn it in to the instructor for feedback.

FEATURES

Each chapter is divided into two parts—cognitive and clinical—and contains:

- Purpose—A brief summary of the material you are learning in the chapter.
- Reading Assignment—The corresponding chapter and page numbers from the *Physical Examination & Health Assessment* textbook.
- Suggested journal articles—All new for the 9th edition, these are current and choice readings for critical thinking and for interventions.
- Glossary—Important or specialized terms with accompanying definitions.
- Study Guide—Specific short-answer and fill-in questions to help you highlight and learn content from the chapter. New critical thinking questions are included to coordinate the reading and video assignments. Important illustrations of human anatomy, in full color, have been reproduced from the textbook with the labels deleted so you can identify and fill in the names of the structures yourself.
- Clinical Judgment Questions—New multiple-choice questions, matching, and all-new Next-Generation NCLEX® (NGN) – Style Questions so you can monitor your own mastery of the material. Take the self-exam and then check the answer key provided in the back of the book.
- Critical Thinking Activities—most are new for the 9th edition.
- Clinical Objectives—behavioral objectives to achieve during your peer practice in the regional examinations.
- Regional Write-Up Sheets—complete yet succinct physical exam forms that you can use in the skills lab. These list key history questions and physical examination steps, and a means of recording data during the patient encounter.
- Narrative Summary Forms—SOAP format, so you learn to chart narrative accounts of the history and physical exam findings. These forms have accompanying sketches of regional anatomy.
- New Chapter 33 includes Next Generation NCLEX®—Style Unfolding Case Studies. These present a new stage for you to practice prioritizing, decision-making, and using clinical judgment skills.

Learning the skills of history taking and physical examination requires two types of practice: cognitive and clinical. It is our hope that this manual will help you achieve both of these learning and practice modalities.

CAROLYN JARVIS
ANN ECKHARDT

Acknowledgments

We are grateful to those on the team at Elsevier who worked on the *Laboratory Manual*. Our thanks extend to Heather Bays-Petrovic, Content Strategist for organizing and reorganizing our new content; Danielle Frazier, Content Development Manager for hunting and acquiring material; Thoufiq Mohammed, Project Manager for patience and planning; Deepthi Unni, Publishing Services Manager; and Brian Salisbury, Book Designer. We are dependent on this wonderful team to bring our vision into print and to make it useful for our students.

Contents

CHAPTER

1

Evidence-Based Assessment

PURPOSE

This chapter discusses the characteristics of evidence-based practice, diagnostic reasoning, the nursing process, clinical judgment, and critical thinking. This chapter also introduces the database and helps you understand that the amount of data gathered during assessment varies with the physical condition and risk factors.

READING ASSIGNMENT

Jarvis: *Physical Examination and Health Assessment*, 9th ed., Chapter 1, pp. 1–8.

Suggested reading:
Robichaux, C., & Sauerland, J. (2021). The social determinants of health, COVID-19, and structural competence. *OJIN: Online J Issues Nurs, 26*(2), 1–13.

GLOSSARY

Study the following terms after completing the reading assignment. You should be able to cover the definition on the right and define the term out loud.

Assessment .... the collection of data about an individual's health state

Clinical Judgment Model .... a way of structuring nursing education to enhance clinical judgment skills of novice practitioners

Complete database .... a complete health history and full physical examination

Critical thinking .... simultaneously problem solving while self-improving one's own thinking ability

Emergency database .... rapid collection of the database, often compiled concurrently with lifesaving measures

Environment .... the total of all the conditions and elements that make up the surroundings and influence the development of a person

Epigenetics .... the study of how environment and behaviors impact gene expression

Evidence-based practice .... a systematic approach emphasizing the best research evidence, the clinician's experience, patient preferences and values, physical examination, and assessment

Focused database .... used for a limited or short-term problem; concerns mainly one problem, one cue complex, or one body system

Follow-up database .... used in all settings to monitor progress of short-term or chronic health problems

Holistic health .... the view that the mind, body, and spirit are interdependent and function as a whole within the environment

Nursing process .... a method of collecting and analyzing clinical information with the following components: (1) assessment, (2) diagnosis, (3) outcome identification, (4) planning, (5) implementation, and (6) evaluation

Objective data .... what the health professional observes by inspecting, palpating, percussing, and auscultating during the physical examination

Prevention .... any action directed toward promoting health and preventing the occurrence of disease

Social Determinants of Health .... factors that influence a person's health and well-being, including the environment, access to health care, community, education, and economic stability

Subjective data .... what the person says during history taking

STUDY GUIDE

After completing the reading assignment, you should be able to answer the following questions in the spaces provided.

1. One of the critical-thinking skills is the ability to identify assumptions. Explain how the following statement contains an assumption. What is a more appropriate response? *"Ellen, you have to break up with your boyfriend. He is too rough with you. He is no good for you."*

2. Another critical-thinking skill involves validation or checking the accuracy and reliability of data. Describe how you would validate the following data.

   Mr. Quinn tells you his weight this morning was 165 lbs.

The primary counselor tells you Ellen is depressed and angry about being admitted to residential treatment in the clinic.

When auscultating the heart, you hear a blowing, swooshing sound between the first and second heart sounds.

The previous RN tells you that Mr. Jones's family is aloof and does not visit regularly.

3. List the barriers to evidence-based practice, both on an individual level and on an organizational level.

4. Differentiate **subjective** data from **objective** data by placing an **S** or an **O** after each of the following: complaint of sore shoulder _____; unconscious _____; blood in urine _____; family has just moved to a new area _____; dizziness _____; sore throat _____; earache _____; weight gain _____.

5. For the following situations, state the type of data collection you would perform (i.e., *complete* database, *focused* or problem-centered database, *follow-up* database, *emergency* database).
    OxyContin overdose _____; ambulatory, apparently well individual who presents at outpatient clinic with a rash _____; first visit to a health care provider for a checkup _____; recently placed on antihypertensive medication _____.

6. Discuss the impact of racial and cultural diversity in individuals on the U.S. health care system.

7. List three health care interactions you have experienced with a person from a culture or ethnicity different from your own. Were they positive or negative? What could or should have been done differently?

8. Using one sentence or group of phrases, how would you describe your own health state to someone you are meeting for the first time?

CLINICAL JUDGMENT QUESTIONS

This test is for you to check your own mastery of the content. Answers are provided in Appendix A.

1. A. S., a 35-year-old, is at your clinic today for a well visit. She recently moved to the area and is establishing with a new primary care provider. What information would you include in the database for this new patient? **Select all that apply.**

   a. Current health state
   b. Lifestyle and risk factors
   c. Only subjective information
   d. Only objective information
   e. Physical examination
   f. Health maintenance behaviors
   g. Your perception of the patient's health
   h. The patient's perception of current health

2. You are reviewing assessment data of a 45-year-old male patient who had recent surgery and rates his pain at 8 on a 10-point scale. As you review the electronic health record, you note which of the following cues related to the patient's pain? **Select all that apply.**

   a. Normal skin turgor
   b. Normal S1, S2 heart sounds
   c. Pale skin
   d. Tachypnea (rapid breathing)
   e. Tachycardia (rapid pulse)
   f. Clear breath sounds

3. You are working in the emergency department and receive a patient who was admitted via ambulance. The patient is alert, but the injuries are severe. What are your priorities when collecting this patient's emergency database?

   a. A complete health history and full physical examination
   b. A full list of medications, allergies, family history, and personal history
   c. Previously identified problems including any current treatments and health promotion
   d. Collect critical information as you begin lifesaving measures

4. You are caring for a patient who was recently diagnosed with type 1 diabetes. She is learning to manage her diabetes and will need support after discharge. Her knowledge deficit is considered a _____ priority problem and will require a collaborative effort with health care professionals.

   a. First-level
   b. Second-level
   c. Third-level

5. You completed the health history and physical examination on your new admission. After completing the assessment phase of the nursing process, the next step includes which of the following?

    a. Interpreting clinical findings and determining a diagnosis
    b. Clustering cues and evaluating assessment data
    c. Collaborating with the patient and reviewing information
    d. Evaluating the information collected and determining next steps

For questions 6–10 use the following information:

G.R. is a 75-year-old male who presents to the emergency department with chest pain, palpitations, and appears pale and diaphoretic. As the history and physical are completed, the following problems emerge. Please label them first-, second-, or third-level priority problems.

6. Blood pressure 74/50, HR 148 _____

7. Serum potassium 2.7 mmol/L (low), Glucose 225 mg/dL (high) _____

8. Lives alone, no family in the area _____

9. Acute chest pain with radiation to jaw _____

10. Unfamiliar with heart-healthy dietary guidelines _____

11. Which of the following are objective data? **Select all that apply.**

    a. 2-cm scar on dorsal surface of the hand
    b. Complaints of nausea
    c. Clear breath sounds
    d. Headache
    e. BP 110/72

12. S.Q. was just admitted because of cellulitis of her lower extremity due to a cat scratch. She was previously treated outpatient but missed multiple appointments and did not take her medication. As you complete the health history, she shares that she is sleeping on her sister's couch because she lost her job. She lives in an area of town considered a food desert and often eats whatever she can find from a local gas station or fast-food restaurant. She missed her last two follow-up visits for her leg due to inadequate transportation and could not afford to purchase the expensive antibiotics prescribed. Which of the following best describes factors that are influencing her well-being?

    a. S.Q. is not motivated to be compliant with health care provider recommendations. She should make sure she attends all appointments.
    b. Social determinants of health, including lack of economic stability and an environment that lacks nutritious food options, are negatively impacting S.Q.
    c. Social determinants of health are important, but she can overcome these barriers if she tries hard enough.
    d. S.Q. should work harder to get a new job so she has improved economic stability and may be able to become self-sufficient.

13. Evidence-based nursing practice is:

    a. Combining clinical expertise with the use of nursing research to provide the best care for patients while considering the patient's values and circumstances
    b. Appraising and looking at the implications of one or two articles as they relate to the culture and ethnicity of the patient
    c. Completing a literature search to find relevant articles that use nursing research to encourage nurses to use good practices
    d. Finding value-based resources to justify nursing actions when working with patients of diverse cultural backgrounds

NOTES

CHAPTER
2
Cultural Assessment

PURPOSE

This chapter reviews the demographic profile of the United States, the National Standards for Culturally and Linguistically Appropriate Services in Health Care, traditional health/illness beliefs and practices, and information on cultural assessment. At the end of the chapter, you will be able to perform a cultural assessment.

READING ASSIGNMENT

Jarvis: *Physical Examination and Health Assessment*, 9th ed., Chapter 2, pp. 9–18.

Suggested reading:
Lopez, L., Hart. L. H., & Katz, M. H. (2021). Racial and ethnic health disparities related to COVID-19. *JAMA, 325*(8), 719–720.
Carron, R. (2020). Health disparities in American Indians/Alaska Natives: Implications for nurse practitioners. *Nurse Pract, 46*(6), 26–32.

GLOSSARY

Study the following terms after completing the reading assignment. You should be able to cover the definition on the right and define the term out loud.

Acculturation .... process of social and psychological exchanges with encounters between persons of different cultures, resulting in changes in either group

Cultural and linguistic competence .... a set of congruent behaviors, attitudes, and policies that come together in a system among professionals that enables work in cross-cultural situations

Cultural care .... professional health care that is culturally sensitive, appropriate, and competent

Culture .... the nonphysical attributes of a person—the thoughts, communications, actions, beliefs, values, and institutions of racial, ethnic, religious, or social groups

Cultural awareness .... recognition of differences and similarities between cultures; recognition and understanding of one's own culture

Cultural humility .... recognition of the value and worth of cultures other than one's own; respect for intracultural variation

Cultural knowledge .... knowledge of different cultural characteristics

Cultural skills .... ability to complete a thorough cultural assessment and recognize potential variations in people based on cultural background

Ethnicity .... a social group within the social system that claims to possess variable traits such as a common geographic origin, migratory status, and religion

Folk healer .... lay healer in the person's culture apart from the biomedical or scientific health care system

Health or illness .... the balance or imbalance of the person, both within one's being (physical, mental, and/or spiritual) and in the outside world (natural, communal, and/or metaphysical)

Religion .... an organized system of beliefs concerning the cause, nature, and purpose of the universe, as well as attendance at regular services

Socialization .... the process of being raised within a culture and acquiring the characteristics of that group

Spirituality .... a broad term focused on a connection to something larger than oneself, and a belief in transcendence

Title VI of the Civil Rights Act of 1964 .... a federal law that mandates that when people with limited English proficiency (LEP) seek health care in health care settings such as hospitals, nursing homes, clinics, daycare centers, and mental health centers, services cannot be denied to them

Values .... a desirable or undesirable state of affairs and a universal feature of all cultures

STUDY GUIDE

After completing the reading assignment, you should be able to answer the following questions in the spaces provided.

1. Describe the provisions of Title VI of the Civil Rights Act of 1964.

2. Describe the rationale for providing culturally appropriate care.

3. List the basic characteristics of culture.

4. List and describe factors related to socialization.

5. List and define three major theories about how people view the causes of illness.

6. Define the *yin yang theory* of health and illness and relate this to different health care beliefs.

7. Define the *hot and cold theory* of health and illness and relate this to different health care beliefs.

8. Describe five methods of complementary interventions.

CLINICAL JUDGMENT QUESTIONS

This test is for you to check your own mastery of the content. Answers are provided in Appendix A.

1. Which statement best describes religion?

   a. An organized system of beliefs concerning the cause, nature, and purpose of the universe
   b. Belief in a divine or superhuman spirit to be obeyed and worshiped
   c. Affiliation with one of the 1200 recognized religions in the United States
   d. The following of established rituals, especially in conjunction with health-seeking behaviors

2. The major factor contributing to the need for cultural care nursing is:

   a. An increasing birth rate.
   b. Limited access to health care services.
   c. Demographic change.
   d. A decreasing rate of immigration.

3. You are the triage nurse in the emergency department and perform the initial intake assessment on a patient who does not speak English. Based on your understanding of linguistic competence, which action would present as a barrier to effective communication?

   a. Maintaining a professional, respectful demeanor
   b. Allowing for additional time to complete the process
   c. Providing the patient with a paper and pencil so answers can be written
   d. Obtaining interpreter services so the family does not need to translate

4. The first step to cultural competency by a nurse is to:

   a. Identify the meaning of health to the patient.
   b. Understand how a health care delivery system works.
   c. Develop a frame of reference to traditional health care practices.
   d. Understand their heritage and its basis in cultural values.

5. Which statement is most appropriate to use when initiating an assessment of cultural beliefs with a patient?

   a. "Are you of the Christian faith?"
   b. "Do you want to see a medicine man?"
   c. "How often do you seek help from medical providers?"
   d. "What cultural or spiritual beliefs are important to you?"

6. Which statement best reflects the biomedical causation of illness?
   a. Each being is only a part of a larger structure in the world of nature as it relates to health and illness.
   b. Causal relationship exists, leading to expression of illness.
   c. Belief in the struggle between good and evil is reflected in the regulation of health and illness.
   d. Illness occurs as a result of disturbances between hot and cold reactions.

7. You are caring for a Jewish patient who needs a leg amputation. The patient is concerned about what will happen to the leg after amputation and becomes visibly distraught when you inform him it will be disposed of by the hospital. What should you do?

   a. Provide information on postoperative prosthetics so he understands that loss of the limb does not limit physical ability.
   b. Provide education on the surgical procedure and what to expect in the immediate post-operative period so he feels more prepared.
   c. Ask if he would like you to contact friends, family, or the hospital chaplain so he can talk about how he feels.
   d. Ask about his cultural beliefs and whether there is anything the hospital can do to support him before, during, and after surgery.

For questions 8–9 use the following information: *You are a nurse in the university health center. You notice that X.L. is on your list for the fourth time in the past three months. Her previous complaints include weight loss and fatigue. Today, she is in the clinic for irregular periods and appears pale with hollow cheekbones. She is a 19-year-old first-year student with an uneventful past medical history. She is a first-generation college student whose parents immigrated from Iran 20 years ago.*

8. What questions should be included in a cultural assessment? **Select all that apply.**

   a. Are there any foods that you are unable to eat due to cultural beliefs?
   b. Are you using any complementary or alternative treatments currently?
   c. Could pregnancy be the reason for your irregular periods and illness?
   d. What is your favorite food to eat?
   e. How are you doing in your classes? Have you been able to make friends?

9. During further investigation you discover that X.L. follows a Halal diet. You know very little about the diet. What is the most appropriate next step?

   a. Ask X.L. about the diet she follows and whether she has access to appropriate food in the university dining facility.
   b. Complete a physical assessment to determine the cause of her progressive symptoms.
   c. Make a note of the diet in her chart and plan to do research on the diet prior to seeing your next patient.
   d. Complete a thorough health history to determine if she has experienced any changes in health since her last appointment.

10. During report on a 39-year-old Hispanic male, you learn that the patient had surgery yesterday but has refused all pain medication and denies any pain. As you assess the patient, you notice an elevated heart rate and blood pressure as well as grimacing with abdominal palpation, but the patient continues to deny pain. You:

    a. continue the assessment believing that if a patient is in pain, they will tell you.
    b. recognize that pain expression may vary based on culture and that all Hispanic men do not take pain medications

    c. recognize that pain expression may vary based on culture and ask appropriate cultural assessment questions
    d. recognize that men do not respond to pain the same way as women, and they may not feel pain the same way

11. You are caring for a patient who requests that a shaman (medicine man) visit him while he is hospitalized. He would like a smudging ritual completed prior to his upcoming treatment. You know that smudging involves the burning of sage. Your best response is:

    a. We cannot allow that ritual in the hospital because we do not allow open flames.
    b. Call your shaman and have him come any time. Just make sure to close the door.
    c. Let's work with the shaman to determine the best way to complete the ritual in a safe manner.
    d. Don't worry. Dr. Smith is the best, so you have nothing to worry about.

CLINICAL JUDGMENT EXERCISE 1

Consider the following clinical examples. What is your reaction to each example? How would you handle the situation if you were a part of the conversation or overheard either conversation?

- **Situation 1:** You receive report on a new admission who is coming in with pancreatitis. During report, you are told that the woman's primary language is Spanish. After you share this information with the admitting physician, the physician states, "Oh, great! I sure hope she has somebody with her who can speak English. You KNOW what a pain it is to set up and use the translator system. What am I saying?! She is sure to have SOMEONE with her who speaks English. Those people ALWAYS come in packs."
- **Situation 2:** You are at the nurses' station and overhear the following conversation:
  Person 1: "I need to know which patient is going home so that I can write discharge orders."
  Person 2: "The Indian family."
  Person 1 (laughing): "Indian how? Red dot or red feather?"
- **Situation 3:** A nurse is visibly upset and crying at the nurses' station. She tells you: "The patient in 3201 is going to die! She is experiencing postpartum hemorrhage but won't accept a blood transfusion because of her religion. I wish I could convince her to get the transfusion. I don't understand why she's worried about it."
- **Situation 4:** The emergency department nurse calls to give report on a new admission. This is the information you receive:
  "John or wait, he goes by something else now—I mean she (snickering). This is a private room, right? He…she…I don't know…I'll just say it has a penis, but boobs. You cannot put this in with a male or female patient!"

CLINICAL JUDGMENT EXERCISE 2

With a partner or a small group, discuss common stereotypes you have heard, seen, or believe. Be open and honest in your discussion. Where do the stereotypes come from? How might a negative stereotype impact the care you provide a patient? How will being aware of stereotypes potentially enhance patient care?

SKILLS LABORATORY AND CLINICAL SETTING

You are now ready for the clinical component of this chapter. The purpose of the clinical component is to collect data for a cultural assessment on a peer in the skills laboratory or on a patient in the clinical setting. Although you may not yet have been assigned chapters on the health history, the questions asked during a cultural assessment are clearly defined and should pose no problem. The best experience would be for you to pair up with a peer from a cultural heritage *different* from your own. If this is not possible, you will still gain insight and sensitivity into the cultural dimensions of health and will gain mastery of cultural assessment. Prior to completing the cultural assessment on a peer, complete a cultural self-assessment. Be honest with yourself as you consider your own cultural beliefs and values. Use the "Becoming a Culturally Sensitive Practitioner" section of your text to guide your self-assessment and the cultural assessment of a peer.

The Interview

PURPOSE

This chapter discusses the process of communication; presents the techniques of interviewing, including open-ended versus closed questions, the 9 types of examiner responses, the 10 "traps" of interviewing, and nonverbal skills; and considers variations in technique that are necessary for individuals of different ages, for those with special needs, and for culturally diverse people.

READING ASSIGNMENT

Jarvis: *Physical Examination and Health Assessment*, 9th ed., Chapter 3, pp. 19–40.

Suggested reading:
Cottrell, D. B. (2019). Fostering sexual and gender minority status disclosure in patients. *Nurse Pract*, 44(7), 43–48.
National Institutes of Health Office of Equity, Diversity, and Inclusion. (n.d.). Sexual and Gender Minority. https://www.edi.nih.gov/people/sep/lgbti/research

GLOSSARY

Study the following terms after completing the reading assignment. You should be able to cover the definition on the right and define the term out loud.

Ad hoc interpreter .... using a patient's family member, friend, or child as interpreter for a patient with limited English proficiency (LEP)

Animism .... imagining that inanimate objects (e.g., a blood pressure cuff) come alive and have human characteristics

Avoidance language .... the use of euphemisms to avoid reality or to hide feelings

Clarification .... examiner's response used when the patient's word choice is ambiguous or confusing

Closed questions .... questions that ask for specific information and elicit a short, one- or two-word answer, a "yes" or "no," or a forced choice

Confrontation .... response in which examiner gives honest feedback about what they have seen or felt after observing a certain patient action, feeling, or statement

Distancing .... the use of impersonal speech to put space between oneself and a threat

Elderspeak .... infantilizing and demeaning language used by a health professional when speaking to an older adult

Empathy .... viewing the world from the other person's inner frame of reference while remaining yourself; recognizing and accepting the other person's feelings without criticism

Explanation .... examiner's statements that inform the patient; examiner shares factual and objective information

Facilitation .... examiner's response that encourages the patient to say more, to continue with the story

Gender identity .... how a person sees themselves in relation to roles and behaviors that are socially assigned to different genders

Geographic privacy .... private room or space with only the examiner and patient present

Interpretation .... examiner's statement that is not based on direct observation, but is based on examiner's inference or conclusion; links events, makes associations, or implies cause

Interview .... meeting between the examiner and patient with the goal of gathering a complete health history

Jargon .... medical vocabulary used with a patient in an exclusionary and paternalistic way

Leading question .... a question implying one answer is better than another

Nonverbal communication .... message conveyed through body language—posture, gestures, facial expression, eye contact, touch, and even where one places the chairs

Open-ended question .... asks for longer narrative information; unbiased; leaves the person free to answer in any way

Reflection .... examiner response that echoes the patient's words; repeats part of what the patient has just said

Sexual orientation .... refers to sexual and emotional attraction to others (i.e., heterosexual, bisexual, gay)

Summary .... final review of what examiner understands patient has said, condenses facts and presents a survey of how the examiner perceives the health problem or need

Telegraphic speech .... speech used by age 3 or 4 years in which three- or four-word sentences contain only the essential words

Verbal communication .... messages sent through spoken words, vocalizations, or tone of voice

STUDY GUIDE

After completing the reading assignment, you should be able to answer the following questions in the spaces provided.

1. List eight items of information that should be communicated to the client concerning the terms or expectations of the interview.

2. Describe points to consider in preparing the physical setting for the interview.

3. List the pros and cons of notetaking during the interview.

4. Contrast open-ended versus closed questions and explain the purpose of each during the interview.

5. List the nine types of examiner responses that could be used during the interview and give a short example of each.

6. List the 10 traps of interviewing and give a short example of each.

7. State at least six types of nonverbal behaviors.

8. State a useful phrase to use as a closing when ending the interview.

9. Discuss special considerations when interviewing an older adult.

10. How would you modify your interviewing technique when working with a hearing-impaired person?

11. Formulate a response you would make to a client who has spoken in a sexually aggressive way.

12. List at least five points to consider when using an interpreter during an interview.

13. List three examples of heterosexist language or behavior that are commonplace in health care.

CLINICAL JUDGMENT QUESTIONS

This test is for you to check your own mastery of the content. Answers are provided in Appendix A.

1. The practitioner, entering the examining room to meet a patient for the first time, states: "Hello, I'm M.M., and I'm here to gather some information from you and to perform your examination. This will take about 30 minutes. D.D. is a student working with me. If it's all right with you, she will remain during the examination." Which of the following must be added to cover all aspects of the interview contract?

    a. A statement regarding confidentiality, patient costs, and the expectations of each person
    b. The purpose of the interview and the role of the interviewer
    c. Time and place of the interview and a confidentiality statement
    d. An explicit purpose of the interview and a description of the physical examination, including diagnostic studies

2. Which of the following are open-ended questions? **Select all that apply.**

    a. Tell me about your headaches.
    b. Describe your chest pain.
    c. Point to where the pain is.
    d. What do you expect from me as your nurse?
    e. Do you want to discuss all your options?

3. M.J., age 85, has been diagnosed with terminal lung cancer. During report you were told that the family does not want her to know the diagnosis. M.J. asks you, "Am I going to die?" Which of the following is the best therapeutic response from you, the nurse?

    a. "Tell me what prompted that question."
    b. "I will ask your physician to discuss this matter with you."
    c. "Let's take each day as it comes."
    d. "I think you should discuss that with your family."

4. When teaching a client how to effectively manage their new medication regimen, the nurse recognizes that the best method of communicating therapeutically with the client is to:

a. Talk to the client in the visitors' lounge
b. Talk to the client within his personal space
c. Communicate with the client using touch
d. Face the client while leaning slightly forward

5. Factors important during an interview include: **Select all that apply.**

a. Equal status seating
b. Leading questions
c. Active listening
d. Distancing
e. Social responses
f. Avoidance language
g. Providing privacy
h. Professional jargon

6. You are preparing to do the initial interview with a 15-year-old patient. In order to establish rapport, you:

a. Begin the interview by immediately discussing the health concern. Adolescents do not want small talk and want to finish as quickly as possible.
b. Begin the interview by completing the full health history and discussing drug/alcohol use. Adolescents want to finish as quickly as possible.
c. Begin the interview by asking open, friendly questions about school and hobbies. Adolescents appreciate the opportunity to discuss themselves.
d. Begin the interview by asking open-ended questions that explore the health history. Adolescents are knowledgeable, and you can speak to them like adults.

7. Which of the following statements/questions need to be rewritten to avoid heterosexist language? **Select all that apply.**

a. What type of birth control do you use?
b. Are you in a relationship?
c. What is your marital status?
d. What is your personal pronoun?
e. Please circle your gender: Male Female

8. You work in the emergency department, and an 88-year-old Spanish-speaking patient was just brought by ambulance with chest pain. You do not speak Spanish and there is no in-person interpreter available. Your best option to ensure communication is:

a. Identify a friend or family member who can provide interpreter services. It's better to have someone in person.
b. Leverage technology to ensure communication. Your hospital recently invested in video interpreter services.
c. Use gestures, simple words, and a loud voice to work through the history and physical exam.
d. Call another floor and see if they have anyone who knows Spanish. The patient can probably wait for a while.

9. Mark each of the following statements as therapeutic or nontherapeutic.

Statement	Therapeutic	Nontherapeutic
I'm sure everything will be fine.		
You sound upset. Please tell me more about what happened today.		
Dr. Daniels knows what he is talking about. Just follow his recommendations.		
What are the pros and cons of surgery?		
If I were you, I would get another opinion before having surgery.		
Why did you wait so long to see the doctor after the symptoms began?		
You must not eat or drink anything after midnight except for small sips of water to take your morning pills.		
No need to cry. Let's move on to a different topic.		

10. Nonverbal behaviors are just as important as verbal behaviors. Please mark the following behaviors as positive or negative.

Behavior	Positive	Negative
Tapping a pen rhythmically on the table.		
Warm smile while leaning slightly forward.		
Moderate tone of voice and rate of speech.		
Frequently crossing and uncrossing legs.		
Arms crossed over chest.		
Standing by the client's bed.		

CRITICAL THINKING ACTIVITY 1

Practice is an important part of developing communication skills. With a partner, record a patient–nurse interaction. Have your partner pretend to be a patient seeking health care at a local clinic. The partner should create a character, such as a single mother describing vague symptoms in an attempt to get a prescription for her uninsured children, an older woman who focuses the interview on the student nurse's personal life instead of answering the questions, a client who is angry about having to wait 30 minutes to be seen, or a young man who thinks he has a sexually transmitted infection but does not want to discuss his symptoms. You can choose your own character, but it should be someone who poses a communication challenge. You may want to ask your instructor for potential vignettes. Entering the interview, you will not know the real reason for the visit and must rely on therapeutic communication skills to determine how to effectively communicate with the patient. The interviews should last no more than 10 minutes and will likely be much shorter. Once you have been the nurse, pick a new scenario and switch roles. After completing the interactions, analyze the interaction with special attention to:
- Therapeutic communication techniques, verbal and nonverbal
- Nontherapeutic communication techniques, verbal and nonverbal
- Areas for improvement
- Skills at which you excelled

A video recording of this exercise is ideal so you can analyze the interaction. Pay special attention to your nonverbals, including a tendency to fidget. Although you may be nervous to record yourself, a recording provides the best opportunity to analyze your skills and will help you in your future interactions with patients. What you say during the interaction is not as important as your analysis of the interaction.

Jarvis, Carolyn and Eckhardt, Ann: PHYSICAL EXAMINATION & HEALTH ASSESSMENT:
Ninth Edition, Study Guide & Laboratory Manual. Copyright © 2024 by Elsevier Inc. All rights reserved.

CRITICAL THINKING ACTIVITY 2

Below is a list of medical terms. Think about different ways to explain them to people with low health literacy, children, and older adults. Likely, your explanations will be different depending on your audience. Take time to discuss your descriptions with a partner or in a group.

Hypertension
Diabetes
Cardiac catheterization
Urinary tract infection
Incontinence
Diarrhea
Nausea
Glaucoma
Anticoagulation

CRITICAL THINKING ACTIVITY 3

Techniques for appropriate communication are important, but knowing yourself is equally important—your beliefs, your culture, your biases. You must quickly establish rapport with patients and you need to make sure that you can adequately meet their needs in a nonjudgmental way. Negative facial expression or other negative nonverbal messages can break communication and shatter the rapport you have established. By knowing yourself and your personal biases, you may be able to control your nonverbal expressions. Most people have beliefs about subjects like teen pregnancy and alcohol or illicit drug use. Awareness of personal prejudices can help you maintain neutrality when faced with difficult patient situations. Answer the following questions or complete the following statements openly and honestly without editing your thoughts in an effort to know yourself better.

1. What do I believe about gender roles?
2. What is my definition of health?
3. When I take care of a person from a different religion, I feel ...
4. When I meet someone new, I make the following assumptions ...
5. I am most fearful of working with ...
6. When I see a same-sex couple, I feel ...
7. I have the following assumptions/stereotypes about people who are
   a. Homeless
   b. Unemployed
   c. Teen parents
   d. Drug addicts
   e. Catholic
   f. Muslim
   g. Christian
   h. Jewish
   i. Transgender

SKILLS LABORATORY AND CLINICAL SETTING

Note that the clinical component of this chapter is the gathering of the complete health history. The history forms are included in Chapter 4.

NOTES

The Complete Health History

PURPOSE

This chapter presents the elements of a complete health history including how to interview the patient to gather data, how to analyze the information, and how to record the history accurately.

READING ASSIGNMENT

Jarvis: *Physical Examination and Health Assessment*, 9th ed., Chapter 4, pp. 41–58.

Suggested reading:
Barbel, P. (2021). Vaccine safety in infants and children. *Nurse Pract, 46*(2), 16–18.
Hunt, D. A., Keefe, J., & Whitehead, T. (2021). Understanding cannabis: Clinical considerations. *J Nurse Pract, 17*, 163–167.

STUDY GUIDE

After completing the reading assignment, you should be able to answer the following questions in the spaces provided.

1. State the purpose of the complete health history.

2. List and define the critical characteristics used to explore each symptom the patient identifies.

3. Define the elements of the health history: reason for seeking care; present health state or present illness; past history, family history; review of systems; functional patterns of living.

4. Discuss the rationale for obtaining a family history.

5. Define a pedigree or genogram.

6. Discuss the rationale for obtaining a review of systems.

7. Describe the items included in a functional assessment.

CLINICAL JUDGMENT QUESTIONS

This test is for you to check your own mastery of the content. Answers are provided in Appendix A.

1. When completing a family history, it is important to ask about the following: **Select all that apply.**

   a. Mental health
   b. Alcohol/drug addiction
   c. Pneumonia
   d. Cancer
   e. High blood pressure
   f. Eczema
   g. Allergies
   h. Diabetes

2. While assessing a patient for allergies, he states he is allergic to penicillin. Which response is best?

   a. "Are you allergic to any other drugs?"
   b. "How often have you received penicillin?"
   c. "I'll write your allergy on your chart so you won't receive any."
   d. "Please describe what happens to you when you take penicillin."

3. The nurse is asking a patient for his reason for seeking care and asks about the signs and symptoms he is experiencing. Which of these is an example of a symptom? **Select all that apply.**

   a. Chest pain
   b. Clammy skin
   c. Fatigue
   d. Serum potassium level 4.2 mEq/L
   e. Cyanosis around lips
   f. A temperature of 100°F
   g. Numbness in fingers

4. The mother of a 2-year-old toddler tells the nurse that her son has an ear infection. What would be the most appropriate response?

   a. "Maybe he is just teething, but we will look in his ears later."
   b. "Does he have a history of frequent ear infections? It could just be teething."
   c. "Are you sure he is really having ear pain and not something else?"
   d. "Describe what he is doing that makes you think he has an ear infection."

5. Underline the signs in the following patient example.

6. Highlight the reason for seeking care in the following patient example.

Patient Example

The client comes to the clinic for "shortness of breath after climbing stairs." He is a 49-year-old male construction worker who, upon further questioning, reports chest pain with exertion, fatigue, and a stomach ache. Upon talking to the patient, you note that he appears pale and clammy. His hands are cool to the touch, and he is audibly wheezing.

7. To fully assess pain, which of the following factors should be included in the assessment? **Select all that apply.**

   a. Onset, frequency, and duration
   b. Probable diagnosis of cause
   c. Alleviating and aggravating factors
   d. Meaning of the pain according to the patient
   e. Vital signs as an objective assessment for pain
   f. Severity of the pain (pain scale rating)

8. As you complete the health history, the patient appears nervous and avoids eye contact. It is unclear whether he is a reliable source of information, and you begin to question whether he is being truthful during the interview. Your best option is:

   a. Continue with the interview but note the nervous appearance and avoidance of eye contact.
   b. Confront the patient. Let him know that you are concerned he is not a reliable source of his health information.
   c. Continue with the interview but ask the same question in a different way to determine reliability.
   d. Ask the person if there is someone else who can serve as a secondary contact to ensure information is correct.

9. When completing the health history on a young child, additional information is collected. Identify whether the following information is collected regardless of age or only collected on children.

Information	Always Collected	Children Only
Perinatal history		
Reason for seeking care		
Immunization status		
Medications		
Developmental milestones		
Family history		

CRITICAL THINKING ACTIVITIES

Complete a genogram using an online tool. After completion, consider the following questions:

1. How difficult was it for you to obtain the information necessary to complete the genogram?
2. Were there questions that you could not answer even after consulting with other family members? How did that make you feel?
3. Did you identify unknown health risks through completion of your personal genogram?
4. How will completing your genogram impact the way in which you describe the importance of family history when interacting with patients?

SKILLS LABORATORY AND CLINICAL SETTING

The purpose of the clinical component is to practice conducting a complete health history on a peer in the skills laboratory and to achieve the following.

Clinical Objectives

1. Demonstrate knowledge of interviewing skills by: arranging a private, quiet, comfortable setting; introducing yourself and stating your goals for the interview; posing open-ended and direct questions appropriately; listening to the patient in an attentive, nonjudgmental manner; and choosing appropriate vocabulary the patient understands.

2. Demonstrate knowledge of the components of a health history by: recording the reason for seeking care in the person's own words; eliciting all the critical characteristics to describe the patient's symptom(s); gathering pertinent data for the past history, family history, and systems review; identifying self-care behaviors and risk factors from the functional assessment.

3. Record the history data accurately and as a reflection of what the patient believes the true health state to be.

Instructions

Work in pairs and obtain a complete health history from a peer. Although you already know each other as student colleagues, play your role straight as examiner or patient for the best learning experience. Be aware that some of the history questions cover personal content. When you are acting as the patient, you have the right to withhold an answer if you do not feel comfortable with the amount of material you will be asked to divulge. Your own rights to privacy must coexist with the goals of the learning experience.

Familiarize yourself with the following history form and practice phrasing your questions ahead of time. Note that the language on this form is intended as a prompt for the examiner and must be translated into clear and appropriate phrases for the patient. As a beginning examiner, you will need to use one copy of the form as a worksheet during the actual interview and use a fresh copy of the form for your rewritten formal record.

WRITE-UP—HEALTH HISTORY

Date _____

Examiner _____

1. Biographic Data

Name _____ Preferred pronoun _____

Occupation _____

Birthdate _____ Birthplace _____

Age _____ Gender _____ Relationship Status _____

Race/ethnic origin _____

2. Source and Reliability

3. Reason for Seeking Care

4. Present Health or History of Present Illness

5. Past Health

Describe general health _____

Childhood illnesses _____

Accidents or injuries (include age) _____

Serious or chronic illnesses (include age) _____

Hospitalizations (what for? Location?) _____

Operations (name procedure, age) _____

Obstetric history: Gravida _____ Term _____ Preterm _____
                    (# Pregnancies)   (# Term pregnancies)   (# Preterm pregnancies)

                    Ab/incomplete _____ Children living _____
                    (# Abortions or miscarriages)

Course of pregnancy _____

(Date delivery, length of pregnancy, length of labor, baby's weight and sex, vaginal delivery or cesarean section, complications, baby's condition)

Immunizations _____

Last examination date: Physical _____ Dental _____ Vision _____

Allergies _____ Reaction _____

Current medications _____

_____

6. Family History—Specify Which Relative(s)

Heart disease_____   Allergies _____

High blood pressure _____   Asthma _____

Stroke _____   Obesity _____

Diabetes _____   Alcoholism or drug addiction _____

Blood disorders_____   Mental illness _____

Breast or ovarian cancer _____   Suicide _____

Cancer (other) _____   Seizure disorder _____

Sickle cell _____   Kidney disease _____

Arthritis _____   Tuberculosis_____

Construct genogram below.

7. Review of Systems

	Describe circled items.
(Circle both past health problems that have been resolved and current problems, including date of onset.)	

General Overall Health State: Present weight (gain or loss, period of time, by diet or other factors), fatigue, weakness or malaise, fever, chills, sweats or night sweats.

Skin: History of skin disease (eczema, psoriasis, hives), pigment or color change, change in mole, excessive dryness or moisture, pruritus, excessive bruising, rash or lesion.

Hair: Recent loss, change in texture.

Nails: Change in shape, color, or brittleness.
  Health Promotion: Amount of sun exposure, method of self-care for skin and hair.

Head: Any unusually frequent or severe headache, any head injury, dizziness (syncope), or vertigo, history of concussions.

Eyes: Difficulty with vision (decreased acuity, blurring, blind spots), eye pain, diplopia (double vision), redness or swelling, watering or discharge, glaucoma or cataracts.
  Health Promotion: Wears glasses or contacts, last vision check, glaucoma test, how coping with loss of vision, if any.

Ears: Earaches, infections, discharge and its characteristics, tympanostomy tubes, tinnitus, or vertigo.
  Health Promotion: Hearing loss, hearing aid use, how loss affects daily life, any exposure to environmental noise, method of cleaning ears

Nose and Sinuses: Discharge and its characteristics, any unusually frequent or severe colds, sinus pain, nasal obstruction, snoring, nosebleeds, allergies or hay fever, or change in sense of smell.

Mouth and Throat: Mouth pain, frequent sore throat, bleeding gums, toothache, lesion in mouth or tongue, dysphagia, hoarseness or voice change, tonsillectomy, altered taste.
  Health Promotion: Pattern of daily dental care, use of prostheses (dentures, bridge), and last dental checkup.

Neck: Pain, limitation of motion, lumps or swelling, enlarged or tender nodes, goiter.

Breast: Pain, lump, nipple discharge, rash, history of breast disease, any surgery on breasts.
  Axilla: Tenderness, lump or swelling, rash.
  Health Promotion: Performs breast self-examination, including frequency and method used, last mammogram and results.

Respiratory System: History of lung disease (asthma, emphysema, bronchitis, pneumonia, tuberculosis), chest pain with breathing, wheezing or noisy breathing, shortness of breath, how much activity produces shortness of breath, cough, sputum (color, amount), hemoptysis, toxin or pollution exposure.
  Health Promotion: Last chest x-ray examination.

(Circle if present.)   Describe circled items.

Cardiovascular System: Precordial or retrosternal pain, palpitation, cyanosis, dyspnea on exertion (specify amount of exertion it takes to produce dyspnea), orthopnea, paroxysmal nocturnal dyspnea, nocturia, edema, history of heart murmur, hypertension, coronary artery disease, anemia.
   Health Promotion: Date of last ECG or other heart tests and results.

Peripheral Vascular System: Coldness, numbness and tingling, swelling of legs (time of day, activity), discoloration in hands or feet (bluish red, pallor, mottling, associated with position, especially around feet and ankles), varicose veins or complications, intermittent claudication, thrombophlebitis, ulcers.
   Health Promotion: If work involves long-term sitting or standing, avoid crossing legs at the knees; wear support hose.

Gastrointestinal System: Appetite, food intolerance, dysphagia, heartburn, indigestion, pain (associated with eating), other abdominal pain, pyrosis (esophageal and stomach burning sensation with sour eructation), nausea and vomiting (character), vomiting blood, history of abdominal disease (ulcer, liver or gallbladder, jaundice, appendicitis, colitis), flatulence, frequency of bowel movement, any recent change, stool characteristics, constipation or diarrhea, black stools, rectal bleeding, rectal conditions, hemorrhoids, fistula.
   Health Promotion: Use of antacids or laxatives.

Urinary System: Frequency, urgency, nocturia (the number of times awakens at night to urinate, recent change), dysuria, polyuria or oliguria, hesitancy or straining, narrowed stream, urine color (cloudy or presence of hematuria), incontinence, history of urinary disease (kidney disease, kidney stones, urinary tract infections, prostate); pain in flank, groin, suprapubic region, or low back.
   Health Promotion: Measures to avoid or treat urinary tract infections, use of Kegel exercises.

Male Genital System: Penis or testicular pain, sores or lesions, penile discharge, lumps, hernia.
   Health Promotion: Perform testicular self-examination? How frequently?

Female Genital System: Menstrual history (age at menarche, last menstrual period, cycle and duration, any amenorrhea or menorrhagia, premenstrual pain or dysmenorrhea, intermenstrual spotting), vaginal itching, discharge and its characteristics, age at menopause, menopausal signs or symptoms, postmenopausal bleeding.
   Health Promotion: Last gynecologic checkup, last Pap test and results.

Sexual Health: Presently in a relationship involving sexual activity? Are aspects of sex satisfactory to you and partner, any dyspareunia (for female), any changes in erection or ejaculation (for male), use of contraceptive (if applicable), is contraceptive method satisfactory? Use of condoms, how frequently? Aware of any contact with partner who has sexually transmitted infection (gonorrhea, herpes, chlamydia, venereal warts, human immunodeficiency virus [HIV]/acquired immunodeficiency syndrome [AIDS], syphilis)?
   Health Promotion. Routine testing for sexually transmitted infections and use of preexposure prophylaxis if applicable.

(Circle if present.) | Describe circled items.

Musculoskeletal System: History of arthritis or gout. In the joints: pain, stiffness, swelling (location, migratory nature), deformity, limitation of motion, noise with joint motion. In the muscles: any pain, cramps, weakness, gait problems or problems with coordinated activities. In the back: any pain (location and radiation to extremities), stiffness, limitation of motion, or history of back pain or disc disease.

    Health Promotion: How much walking per day? What is the effect of limited range of motion on daily activities, such as on grooming, feeding, toileting, dressing? Any mobility aids used?

Neurologic System: History of seizure disorder, stroke, fainting, blackouts. In motor function: weakness, tic or tremor, paralysis, coordination problems. In sensory function: numbness and tingling (paresthesia). In cognitive function: memory disorder (recent or distant, disorientation). In mental status: any nervousness, mood change, depression, or any history of mental health dysfunction or hallucinations.

Hematologic System: Bleeding tendency of skin or mucous membranes, excessive bruising, lymph node swelling, exposure to toxic agents or radiation, blood transfusion and reactions.

Endocrine System: History of diabetes or diabetic symptoms (polyuria, polydipsia, polyphagia), history of thyroid disease, intolerance to heat or cold, change in skin pigmentation or texture, excessive sweating, relationship between appetite and weight, abnormal hair distribution, nervousness, tremors, need for hormone therapy.

Functional Assessment (Including Activities of Daily Living)

Self-Esteem, Self-Concept: Education (last grade completed, other significant training) _____

_____

Financial status (income adequate for lifestyle and/or health concerns) _____

_____

Value-belief system (religious practices and perception of personal strengths) _____

_____

Self-care behaviors _____

_____

Activity and Exercise: Daily profile, usual pattern of a typical day _____

_____

Independent or needs assistance with activities of daily living (ADLs), feeding, bathing, hygiene, dressing, toileting, bed-to-chair transfer, walking, standing, climbing stairs _____

_____

Leisure activities _____

Exercise pattern (type, amount per day or week, method of warm-up session, method of monitoring body's response to exercise) _____

_____

Other self-care behaviors _____

Sleep and Rest: Sleep patterns, daytime naps, any sleep aids used _____

_____

Other self-care behavior _____

Nutrition and Elimination: Record 24-hour diet recall. _____

_____

Is this menu pattern typical of most days? _____

Who buys food? _____ Who prepares food? _____

Finances adequate for food? _____

Who is present at mealtimes? _____

Other self-care behaviors _____

Interpersonal Relationships and Resources: Describe own role in family _____

Do you get along with family, friends, coworkers, classmates? _____

_____

Get support with a problem from _____

How much daily time spent alone? _____

Is this pleasurable or isolating? _____

Other self-care behaviors _____

Coping and Stress Management: Describe stresses in life now _____

_____

Change(s) in past year _____

Methods used to relieve stress _____

Are these methods helpful? _____

Personal Habits: Daily intake caffeine (coffee, tea, colas) _____

Smoke cigarettes? _____ Number packs per day _____

Daily use for how many years _____ Age started _____

Ever tried to quit? _____ How did it go? _____

Drink alcohol? _____ Date of last alcohol use _____

Amount of alcohol that episode _____

Out of last 30 days, on how many days have you had alcohol? _____

Ever told you had a drinking problem? _____

Use marijuana? _____ Form (e.g., smoked, ingested)? _____

Frequency of use? _____ Recreational or medicinal? _____

If medicinal, name of healthcare provider. _____

Out of the last 30 days, how many days did you use marijuana? _____

Any use of illicit drugs? _____

Cocaine? _____

Crack cocaine? _____ Amphetamines? _____

Heroin? _____ Prescription painkillers? _____

Barbiturates? _____ LSD? _____

Ever been in treatment for drugs or alcohol? _____

Environment and Hazards: Housing and neighborhood (type of structure, live alone, know neighbors) __
_____
_____

Safety of area _____

Adequate heat and utilities _____

Access to transportation _____

Involvement in community services _____

Hazards at workplace or home _____

Experiences with racism or discrimination where you live or work? Safety of environment? _____

Use of seatbelts _____

Travel to or residence in other countries _____

Military service in other countries _____

Self-care behaviors _____

Intimate Partner Violence: How are things at home? Do you feel safe? _____
_____

Ever been emotionally or physically abused by your partner or someone important to you? _____
_____

Ever been hit, slapped, kicked, pushed, or shoved or otherwise physically hurt by your partner or ex-partner?
_____

Partner or ex-partner ever force you into having sex? _____

Are you afraid of your partner or ex-partner? _____

Occupational Health: Please describe your job. _____

Work with any health hazards (e.g., asbestos, inhalants, chemicals, repetitive motion)? _____

_____

Any equipment at work designed to reduce your exposure? _____

Any work programs designed to monitor your exposure? _____

Any health problems that you think are related to your job? _____

What do you like or dislike about your job? _____

Perception of Own Health: How do you define health? _____

View of own health now _____

What are your concerns? _____

What do you expect will happen to your health in future? _____

_____

Your health goals _____

Your expectations of nurses, physicians _____

PURPOSE

This chapter presents the components of the mental status examination, including assessing a person's appearance, behavior, cognitive functions, and thought processes and perceptions; understanding the rationale and methods of examination of mental status; and recording the assessment accurately.

READING ASSIGNMENT

Jarvis: *Physical Examination and Health Assessment,* 9th ed., Chapter 5, pp. 59–80.

Suggested reading:
Dunlap, J. J., & Filipek, P. A. (2020). Autism spectrum disorder: The nurse's role. *Am J Nurs, 120*(11), 40–50.
Fazel, S., & Runeson, B. (2020). Suicide. *N Engl J Med, 382,* 266–274.

GLOSSARY

Study the following terms after completing the reading assignment. You should be able to cover the definition on the right and define the term out loud.

Abstract reasoning .... pondering a deeper meaning beyond the concrete and literal

Attention .... concentration, ability to focus on one specific thing

Bereavement .... state of loss, sorrow, and/or grief due to the death of a loved one, decline in personal or a loved one's health, or the end of an important relationship

Consciousness .... being aware of one's own existence, feelings, and thoughts and being aware of the environment

Delirium .... an acute confusional change or loss of consciousness and perceptual disturbance that may accompany acute illness; usually resolves when the underlying cause is treated

Dementia .... a gradual progressive process, causing decreased cognitive function even though the person is fully conscious and awake; not reversible

Executive function .... high-level cognitive skills, including organizational and regulatory ability

Language .... using the voice to communicate one's thoughts and feelings

Memory .... ability to lay down and store experiences and perceptions for later recall

Mood .... prolonged display of a person's feelings

Orientation .... awareness of the objective world in relation to the self

Perceptions .... awareness of objects through any of the five senses

Thought content .... what the person thinks—specific ideas, beliefs, the use of words

Thought process .... the way a person thinks, the logical train of thought

Visuospatial .... ability to process visual information and perceive relationships between objects in space

STUDY GUIDE

After completing the reading assignment, you should be able to answer the following questions in the spaces provided.

1. Define the term *mental disorder*.

2. Differentiate *organic brain disorder* from *psychiatric mental disorder*.

3. List four situations in which it would be necessary to perform a complete mental status examination.

4. Explain four factors that could affect a patient's response to the mental status examination but have nothing to do with mental disorders.

5. State convenient ways to assess a person's recent memory within the context of the initial health history.

6. Which mental function is the Four Unrelated Words Test intended to test?

7. List at least four risk factors and four warning signs of suicide.

8. Describe the patient response level of consciousness that would be graded as:

Lethargic or somnolent _____

Obtunded _____

Stupor or semicoma _____

Coma _____

Delirium _____

9. Describe the primary differences between delirium, dementia, and depression.

10. Describe how the mental status exam is adapted to different age groups (e.g., children, older adults).

CRITICAL THINKING ACTIVITIES

Use the Montreal Cognitive Assessment (MoCA) on the next page to complete a cognitive screen on a partner. Switch partners, and complete the Mini-Cog (http://mini-cog.com/mini-cog-instrument/standardized-mini-cog-instrument/) on a different partner. Compare and contrast the differences between the screening tools. Which seemed more appropriate for use in an outpatient clinic? The hospital? Were you comfortable providing instructions and scoring each instrument? What questions do you have about scoring?

Next, use the MoCA and Mini-Cog in a clinical setting. Complete the MoCA and Mini-Cog on different older adults (>65 years). Did you have to change your delivery with an older person? Discuss the experience with classmates to identify differences found with different patients and in different settings.

MONTREAL COGNITIVE ASSESSMENT (MOCA)
Version 7.1 Original Version

NAME :
Education :   Date of birth :
Sex :   DATE :

VISUOSPATIAL / EXECUTIVE

Copy cube

Draw CLOCK (Ten past eleven)
(3 points)

POINTS

[ ]   [ ]   [ ]   [ ]   [ ]   __/5
                              Contour   Numbers   Hands

NAMING

[ ]   [ ]   [ ]   __/3

MEMORY

Read list of words, subject must repeat them. Do 2 trials, even if 1st trial is successful. Do a recall after 5 minutes.

	FACE	VELVET	CHURCH	DAISY	RED	No points
1st trial						
2nd trial						

ATTENTION

Read list of digits (1 digit/ sec.).

Subject has to repeat them in the forward order   [ ] 2 1 8 5 4

Subject has to repeat them in the backward order   [ ] 7 4 2   __/2

Read list of letters. The subject must tap with his hand at each letter A. No points if ≥ 2 errors

[ ] F B A C M N A A J K L B A F A K D E A A A J A M O F A A B   __/1

Serial 7 subtraction starting at 100   [ ] 93   [ ] 86   [ ] 79   [ ] 72   [ ] 65

4 or 5 correct subtractions: **3 pts**, 2 or 3 correct: **2 pts**, 1 correct: **1 pt**, 0 correct: **0 pt**   __/3

LANGUAGE

Repeat : I only know that John is the one to help today. [ ]
The cat always hid under the couch when dogs were in the room. [ ]   __/2

Fluency / Name maximum number of words in one minute that begin with the letter F   [ ] _____ (N ≥ 11 words)   __/1

ABSTRACTION

Similarity between e.g. banana - orange = fruit   [ ] train – bicycle   [ ] watch - ruler   __/2

DELAYED RECALL

Has to recall words **WITH NO CUE**	FACE [ ]	VELVET [ ]	CHURCH [ ]	DAISY [ ]	RED [ ]	Points for UNCUED recall only	__/5
Optional Category cue							
Multiple choice cue							

ORIENTATION

[ ] Date   [ ] Month   [ ] Year   [ ] Day   [ ] Place   [ ] City   __/6

© Z.Nasreddine MD   www.mocatest.org   Normal ≥ 26 / 30

TOTAL   __/30
Add 1 point if ≤ 12 yr edu

Administered by: _____

CLINICAL JUDGMENT QUESTIONS

This test is for you to check your own mastery of the content. Answers are provided in Appendix A.

1. Select the finding that most accurately describes appearance of a patient.

   a. Tense posture and restless activity. Clothing clean but not appropriate for season.
   b. Oriented × 3. Affect appropriate for circumstances.
   c. Alert and responds to verbal stimuli. Tearful when diagnosis discussed.
   d. Laughing inappropriately, oriented × 3.

2. During an interview with a patient diagnosed with a seizure disorder, the patient states, "I plan to be an airline pilot." If the patient continues to have this as a career goal after teaching regarding seizure disorders has been provided, you might question the patient's:

   a. Thought processes.
   b. Judgment.
   c. Attention span.
   d. Recent memory.

3. You are assessing a 75-year-old man. What is an expected finding?

   a. He will have no decrease in any of his abilities, including response time.
   b. He will have difficulty on tests of remote memory because this typically decreases with age.
   c. It may take him a little longer to respond, but his general knowledge and abilities should not have declined.
   d. He will have had a decrease in his response time due to language loss and a decrease in general knowledge.

4. You are completing a mental status examination on a patient who had a stroke 3 days ago. He is alert and oriented × 3. During the exam, you note agraphia and agrammatic speech. Upon talking to his partner, you learn he is well educated and had no speech difficulty prior to his stroke. Given this information, you know the stroke likely impacted:

   a. Broca area.
   b. Wernicke area.
   c. Posterior language area.
   d. Frontal language area.

For questions 5–7 use the following information: *Mr. Smith is a 63-year-old man who is in the clinic for a new patient appointment. He has a history of depression, hypertension, and diabetes. Mr. Smith tells you he was medically discharged from the military after a traumatic brain injury during his service in Iraq in 2000 and that he recently retired from his job as an insurance agent after more than 20 years in the business. He does not report any deficits from his traumatic brain injury. His family history is positive for depression (brother), suicide (brother), heart disease (father and paternal grandfather), and diabetes (mother). Both of his parents are still living and in reportedly "good" health. He lives with his wife and dog.*

5. What information provided by Mr. Smith puts him at higher risk for suicide? **Select all that apply.**

   a. Family history of suicide
   b. Hypertension
   c. Family history of heart disease
   d. History of traumatic brain injury
   e. Diabetes
   f. Depression

6. Given Mr. Smith's history, what screening(s) should be completed? **Select all that apply.**

   a. Patient Health Questionnaire-2
   b. Generalized Anxiety Disorder-2
   c. Ask Suicide-Screening Questions
   d. Mini-Mental State Examination
   e. Mini-cog

7. Write a narrative account of a mental status assessment for an 88-year-old female with mild cognitive impairment. How would this narrative be different if the patient were cognitively intact?

For questions 8–15, match column B to column A.

Column A—Definition

8. _____ Lack of emotional response
9. _____ Loss of identity
10. _____ Excessive well-being
11. _____ Annoyed, easily provoked
12. _____ Loss of control
13. _____ Sad, gloomy, dejected
14. _____ Rapid shift of emotions
15. _____ Worried about known external danger

Column B—Type of Mood and Affect

a. Depression
b. Flat affect
c. Euphoria
d. Lability
e. Rage
f. Irritability
g. Fear
h. Depersonalization

16. You are asked to complete a full mental status examination of a patient who is being seen for increasing "forgetfulness." Put the following steps in the correct order by numbering 1–5.

   _____ Check hearing and vision.
   _____ Ask orientation questions.
   _____ Supplemental mental status examination (e.g., Mini-Cog, MMSE, MoCA)
   _____ Note general appearance
   _____ Give patient four words to remember for the Four Unrelated Words Test

17. For each item below, specify whether it is a characteristic of dementia, delirium, or depression. Some characteristics may describe more than one disease process.

Characteristic	Delirium	Dementia	Depression
Sudden onset			
Impaired memory			
Level of consciousness not altered			
Characterized by rapid emotional swings			
Reversible with proper treatment			

SKILLS LABORATORY AND CLINICAL SETTING

The purpose of the clinical component is to achieve beginning competency with the administration of the mental status examination. You will also screen your patient for anxiety (GAD-7), depression (PHQ-9), and suicidality (ASQ). The GAD-7, PHQ-9, and ASQ are available in your textbook.

Practice steps of the full mental status examination, screening for anxiety, and screening for depression on a peer or patient in the clinical setting. Give appropriate instructions throughout the examination. Use the regional write-up sheet that follows to record your findings.

REGIONAL WRITE-UP—MENTAL STATUS EXAMINATION

Date _____

Examiner _____

Patient _____ Age _____ Gender _____

Occupation _____

MENTAL STATUS

(Before testing, tell the person the four words you want them to remember and recall in a few minutes for the Four Unrelated Words Test.)

1. Appearance

   Posture _____
   Body movements _____
   Dress _____
   Grooming and hygiene _____

2. Behavior

   Level of consciousness _____
   Facial expression _____
   Speech:
      Quality _____
      Pace _____
      Word choice _____
   Mood and affect _____

3. Cognitive Functions

   Orientation:
      Time _____ Place_____ Person_____
   Attention span _____
   Recent memory _____
   Remote memory _____
   New learning—Four Unrelated Words Test _____
   Additional testing for aphasia:
      Word comprehension _____
      Reading _____
      Writing _____
   Judgment _____

4. Thought Processes and Perceptions

   Thought processes _____
   Thought content _____
   Perceptions _____
   Suicidal thoughts _____

NOTES

Substance Use Assessment

PURPOSE

This chapter presents the scope of the problem regarding primary care and hospital patients who drink excessive alcohol and use illicit drugs. Screening tools and interview approaches are presented.

READING ASSIGNMENT

Jarvis: *Physical Examination and Health Assessment,* 9th ed., Chapter 6, pp. 81–94.

Suggested reading:
Mackavey, C., & Kearney, K. (2020). Substance use disorder: Screening adolescents in primary care. *Nurse Pract, 45*(5), 25–33.

GLOSSARY

Study the following terms after completing the reading assignment. You should be able to cover the definition on the right and define the term out loud.

Alcohol abuse .... one or more of the following events in a year: recurrent use resulting in failure to fulfill major role obligations; recurrent use in hazardous situations; recurrent alcohol-related legal problems (e.g., DUI); continued use despite social or interpersonal problems caused or exacerbated by alcohol

Alcohol use disorder .... two or more of the following events in a year: tolerance (increased amounts to achieve effect; diminished effect from same amount); withdrawal; a great deal of time spent obtaining alcohol, using it, or recovering from its effect; important activities given up or reduced because of alcohol; drinking more or longer than intended; persistent desire or unsuccessful efforts to cut down or control alcohol use; use continued despite knowledge of having a psychological problem caused or exacerbated by alcohol

Binge drinking .... on one occasion: five or more standard alcohol drinks for men; four or more standard alcohol drinks for women

Heavy alcohol use .... binge drinking on 5 or more days in the past month (SAMHSA). Or for men, 15 or more drinks per week; for women, 8 or more drinks per week (CDC)

Standard alcohol drink .... 14 grams of pure alcohol as found in one 12-ounce beer (5% alcohol); one 8-ounce malt liquor (7% alcohol); one 5-ounce glass of wine (12% alcohol); or 1.5 ounces of spirits (gin, vodka, whiskey, rum) (40% alcohol)

STUDY GUIDE

After completing the reading assignment, you should be able to answer the following questions in the space provided.

1. What proportion of Americans ages 12 and older report drinking alcohol in the past year? And report binge drinking (≥5 drinks/occasion)?

2. List the effects of alcohol.

3. Define the use of prescription opioid pain relievers for a nonmedical use.

4. Discuss the extra risk alcohol drinking poses to the aging adult. Discuss the same for an adolescent.

5. Contrast the use and settings for the following alcohol screening tools: AUDIT; AUDIT-C; CAGE questionnaire.

6. State three clinical laboratory findings that are used to detect or monitor alcohol use.

CRITICAL THINKING ACTIVITIES

1. Read your daily newspaper for 4 days, making a list of all news stories (e.g., auto accidents, drowning, personal injury) that are or possibly could be alcohol or drug related.
2. In a group of three or four students, interview a primary care provider, emergency department provider, and intensive care unit provider. Ask each one for clinical examples of alcohol-related cases in their units.
3. Review your school or university alcohol policy in the student handbook. How does the handbook statement differ from the actual situation on campus or is it different?

CLINICAL JUDGMENT QUESTIONS

This test is for you to check your own mastery of the content. Answers are provided in Appendix A.

1. A pregnant woman explains that she does not intend to stop drinking because her friends continued to drink during pregnancy and "nothing happened to them or their kids." How should the clinician respond to this statement?

   a. "While it's true that there is no scientific evidence that alcohol harms the fetus, abstinence is recommended because of the physical effects on your body."
   b. "No amount of alcohol has been determined to be safe for a pregnant woman so I would recommend you stop drinking alcohol completely."
   c. "Maybe you could cut back on your alcohol intake, at least until you're in the third trimester, when the effects on the fetus are minimal."
   d. "If you can limit yourself to only one drink per day, you will be helping yourself and your baby."

2. You are screening for alcohol use in a 45-year-old male who reports an increase in drinking after being laid off. Which of the following statements would be indicative of exceeding the recommended limit?

   a. "I used to go out after work on Fridays with my friends. Now I drink a beer most nights of the week."
   b. "I used to go out after work on Fridays with my friends. Now I have three or four beers most nights."
   c. "I used to go out after work on Fridays with my friends. Now I don't drink at all since I don't go out after work."
   d. "I used to go out after work on Fridays with my friends. Now I have two beers most nights."

3. You are assessing a male patient's alcohol consumption. Which statement would alert you to investigate further?

   a. "I drink at wedding and holidays."
   b. "I enjoy a few beers on the weekend."
   c. "No matter how much I drink I don't get drunk."
   d. "I drink a beer with dinner every day."

4. You are screening your patient for alcohol and substance use. The patient reports drinking alcohol but reports abstaining from illicit substance use. When you complete the CAGE questionnaire, the patient reports that he sometimes thinks he should cut down on his drinking and that he finds himself occasionally needing to have a drink in the morning to get going. Based on this assessment you tell the patient:

   a. While I don't think you should drink in the morning, your drinking does not seem to be impacting your work or home life. You might consider cutting down, though.
   b. I would recommend keeping a journal of how much you drink. That way, when you come back, we can have a discussion of drinking patterns.
   c. I believe you may have an alcohol use disorder. I am here to help and would like to identify some treatment options.
   d. I believe you have an alcohol use disorder. You must stop drinking now or you will likely die early.

5. Which of the following physiologic changes put older adults at higher risk when consuming alcohol? **Select all that apply.**

   a. Decrease muscle mass
   b. Increase body water
   c. Decrease body water
   d. Decreased kidney function
   e. Increase in liver metabolism
   f. Higher metabolism

6. You are caring for a newly admitted patient in the intensive care unit. He is alert and oriented after being in a car accident. He has multiple injuries including bilateral broken femurs, fracture of T10, and multiple lacerations. While completing his intake questionnaire, you recognize the importance of screening for alcohol use and will proceed in the following manner:

   a. Ask how often and how much he drinks. This is not the time to ask any further questions.
   b. Recognize that alcohol withdrawal is a potential complication, and ask him the AUDIT-C questionnaire.
   c. Recognize that alcohol withdrawal is a potential complication, and ask him the AUDIT questionnaire.
   d. Proactively place him on CIWA-Ar precautions because he was in a car accident and is likely unreliable.

7. Which of the following is a standard drink? **Select all that apply.**

   a. 5 oz of table wine
   b. 1.5 oz of hard liquor (e.g., gin, vodka)
   c. 12 oz can of malt liquor (12% ABV)
   d. One martini
   e. 12 oz can of beer (5% ABV)
   f. Pint of beer
   g. ½ bottle of a standard table wine

8. For each of the following items, specify whether it is a characteristic of intoxication with each substance. Some characteristics may describe more than one.

Characteristic	Alcohol	Marijana	Opiates	Cocaine
Pinpoint pupils				
Reddened eyes				
Pupillary dilation				
Loss of balance				
Slurred speech				
Talkativeness				

9. For each item below, specify whether it is a characteristic of withdrawal from each substance. Some characteristics may describe more than one.

Characteristic	Alcohol	Marijuana	Opiates	Cocaine
Irritability				
Dilated pupils				
Hallucinations				
Fatigue				
Hand tremors				

SKILLS LABORATORY AND CLINICAL SETTING

Pair up with a classmate and interview each other using the AUDIT questionnaire. Keep your answers confidential and share the questionnaire after use—this is not to turn in to the instructor. Note that questions 1 to 3 cover alcohol consumption, questions 4 to 6 cover drinking behavior, and questions 7 to 10 cover adverse consequences from alcohol. Record the score at the end of each line and the total; the maximum score is 40. A cutpoint of 8 or more indicates hazardous alcohol consumption.

Now role-play, and one of you take the role of the nurse and the other take the role of the hospitalized person in possible alcohol withdrawal. Proceed through the CIWA assessment guide. A complete assessment takes about 5 minutes. Note the points at which medication by protocol is recommended as needed or is ordered.

THE ALCOHOL USE DISORDERS IDENTIFICATION TEST—AUDIT*

Questions	0	1	2	3	4
1. How often do you have a drink containing alcohol?	Never	Monthly or less	2 to 4 times a month	2 to 3 times a week	4 or more times a week
2. How many drinks containing alcohol do you have on a typical day when you are drinking?	1 or 2	3 or 4	5 or 6	7 to 9	10 or more
3. How often do you have five or more drinks on one occasion?	Never	Less than monthly	Monthly	Weekly	Daily or almost daily
4. How often during the last year have you found that you were not able to stop drinking once you had started?	Never	Less than monthly	Monthly	Weekly	Daily or almost daily
5. How often during the last year have you failed to do what was normally expected of you because of drinking?	Never	Less than monthly	Monthly	Weekly	Daily or almost daily
6. How often during the last year have you needed a first drink in the morning to get yourself going after a heavy drinking session?	Never	Less than monthly	Monthly	Weekly	Daily or almost daily
7. How often during the last year have you had a feeling of guilt or remorse after drinking?	Never	Less than monthly	Monthly	Weekly	Daily or almost daily
8. How often during the last year have you been unable to remember what happened the night before because of your drinking?	Never	Less than monthly	Monthly	Weekly	Daily or almost daily
9. Have you or someone else been injured because of your drinking?	No		Yes, but not in the last year		Yes, during the last year
10. Has a relative, friend, doctor, or other health care worker been concerned about your drinking or suggested you cut down?	No		Yes, but not in the last year		Yes, during the last year
					Total

***Note:** This questionnaire (the AUDIT) is reprinted with permission from the World Health Organization. To reflect standard drink sizes in the United States, the number of drinks in question 3 was changed from six to five. A free AUDIT manual with guidelines for use in primary care settings is available online at www.who.org.

Alcohol Withdrawal Assessment Scoring Guidelines (CIWA - Ar)

Nausea/Vomiting - Rate on scale 0–7.
0 - None
1 - Mild nausea with no vomiting
2
3
4 - Intermittent nausea
5
6
7 - Constant nausea and frequent dry heaves and vomiting

Tremors - Have patient extend arms and spread fingers.
Rate on scale 0–7.
0 - No tremor
1 - Not visible, but can be felt fingertip to fingertip
2
3
4 - Moderate, with patient's arms extended
5
6
7 - Severe, even w/arms not extended

Anxiety - Rate on scale 0–7.
0 - No anxiety, patient at ease
1- Mildly anxious
2
3
4 - Moderately anxious or guarded, so anxiety is inferred
5
6
7 - Equivalent to acute panic states seen in severe delirium or acute schizophrenic reactions

Agitation - Rate on scale 0–7.
0 - Normal activity
1 - Somewhat normal activity
2
3
4 - Moderately fidgety and restless
5
6
7 - Paces back and forth, or constantly thrashes about

Paroxysmal Sweats - Rate on scale 0–7.
0 - No sweats
1 - Barely perceptible sweating, palms moist
2
3
4 - Beads of sweat obvious on forehead
5
6
7 - Drenching sweats

Orientation and Clouding of Sensorium - Ask, "What day is this? Where are you? Who am I?" Rate on scale 0-4.
0 - Oriented
1 - Cannot do serial additions or is uncertain about date

2 - Disoriented to date by no more than 2 calendar days

3 - Disoriented to date by more than 2 calendar days
4 - Disoriented to place and/or person

Tactile Disturbances - Ask, "Have you experienced any itching, pins and needles sensation, burning or numbness, or a feeling of bugs crawling on or under your skin?"
Rate on scale 0–7.
0 - None
1 - Very mild itching, pins and needles, burning, or numbness
2 - Mild itching, pins and needles, burning, or numbness
3 - Moderate itching, pins and needles, burning, or numbness
4 - Moderate hallucinations
5 - Severe hallucinations
6 - Extremely severe hallucinations
7 - Continuous hallucinations

Auditory Disturbances - Ask, "Are you more aware of sounds around you? Are they harsh? Do they startle you? Do you hear anything that disturbs you or that you know isn't there?"
Rate on scale 0–7.
0 - Not present
1 - Very mild harshness or ability to startle
2 - Mild harshness or ability to startle
3 - Moderate harshness or ability to startle
4 - Moderate hallucinations
5 - Severe hallucinations
6 - Extremely severe hallucinations
7 - Continuous hallucinations

Visual Disturbances - Ask, "Does the light appear to be too bright? Is its color different than normal? Does it hurt your eyes? Are you seeing anything that disturbs you or that you know isn't there?" Rate on scale 0–7.
0 - Not present
1 - Very mild sensitivity
2 - Mild sensitivity
3 - Moderate sensitivity
4 - Moderate hallucinations
5 - Severe hallucinations
6 - Extremely severe hallucinations
7 - Continuous hallucinations

Headache - Ask, "Does your head feel different than usual? Does it feel like there is a band around your head?" Do not rate dizziness or lightheadedness. Rate on scale 0–7.
0 - Not present
1 - Very mild
2 - Mild
3 - Moderate
4 - Moderately severe
5 - Severe
6 - Very severe
7 - Extremely severe

Procedure:
1. Assess and rate each of the 10 criteria of the CIWA scale. Each criterion is rated on a scale from 0 to 7, except for "Orientation and clouding of sensorium," which is rated on a scale from 0 to 4. Add up the scores for all ten criteria. This is the total CIWA-Ar score for the patient at that time. Document vitals and CIWA-Ar assessment on the Withdrawal Assessment Sheet. Document administration of PRN medications on the assessment sheet as well.
2. The CIWA-Ar scale is the most sensitive tool for assessment of the patient experiencing alcohol withdrawal. Nursing assessment is vitally important. Early intervention for a CIWA-Ar score of 8 or greater provides the best means to prevent the progression of withdrawal.

Jarvis, Carolyn and Eckhardt, Ann: PHYSICAL EXAMINATION & HEALTH ASSESSMENT:
Ninth Edition, Study Guide & Laboratory Manual. Copyright © 2024 by Elsevier Inc. All rights reserved.

Assessment Protocol		Date											
a. Vitals, Assessment Now.		Time											
b. If initial score ≥ 8 repeat q1h x 8 hrs, then if stable q2h x 8 hrs, then if stable q4h.		Pulse											
		RR											
c. If initial score < 8, assess q4h x 72 hrs.		O₂ sat											
If score < 8 for 72 hrs, d/c assessment. If score ≥ 8 at any time, go to (b) above.		BP											
d. If indicated (see indications below), administer PRN medications as ordered and record on MAR and below.													

Assess and rate each of the following (CIWA-Ar Scale):   Refer to reverse for detailed instructions in use of the CIWA-Ar scale.

Nausea/Vomiting (0–7) 0 - none; 1 - mild nausea, no vomiting; 4 - intermittent nausea; 7 - constant nausea, frequent dry heaves & vomiting.												
Tremors (0–7) 0 - no tremor; 1 - not visible but can be felt; 4 - moderate w/ arms extended; 7 - severe, even w/ arms not extended.												
Anxiety (0–7) 0 - none, at ease; 1 - mildly anxious; 4 - moderately anxious or guarded; 7 - equivalent to acute panic state.												
Agitation (0–7) 0 - normal activity; 1 - somewhat normal activity; 4 - moderately fidgety/restless; 7 - paces or constantly thrashes about.												
Paroxysmal Sweats (0–7) 0 - no sweats; 1 - barely perceptible sweating, palms moist; 4 - beads of sweat obvious on forehead; 7 - drenching sweat.												
Orientation (0–4) 0 - oriented; 1 - uncertain about date; 2 - disoriented to date by no more than 2 days; 3 - disoriented to date by > 2 days; 4 - disoriented to place and / or person.												
Tactile Disturbances (0–7) 0 - none; 1 - very mild itch, P&N, numbness; 2-mild itch, P&N, burning, numbness; 3 - moderate itch, P&N, burning, numbness; 4 - moderate hallucinations; 5 - severe hallucinations; 6 – extremely severe hallucinations; 7 - continuous hallucinations.												
Auditory Disturbances (0–7) 0 - not present; 1 - very mild harshness/ability to startle; 2 - mild harshness, ability to startle; 3 - moderate harshness, ability to startle; 4 - moderate hallucinations; 5 - severe hallucinations; 6 - extremely severe hallucinations; 7 - continuous hallucinations.												
Visual Disturbances (0–7) 0 - not present; 1 - very mild sensitivity; 2 - mild sensitivity; 3 - moderate sensitivity; 4 - moderate hallucinations; 5 - severe hallucinations; 6 - extremely severe hallucinations; 7 - continuous hallucinations.												
Headache (0-7) 0 - not present; 1 - very mild; 2 - mild; 3 - moderate; 4 - moderately severe; 5 - severe; 6 - very severe; 7 - extremely severe.												
Total CIWA-Ar score:												

PRN med: (circle one)	Dose given (mg):												
Diazepam Lorazepam	Route:												
Time of PRN medication administration:													
Assessment of response (CIWA-Ar score 30-60 minutes after medication administered)													
RN Initials													

Scale for Scoring:
 Total Score =
   0–9: absent or minimal withdrawal
   10–19: mild to moderate withdrawal
   More than 20: severe withdrawal
	Indications for PRN medication:
	 a. Total CIWA-Ar score 8 or higher if ordered PRN only (symptom-triggered method).
	 b. Total CIWA-Ar score 15 or higher if on scheduled medication (scheduled + PRN method).
	 Consider transfer to ICU for any of the following: Total score above 35, q1h assess. x more than 8 hrs required, more than 4 mg/hr lorazepam x 3 hr **or** 20 mg/hr diazepam x 3 hr required, or resp. distress.

Patient Identification (Addressograph)

Signature/Title	Initials	Signature/Title	Initials

This scale is not copyrighted and may be used freely.
Adapted from Sullivan, J. T., Sykora, K., Schneiderman, J., Naranjo, C. A., Sellers, E. M. (1989). Assessment of alcohol withdrawal: The revised Clinical Institute Withdrawal Assessment for Alcohol scale (CIWA-Ar). *Br J Addict 84*:1353-1357. Reprinted from www.ihs.gov, revised 2003.

NOTES

Family Violence and Human Trafficking

PURPOSE

This chapter presents information about intimate partner violence, elder abuse, child abuse, and human trafficking. The content includes how to assess the extent of the abuse, how to assess the extent of physical and psychological harm, and how to document appropriately.

READING ASSIGNMENT

Jarvis: *Physical Examination and Health Assessment*, 9th ed., Chapter 7, pp. 95–110.

Suggested readings:
Roney, L. N., & Villano, C. E. (2020). Recognizing victims of a hidden crime: Human trafficking victims in your pediatric trauma bay. *J Trauma Nurs, 27*(1), 37–41.

GLOSSARY

Study the following terms after completing the reading assignment. You should be able to cover the definition on the right and define the term out loud.

Child emotional abuse .... any pattern of behavior that harms a child's emotional development or sense of self-worth. It includes frequent belittling, rejection, threats, and withholding love and support.

Child neglect .... failure to provide for a child's basic needs (physical, educational, medical, and emotional)

Child physical abuse .... physical injury resulting from punching, beating, kicking, biting, burning, shaking, or otherwise harming a child. Even if the parent or caregiver did not intend to harm the child, such acts are considered abuse when done purposefully.

Child sexual abuse .... includes fondling a child's genitals, incest, penetration, rape, sodomy, indecent exposure, and commercial exploitation through prostitution or the production of pornographic materials

Elder abuse .... infliction of harm on adults over the age of 60 years. Forms include physical abuse, sexual abuse, emotional abuse, neglect, and financial abuse.

Elder neglect .... failure of a caregiver to prevent harm to an adult over 60 years old. Examples include inadequate feeding and hydration, unsanitary living conditions, and poor personal hygiene.

Human trafficking .... "compelling or coercing a person to provide labor or services, or to engage in commercial sex acts" (US Department of Justice, 2020). If the victim is a minor, commercial sex acts are considered trafficking whether coercion is present. Human trafficking does not require movement of the person from one place to another.

Intimate partner violence (IPV) .... physical and/or sexual violence (use of physical force) or threat of such violence; also psychological or emotional abuse and/or coercive tactics when there has been prior physical and/or sexual violence between spouses or nonmarital partners (e.g., dating) or former spouses or nonmarital partners

Mandatory reporter .... a specified group of people (e.g., health care providers) required by law to report abuse (of a specified nature against specified people) to a governmental agency (e.g., protective services, the police)

Psychological abuse .... infliction of emotional and/or mental anguish by humiliation, coercion, and threats and/or lack of social stimulation. Examples include yelling, threats of harm, threats of withholding basic medical and/or personal care, and leaving the person alone for long periods.

Routine universal screening for IPV .... asking all adult patients each time they are in the health care system, no matter what their problem or concern, whether they have experienced IPV

STUDY GUIDE

After completing the reading assignment, you should be able to answer the following questions in the spaces provided.

1. Identify the most common physical health problems that result from intimate partner violence.

2. Identify the most common mental health problems that result from intimate partner violence.

3. Differentiate abuse from neglect.

4. Identify commonly used screening tools for intimate partner violence.

5. Identify commonly used screening questions for older adult abuse.

6. Identify important elements of assessment for an abused person.

7. Discuss bruising in children and how it relates to their development level.

8. Identify some of the important elements of the child's medical history when assessing for suspected child maltreatment.

9. Discuss some of the long-term consequences of child maltreatment.

10. Identify risk factors that may contribute to child maltreatment.

11. Identify risk factors, protective factors, and signs of human trafficking.

CRITICAL THINKING ACTIVITIES

1. Review laws in your state and at least one other state related to intimate partner violence, elder abuse, and child maltreatment. Do the laws between the states differ? Were you surprised by any of the laws or mandatory reporting regulations? Talk with at least one classmate and compare notes.
2. Identify community resources that help victims of intimate partner violence, elder abuse, child maltreatment, and human trafficking. Create a list of resources and identify any gaps. For example, your community may have a shelter for abused women and children yet lack adequate community resources for male or elderly victims of abuse.
3. During your clinical, screen at least one adult patient for intimate partner violence using a screening tool recommended by the US Preventive Services Task Force. How did the interaction make you feel? Was the client willing to answer the questions? What therapeutic communication techniques did you use during the encounter?
4. Ask health care providers you know whether they have received education on human trafficking and whether the health care facility where they work has a screening protocol. Try to talk to providers in various specialties. Discuss your findings with classmates. Did health care providers receive standardized education? Did most health care facilities have screening protocols in place?
5. List three risk factors for human trafficking and identify why each is a risk factor.

CLINICAL JUDGMENT QUESTIONS

This test is for you to check your own mastery of the content. Answers are provided in Appendix A.

1. Bruising on a nonwalking or noncruising child:

   a. Is a common finding from normal infant activity.
   b. Needs to be further evaluated for either an abusive or medical explanation.
   c. Is commonly seen on the buttocks.
   d. Is not uncommon because infants bruise easily.

2. During an examination, you notice a patterned injury on a 10-year-old patient's back. There are linear ecchymoses on the back but no other signs of bruising and no history of blood dyscrasia. Upon discussion with the parents, they tell you that their child has a bad cold with a high fever and they have been working to release the negative energies associated with the illness by using coining. Given your knowledge of cultural practices, you recognize that:

   a. Coining is practiced in Chinese and Southeast Asian cultures and is not considered effective unless it leaves bruises.
   b. Coining is a form of child abuse because it has no medical benefit so the parents should be reported immediately for abuse.
   c. Coining is a cultural practice but should not leave bruises on the skin. The child needs to be evaluated for abuse.
   d. Coining is a common practice that is safe and effective in treating fever and colds.

3. During an interview, a woman received a score of 11 on the Hurt, Insult, Threaten, Scream (HITS). What is the best way to proceed with the interview and subsequent assessment?

   a. Ask the patient if she is being abused and whether she has contacted the authorities.
   b. Proceed by asking more questions about potential abuse and refer to appropriate social support services.
   c. Tell the patient you believe she is being abused and tell her you will call the police to file a report.
   d. Interview the woman's partner so you have both sides of the story and can ensure trustworthiness of data.

4. You are working the night shift in the emergency room and just received an unconscious 23-year-old female victim of suspected abuse. Because she is unable to answer questions about her injuries, you should:

    a. Provide life-saving measures but delay any assessment of injuries until she can answer questions.
    b. Provide life-saving measures but delay any photographic evidence documentation until she can provide consent.
    c. Provide life-saving measures and include photographic evidence per hospital protocol even without consent.
    d. Provide life-saving measures and try to determine the cause of each individual injury as you chart your full assessment.

5. You are caring for an adolescent female in an urgent care clinic. Her boyfriend checked her in and filled out paperwork. You note that she is listed as 18 years old but appears younger. She is at the clinic due to pelvic pain, and her boyfriend has requested a pregnancy test. You notice that the person she is with appears be in his late 20s or early 30s. She is withdrawn, does not answer questions, and seems unable to answer basic demographic information, including her address and phone number. To complete a full assessment, you do the following. **Select all that apply.**

    a. Defer to the boyfriend to answer questions because he seems to know what is happening.
    b. Complete a physical assessment noting any bruising or other signs of trauma.
    c. Provide a pregnancy test.
    d. Screen for sexually transmitted infection.
    e. Separate the patient and her companion to get a more thorough history from the patient.
    f. Allow the companion to stay in the room to avoid making the patient uncomfortable.

6. You are caring for a 75-year-old male who was hospitalized with pneumonia. As you complete his intake assessment, you ask the standard screening questions, including "Do you feel safe in your home?" and "Do you have adequate income to care for yourself?" He reports feeling safe at home but states that he has been unable to find his checkbook and recently received a bank statement that was missing $5000. He also had his credit card declined last week when he was out to dinner. He lives independently and is cognitively intact. His son and daughter stop by each week to help around the house since his wife passed away last year. As you discuss his family, he shares that his daughter has been through a rough patch since her recent divorce and is having trouble paying her son's college tuition. You:

    a. Contact social work to help with his financial concerns and neurology because he may have dementia because he cannot find his checkbook.
    b. Follow hospital policy to report suspected elder abuse due to potential financial abuse/exploitation.
    c. Provide reassurance that he will be discharged soon, and you are sure his checkbook will turn up.
    d. Encourage him to talk to his daughter about her problems and see if there is anything he can do to help.

7. Documentation of suspected abuse should include which of the following. **Select all that apply.**

    a. photographic evidence
    b. subjective descriptions of injuries
    c. objective descriptions of injuries
    d. appropriate forensic terminology
    e. paraphrased account of victim statement without direct quotes
    f. appropriate direct quotes with some paraphrasing
    g. direct quotes that remove expletives or potentially offensive language

8. Upon your initial assessment, you note the following: minute, pinpoint, nonraised round spots behind the ear; dark purple discoloration of the right eye and cheek; a burn that encompasses the entire right hand; and a 2-inch cut on the right cheek. The appropriate forensic terms that you will use in documentation are: **Select all that apply.**

   a. incision
   b. puncture
   c. alopecia
   d. patterned injury
   e. avulsion
   f. ecchymosis
   g. abrasion
   h. petechiae

9. You are completing an intake assessment of an 18-month-old male who is in the clinic for his well-baby check. You note that he is walking around the chairs in the exam room, smiling, laughing, and appears at ease with his caregiver. He is able to walk without assistance but falls when he gets excited and tries to run. Upon physical examination you notice bruises on his legs bilaterally and his arms. He also has a bruise in the middle of his forehead. The caregiver reports that he ran into the coffee table 2 days ago and he has since moved it out of the living room to avoid future accidents.

   You should recognize that the bruises _(are/are not)_____a sign of abuse. Because the toddler is walking, he is __(likely/unlikely)____to have bruises. Noting how the child acts with the caregiver is an _____(effective/ineffective)_____way to assess the caregiver/child relationship.

CHAPTER
8

Assessment Techniques and Safety in the Clinical Setting

PURPOSE

This chapter presents the assessment techniques of inspection, palpation, percussion, and auscultation; learn the items of equipment needed for a complete physical examination; and consider age-specific modifications you would make for the examination of individuals throughout the life cycle.

READING ASSIGNMENT

Jarvis: *Physical Examination and Health Assessment,* 9th ed., Chapter 8, pp. 111–126.

Suggested reading:
Perkins, R., Ingebretson, E., Holifield, L., & Bergeron, A. (2021). A nurse's guide to COVID-19: An evidence-based review of the care of hospitalized adults with this disease. *Am J Nurs, 121*(3), 28–38.

GLOSSARY

Study the following terms after completing the reading assignment. You should be able to cover the definition on the right and define the term out loud.

Amplitude .... (or intensity) how loud or soft a sound is

Duration .... the length of time a note lingers

Ophthalmoscope .... an instrument that illuminates the internal eye structures, enabling the examiner to look through the pupil at the fundus (background) of the eye

Otoscope .... an instrument that illuminates the ear canal, enabling the examiner to look at the ear canal and tympanic membrane

Pitch .... (or frequency) the number of vibrations (or cycles) per second of a note

Quality .... (or timbre) a subjective difference in a sound as a result of the sound's distinctive overtones

STUDY GUIDE

After completing the reading assignment, you should be able to answer the following questions in the spaces provided.

1. Define and describe the technique of the four physical examination skills:

   Inspection_____

   Palpation_____

   Percussion_____

   Auscultation_____

2. Define the characteristics of the following percussion notes:

	Pitch	Amplitude	Quality	Duration
Resonance				
Hyperresonance				
Tympany				
Dull				

3. Differentiate among light, deep, and bimanual palpation.

4. List the two end pieces of the stethoscope and the conditions for which each is best suited.

5. Describe the environmental conditions to consider in preparing the examination setting.

6. List four situations in which you clean your hands promptly and thoroughly.

7. Describe your own preparation as you encounter the patient for examination: your own dress, your demeanor, safety/universal precautions, sequence of examination steps, instructions to patient.

8. Differentiate standard and transmission-based precautions. Provide examples of when to use each.

9. What age-specific considerations would you make for the examination of the:

Infant? _____

Toddler? _____

Preschooler? _____

School-age child? _____

Adolescent? _____

Older adult? _____

Acutely ill person? _____

CLINICAL JUDGMENT QUESTIONS

This test is for you to check your own mastery of the content. Answers are provided in Appendix A.

1. You are preparing to assess a 1-month-old who is awake and fussy. Given what you know of development, you begin the assessment by:

   a. moving in a head-to-toe fashion so you do not forget anything.
   b. listening to the heart and lungs first while the infant is being held.
   c. personalizing the assessment based on the infant's temperament.
   d. avoiding eye contact because the infant has stranger anxiety.

2. The nurse is assessing a patient's skin for swelling during an office visit. What is the best technique to use to assess the patient's skin for lumps and swelling? Use the:

   a. fingertips because they have better tactile discrimination than the rest of the hand.
   b. dorsal surface of the hand because the skin is thinner than on the palms of the hand.
   c. ulnar portion of the hand because there is increased blood supply that enhances temperature sensitivity.
   d. palmar surface of the hand because it is most sensitive to temperature variations.

3. Palpation can be used for which of the following? **Select all that apply.**

   a. Position of an organ
   b. Size of a mass
   c. Density of an organ
   d. Deep tendon reflex
   e. Pulsation
   f. Vibration

4. When percussing over the lungs of a patient, the nurse notices a dull sound. The nurse should:

   a. consider this a normal finding and continue the assessment.
   b. palpate this area for an underlying mass.
   c. reposition the hands and attempt to percuss in this area again to confirm the finding.
   d. move on with the assessment so as not to alarm the patient.

5. You are preparing to assess a patient who reports changes in skin pigmentation. The best option for lighting is:

   a. Natural daylight
   b. Overhead lighting
   c. Tangential lighting
   d. Sun lamp

6. Extra heart sounds and murmurs are described as low-pitched sounds. Given your knowledge of the stethoscope, you know that low-pitched sounds are best heard with the:

   a. bell end piece held firmly to the skin
   b. bell end piece held lightly against the skin
   c. diaphragm end piece held firmly to the skin
   d. diaphragm end piece held lightly to the skin

7. You are preparing to enter the room of a patient with suspected pertussis. To protect yourself and others you will: **Select all that apply.**

   a. use standard precautions
   b. use contact precautions
   c. use droplet precautions
   d. use airborne precautions
   e. use hand sanitizer
   f. wash your hands with soap and water if visibly soiled
   g. always wash your hands instead of using hand sanitizer

8. To assess a patient's abdomen by palpation, how should the nurse proceed?

   a. Avoid palpation of reported "tender" areas because this may cause the patient pain.
   b. Quickly palpate a tender area to avoid any discomfort that the patient may experience.
   c. Begin the assessment with deep palpation, encouraging the patient to relax and take deep breaths.
   d. Start with light palpation to detect surface characteristics and to accustom the patient to being touched.

9. You are preparing to assess a 99-year-old man who is in the emergency room due to shortness of breath. His respirations appear rapid and labored.

   The best position for this patient is _____. To complete the assessment, you should _____ and _____.

   Select the correct phrases/words for blanks from the following list.
   Supine
   High Fowler's
   Dorsal recumbent
   Proceed in head-to-toe format
   Complete a focused assessment
   Pause as necessary and provide breaks
   Complete the assessment as quickly as possible
   Complete a full head to toe assessment
   Avoid taking breaks so the exam is completed quickly

10. Identify whether the following patient positions are typically used in the inpatient setting, outpatient setting, or both.

Position	Inpatient	Outpatient	Both
Supine			
Lithotomy			
Semi-Fowler's			
Sims			
Dorsal recumbent			

SKILLS LABORATORY AND CLINICAL SETTING

You are now ready for the clinical component of Chapter 8. The purpose of the clinical component is to familiarize yourself with the equipment used in the clinical setting and to achieve the following:

Clinical Objectives

1. Practice inspection, percussion, palpation, and auscultation.
2. Practice using common assessment equipment (e.g., stethoscope).
3. Demonstrate appropriate universal precautions.

Instructions

Practice assessment techniques with partners in the skills laboratory. Because each person is unique, practice on multiple people. The goal is to familiarize yourself with the equipment and techniques so that you are prepared when it is time to apply the skills to specific body systems.

NOTES

General Survey and Measurement

PURPOSE

This chapter presents the method of gathering data for a general survey on a patient and the techniques for measuring height and weight and calculating body mass index.

READING ASSIGNMENT

Jarvis: *Physical Examination and Health Assessment*, 9th ed., Chapter 9, pp. 127–140.

Suggested readings:
Centers for Disease Control and Prevention. (2021). *Overweight and obesity.* https://www.cdc.gov/obesity/index.html
Komar, E., & Kameg, B. (2020). Anorexia nervosa: An overview for primary care providers. *Nurse Pract*, *45*(8), 8–10.

STUDY GUIDE

After completing the reading assignment, write or draw the answer in the spaces provided.

1. List the significant information considered in each of the four areas of a general survey—physical appearance, body structure, mobility, and behavior.

2. Describe the normal posture, body build, and proportions.

3. Note aspects of normal gait.

4. Describe the clinical appearance of the following variations in stature:

Hypopituitary dwarfism_____

Gigantism_____

Acromegaly_____

Achondroplastic dwarfism_____

Marfan syndrome_____

Endogenous obesity (Cushing syndrome)_____

Anorexia nervosa_____

Bulimia nervosa_____

5. State the body mass index of a male weighing 190 lb who is 5′10″ tall _____ and for a female weighing 136 lb who is 5′4″ tall _____.

6. For serial weight measurements, what instructions would you give the patient?

7. Describe the technique for measuring head circumference and chest circumference of an infant.

8. What changes in height and weight distribution would you expect for patients in their 80s or 90s?

CLINICAL JUDGMENT QUESTIONS

This test is for you to check your own mastery of the content. Answers are provided in Appendix A.

1. You are assessing a 5-month-old with known increased intracranial pressure and cranial enlargement. Which finding would you expect?

   a. The infant's head is 2 cm larger than his chest.
   b. The infant's head and chest measure equally.
   c. The infant's head is 5 cm larger than his chest.
   d. The infant's head is 2 cm smaller than his chest.

   Underline the abnormal findings in the general surveys for questions 2–4.

2. E.K. is a 39-year-old female who appears stated age, is alert and oriented, and appears well nourished. Facial grimace with movement. Pronounced limp with walking. Height and weight appear normal for age and gender. No body odor. Good personal hygiene.

3. L.M. is an 89-year-old male who appears stated age, is alert and oriented to person and place only, and able to answer questions. Wide, shuffling gait noted. Kyphosis. No body odor noted. Clothing appropriate for season and age.

4. D.F. is an 18-month-old female. Appears stated age. Pronounced lordosis. Wide, unsteady gait. Arm span shorter than height. Frontal bossing noted.

5. Underline the correct option in the following: The nurse should recognize that lordosis/kyphosis is normal for toddlers, while lordosis/kyphosis is normal for older adults. Other changes with aging include loss/gain of subcutaneous fat in the face and extremities. Older adults lose height due to changes in the long bones/vertebrae.

6. M.L. is a 16-year-old male who is 6' 9" tall with an arm span that is greater than his height and a long pubis-to-sole measurement. He is thin, with a narrow face and hyperextensible joints. Based on the general survey, you know M.L. may have:

   a. Marfan's syndrome
   b. Gigantism
   c. Acromegaly
   d. Hyperpituitarism

CRITICAL THINKING ACTIVITIES

1. Your next patient is a 55-year-old man who has experienced shortness of breath for the past 2 days. When you walk into the room, you hear audible, labored breathing. Based on the picture below, write a general survey.

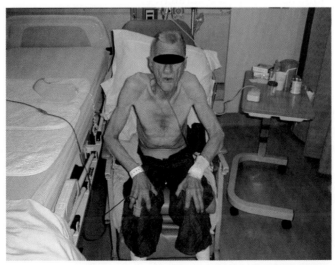

(From Goldman, L. & Schafer, A. I. [2012]. *Goldman's Cecil medicine* [24th ed.]. Philadelphia: Saunders.)

2. H.Y. is at your clinic with her mother for a well-child appointment. She is new to your clinic, and you have no history other than she recently turned 1 year old. Based on the picture below, write a general survey.

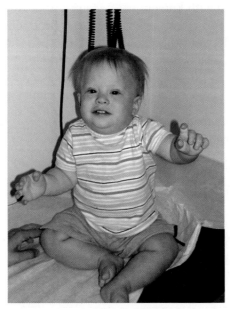

(From Zitelli, B. J., McIntire, S. C., & Nowalk, A. J. [2012]. *Atlas of pediatric physical diagnosis* [6th ed.]. Philadelphia, Saunders.)

SKILLS LABORATORY AND CLINICAL SETTING

You are now ready for the clinical component of Chapter 9. The purpose of the clinical component is to observe and describe the regional examination on a peer in the skills laboratory and to achieve the following:

Clinical Objectives

1. Observe and describe the significant characteristics of a general survey.
2. Measure height, weight, and waist circumference and determine if findings are within normal range.
3. Record the physical examination findings accurately.

Instructions

Practice the steps of gathering data for a general survey and for height, weight, and waist circumference on a peer. Make sure you are familiar with the equipment you will be using. If available, practice with both a balance scale and a digital scale. Record your findings using the regional write-up sheet that follows. The first section of the sheet is intended as a worksheet. It includes points for you to note that add up to the general survey. The bottom of the sheet has instructions for you to write the general survey statement; this is the topic sentence that will serve as an introduction for the complete physical examination write-up.

REGIONAL WRITE-UP—GENERAL SURVEY, VITAL SIGNS

Date _____

Examiner _____

Patient _____ Age _____ Gender _____

Occupation _____

I. Physical Examination
   A. General survey
      1. Physical appearance
         Gender_____
         Level of consciousness _____
         Skin color _____
         Facial features _____
      2. Body structure
         Stature _____
         Nutrition _____
         Symmetry _____
         Posture _____
         Position _____
         Body build, contour _____
         Any physical deformity _____
      3. Mobility
         Gait _____
         Range of motion _____
      4. Behavior
         Facial expression _____
         Mood and affect _____
         Speech _____
         Dress _____
         Personal hygiene _____
   B. Measurement
      1. Height: _____ cm; _____ ft/inches   3. Body mass index _____
      2. Weight: _____ kg; _____ lb   4. Waist circumference _____ inches

II. Summary
Write a summary of the general survey, including height and weight. This will serve as an introduction to the complete physical examination write-up.

Table 9.1 Body Mass Index

BMI	NORMAL								OVERWEIGHT					OBESE							
	19	20	21	22	23	24	25	26	27	28	29	30	31	32	33	34	35	36	37	38	39
HEIGHT (INCHES)	BODY WEIGHT (POUNDS)																				
58	91	96	100	105	110	115	119	124	129	134	138	143	148	153	158	162	167	172	177	181	186
59	94	99	104	109	114	119	124	128	133	138	143	148	153	158	163	168	173	178	183	188	193
60	97	102	107	112	118	123	128	133	138	143	148	153	158	163	168	174	179	184	189	194	199
61	100	106	111	116	122	127	132	137	143	148	153	158	164	169	174	180	185	190	195	201	206
62	104	109	115	120	126	131	136	142	147	153	158	164	169	175	180	186	191	196	202	207	213
63	107	113	118	124	130	135	141	146	152	158	163	169	175	180	186	191	197	203	208	214	220
64	110	116	122	128	134	140	145	151	157	163	169	174	180	186	192	197	204	209	215	221	227
65	114	120	126	132	138	144	150	156	162	168	174	180	186	192	198	204	210	216	222	228	234
66	118	124	130	136	142	148	155	161	167	173	179	186	192	198	204	210	216	223	229	235	241
67	121	127	134	140	146	153	159	166	172	178	185	191	198	204	211	217	223	230	236	242	249
68	125	131	138	144	151	158	164	171	177	184	190	197	203	210	216	223	230	236	243	249	256
69	128	135	142	149	155	162	169	176	182	189	196	203	209	216	223	230	236	243	250	257	263
70	132	139	146	153	160	167	174	181	188	195	202	209	216	222	229	236	243	250	257	264	271
71	136	143	150	157	165	172	179	186	193	200	208	215	222	229	236	243	250	257	265	272	279
72	140	147	154	162	169	177	184	191	199	206	213	221	228	235	242	250	258	265	272	279	287
73	144	151	159	166	174	182	189	197	204	212	219	227	235	242	250	257	265	272	280	288	295
74	148	155	163	171	179	186	194	202	210	218	225	233	241	249	256	264	272	280	287	295	303
75	152	160	168	176	184	192	200	208	216	224	232	240	248	256	264	272	279	287	295	303	311
76	156	164	172	180	189	197	205	213	221	230	238	246	254	263	271	279	287	295	304	312	320

BMI	EXTREME OBESITY														
	40	41	42	43	44	45	46	47	48	49	50	51	52	53	54
HEIGHT (INCHES)	BODY WEIGHT (POUNDS)														
58	191	196	201	205	210	215	220	224	229	234	239	244	248	253	258
59	198	203	208	212	217	222	227	232	237	242	247	252	257	262	267
60	204	209	215	220	225	230	235	240	245	250	255	261	266	271	276
61	211	217	222	227	232	238	243	248	254	259	264	269	275	280	285
62	218	224	229	235	240	246	251	256	262	267	273	278	284	289	295
63	225	231	237	242	248	254	259	265	270	278	282	287	293	299	304
64	232	238	244	250	256	262	267	273	279	285	291	296	302	308	314
65	240	246	252	258	264	270	276	282	288	294	300	306	312	318	324
66	247	253	260	266	272	278	284	291	297	303	309	315	322	328	334
67	255	261	268	274	280	287	293	299	306	312	319	325	331	338	344
68	262	269	276	282	289	295	302	308	315	322	328	335	341	348	354
69	270	277	284	291	297	304	311	318	324	331	338	345	351	358	365
70	278	285	292	299	306	313	320	327	334	341	348	355	362	369	376
71	286	293	301	308	315	322	329	338	343	351	358	365	372	379	386
72	294	302	309	316	324	331	338	346	353	361	368	375	383	390	397
73	302	310	318	325	333	340	348	355	363	371	378	386	393	401	408
74	311	319	326	334	342	350	358	365	373	381	389	396	404	412	420
75	319	327	335	343	351	359	367	375	383	391	399	407	415	423	431
76	328	336	344	353	361	369	377	385	394	402	410	418	426	435	443

Modified from Clinical guidelines on the identification, evaluation, and treatment of overweight and obesity in adults: The evidence report. June 2009. http://www.nhlbi.nih.gov/guidelines/obesity/bmi_tbl.pdf.

PURPOSE

This chapter reviews how to measure and interpret vital signs.

READING ASSIGNMENT

Jarvis: *Physical Examination and Health Assessment*, 9th ed., Chapter 10, pp. 141–162.

Suggested readings:
Elias, M. F., & Goodless, A. L. (2021). Human errors in automated office blood pressure measurement: Still room for improvement. *Hypertension, 77*, 6–15.

GLOSSARY

Study the following terms after completing the reading assignment. You should be able to cover the definition on the right and define the term out loud.

Auscultatory gap .... a brief period when Korotkoff sounds disappear during auscultation of blood pressure; may occur with hypertension

Bradycardia .... heart rate fewer than 50 or 60 beats/min in the adult (depending on agency)

Bradypnea .... decreased respiratory rate; typically, fewer than 8–12 breaths/min in the adult depending on agency

Sphygmomanometer .... instrument for measuring arterial blood pressure

Stroke volume .... amount of blood pumped out of the heart with each heartbeat

Tachycardia .... heart rate greater than 95 beats/min in the adult

Tachypnea .... rapid respiratory rate; respiratory rate above 25 breaths/min in the adult

STUDY GUIDE

After completing the reading assignment, write or draw the answer in the spaces provided.

1. Describe the tympanic membrane and temporal artery thermometers, and compare their use with other forms of temperature measurement.

2. Describe three qualities to consider when assessing the pulse.

3. Describe the qualities of normal respiration and the appropriate approach for counting the respiratory rate.

4. Define and describe the relationships among the terms *blood pressure, systolic pressure, diastolic pressure, pulse pressure,* and *mean arterial pressure.*

5. List factors that affect blood pressure.

6. Relate the use of the wrong size blood pressure cuff to the possible findings that might be obtained.

7. Explain the significance of phase I, phase IV, and phase V Korotkoff sounds during blood pressure measurement.

8. Given an apparently healthy 20-year-old adult, state the expected range for pulse, respirations, and blood pressure.

CLINICAL JUDGMENT QUESTIONS

This test is for you to check your own mastery of the content. Answers are provided in Appendix A.

1. A patient is being seen in the clinic for complaints of "fainting episodes that started last week." How should you proceed with the examination?

   a. Take the blood pressure in both arms and thighs to determine if coarctation of the aorta is present.
   b. Ask the person to walk a few paces and then take their blood pressure. Compare the reading to the resting blood pressure.
   c. Record the blood pressure in the lying, sitting, and standing positions to determine if orthostatic hypotension is the cause.
   d. Record the blood pressure in the lying and sitting positions and average these numbers to obtain a mean blood pressure.

2. J.L., a 69-year-old, was brought to the emergency department due to syncopal episodes following 3 days of nausea and vomiting. Given your knowledge of vital signs, identify what findings you might expect. **Select all that apply**.

   a. Decreased BP with position change from laying to sitting.
   b. Increased BP with position change from laying to sitting.
   c. Increased pulse with position change from laying to sitting.
   d. Decreased pulse with position change from laying to sitting.
   e. Increased respiratory rate due to hypovolemia.
   f. Increased temperature.

3. You are caring for a new admission to the emergency department. He was found asleep on a park bench on a cold winter night, and his temperature is currently 96°F. His extremities are cool and his digits are cyanotic. The provider has asked for an SpO_2 reading. Given his condition, the best option for an accurate SpO_2 is:

   a. Place a probe on his index finger. Hold the probe around the finger. The SpO_2 is likely accurate even if the heart rate does not correlate.
   b. Place the probe on his earlobe. The SpO_2 is likely accurate even if the heart rate does not correlate because the earlobe is a more central location.
   c. Use a finger clip type of probe on his earlobe since you do not have the appropriate type of probe available, but the finger is not working.
   d. Place forehead probe in the middle of his forehead. If the heart rate correlates and the waveform is good, the reading is likely accurate.

4. Circle the correct word in each pair. The nurse should recognize that temperature regulation improves/declines with normal aging. Elderly patients often have lower/higher normal temperatures than their younger counterparts and are more/less likely to have a fever with an infection.

5. E.W. is a 2-month-old at your clinic for a routine check-up. Given your knowledge of developmental needs, you know the best way to proceed with vital signs is:

   a. Proceed in the same order for all patients: temperature, pulse, respiratory rate, and BP. Make sure to count the pulse for a full minute.
   b. Consider the infant's age and begin with the respiratory rate and pulse, counting each for a minute, then take the BP and temperature.
   c. Consider the infant's age and begin with respiratory rate and pulse, counting each for a minute, then take the temperature. BP is not routinely assessed in infants.
   d. Disrobe the infant and lay him on the table to make counting respirations easier. Count respiratory rate and pulse, followed by taking the temperature.

6. You are assessing the vital signs of a 22-year-old male college athlete who reports playing soccer since he was 3 years old. You record the following vital signs: temperature—97°F; pulse—50 beats per minute; respirations—16 per minute; blood pressure—100/64 mm Hg. Which statement is true about these results?

    a. The patient is experiencing tachycardia and tachypnea.
    b. These are normal vital signs for a healthy, athletic adult.
    c. The patient's pulse rate is bradycardic—his physician should be notified.
    d. On the basis of today's readings, the patient should return for follow-up.
    e. Follow-up is needed due to low BP and pulse in this patient.

7. A 4-year-old female presents to the office for a physical. Her parents recently moved to the area. She reports she has not visited a doctor in a few years. Her mother reports an uneventful perinatal course. She was born at term and does not have any preexisting conditions. You obtain the following VS: T 37°C, P 90, RR 26, BP 158/78 right arm, sitting. Given the vital signs, the best next steps include:

    a. Notify the physician immediately. Consider possible essential hypertension.
    b. Obtain a BP in the left arm and a thigh pressure before notifying the provider.
    c. Obtain a BP in the left arm and repeat the right arm pressure then notify the provider.
    d. Check instrument calibration and get a different BP cuff. She should not have a high BP.
    e. The most likely explanation is user error. Have another nurse obtain bilateral BPs.

8. A 45-year-old male with a BMI of 28 is at your clinic for a routine checkup. His BP is 132/82, 134/80, and 132/84 on serial readings, all in the right arm with the patient sitting. His left arm BP is 130/84. His 10-year CVD risk is less than 10%. Given your knowledge of current recommendations, you know the patient should **Select all that apply**:

    a. Be placed on antihypertensive medication
    b. Lose weight
    c. Decrease sodium intake
    d. Increase physical activity
    e. Follow up to repeat BP readings annually
    f. Follow up to repeat BP readings in 6 months
    g. Decrease dietary potassium intake
    h. Limit alcohol intake

9. For each finding, identify whether it is normal or abnormal.

Finding	Normal	Abnormal
Rectal temperature 37.7°C		
Respiratory rate 20 bpm, even		
Respiratory rate 9 bpm		
Pulse 80 bpm, 2+, irregular		
Temperature 35°C		

10. Put the following steps for completing a BP reading using a Doppler in the correct order. Assume the cuff is already in place. Not all steps will be used.

Turn on Doppler flowmeter.
Apply coupling gel to the transducer probe.
Palpate the artery if possible and apply coupling gel. If the artery is not palpable, apply gel to the correct anatomical position.
Slowly deflate the cuff, noting the point at which sound is first heard. This is the systolic pressure.
Rapidly deflate the cuff allowing the blood to dissipate.
Touch the probe to skin, holding it perpendicular to the artery.
Rapidly deflate the cuff, then reinflate to 20–30 mm Hg beyond the point at which the sound disappeared.
Continue inflation 20–30 mm Hg beyond the point at which the sound disappears.
Once you hear the pulsatile whooshing, inflate the cuff until the sound disappears.
Note the point at which sound muffles and disappears. These represent Korotkoff sounds IV and V.

CRITICAL THINKING ACTIVITIES

1. Analyze the following vital sign values. Make sure to note any additional information you need to fully analyze the values:

   55-year-old woman: T 37°C, R 18 breaths/min, P 160 bpm, BP 90/60 mmHg

   2-year-old boy: T 37°C, R 18 breaths/min, P 130 bpm

   89-year-old woman: T 36°C, R 12 breaths/min, P 55 bpm, BP 140/98 mmHg

   25-year-old man: T 39°C, R 26 breaths/min, P 113 bpm, BP 100/60 mmHg

SKILLS LABORATORY AND CLINICAL SETTING

You are now ready for the clinical component of Chapter 10. The purpose of the clinical component is to perform vital signs measurements to achieve the following:

Clinical Objectives

1. Demonstrate temperature measurement using oral, tympanic, and temporal artery thermometers.
2. Describe the procedure for taking a rectal temperature and demonstrate it on a manikin in the skills lab, if available.
3. Correctly take a radial pulse and describe associated characteristics.
4. Correctly take the respiratory rate and describe associated characteristics.
5. Measure blood pressure.
6. Record the vital sign findings accurately.

Instructions

Practice taking a full set of vital signs on at least five peers in the laboratory setting. For each person, note the following:
1. Temperature _____
2. Pulse
   a. Rate _____
   b. Rhythm _____
   c. Force _____
3. Respiratory rate _____; description _____
4. Blood pressure _____ R arm; _____ L arm

NOTES

PURPOSE

This chapter presents the structure and function of pain pathways, understand the process of nociception, understand the rationale and methods of pain assessment, and accurately record the findings.

READING ASSIGNMENT

Jarvis: *Physical Examination and Health Assessment*, 9th ed., Chapter 11, pp. 163–180.

Suggested readings:
Delgado, S. A. (2020). Managing pain in critically ill adults: A holistic approach. *Am J Nurs, 120*(5), 34–43.

GLOSSARY

Study the following terms after completing the reading assignment. You should be able to cover the definition on the right and define the term out loud.

Acute pain .... short-term, self-limiting, often predictable trajectory; stops after injury heals

Allodynia .... experience of pain after a normally nonpainful tactile (e.g., from clothing) or thermal stimulus

Breakthrough pain .... pain restarts or escalates before next scheduled analgesic dose

Chronic (persistent) pain .... pain continues for 6 months or longer after initial injury

Cutaneous pain .... pain originating from skin surface or subcutaneous structures

Incident pain .... occurs predictably after specific movements

Modulation .... pain message inhibited during this last phase of nociception

Neuropathic pain .... abnormal processing of pain message; burning, shooting in nature

Nociception .... process whereby noxious stimuli are perceived as pain; central and peripheral nervous systems intact

Nociceptors .... specialized nerve endings that detect painful sensations

Pain .... "An unpleasant sensory and emotional experience associated with, or resembling that associated with, actual or potential tissue damage." (International Association for the Study of Pain)

Perception ....conscious awareness of painful sensation

Referred pain ....pain felt at a particular site but originates from another location

Somatic pain ....originating from muscle, bone, joints, tendons, or blood vessels

Transduction ....first phase of nociception whereby the painful stimulus is changed into an action potential

Transmission ....second phase of nociception whereby the pain impulse moves from the spinal cord to the brain

Visceral pain ....originating from internal organs such as the gallbladder or stomach

STUDY GUIDE

After completing the reading assignment, write or draw the answers in the spaces provided.

1. Describe the process of nociception using the four phases of:
   Transduction _____
   Transmission _____
   Perception _____
   Modulation _____

2. Identify the differences between nociceptive and neuropathic pain. Which words may typically be used to describe nociceptive pain and neuropathic pain?

3. List various sources of pain.

4. Explain how acute and chronic pain differ in terms of nonverbal behaviors.

5. Identify the most reliable indicator of a person's pain.

6. What does the mnemonic *PQRST* stand for, and how can it be used to guide pain assessment?

7. Describe physical examination findings that might indicate pain.

CRITICAL THINKING ACTIVITIES

1. What conditions are more likely to produce pain in an aging adult?

2. How would you modify your examination when the patient reports having abdominal pain?

3. How would you assess for pain in an individual with dementia?

4. What would you say to someone who tells you that infants do not remember pain and that they are too young for the pain to have any damaging effects?

5. What would you say to a colleague who remarks that the individual with Alzheimer disease does not feel pain and therefore does not require an analgesic?

6. A patient has both chemotherapy-induced peripheral neuropathy and pain related to metastatic bone cancer. Given what you know about pain treatment, should the patient be treated with opioid medication? Why or why not? What other therapy, if any, should be considered?

Fill in the labels indicated on the following illustration:

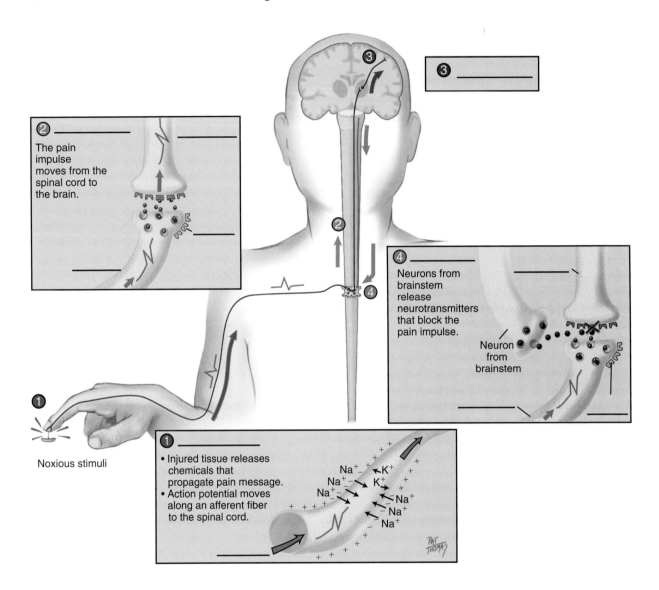

② _____

The pain impulse moves from the spinal cord to the brain.

③ _____

④ _____

Neurons from brainstem release neurotransmitters that block the pain impulse.

Neuron from brainstem

① _____

• Injured tissue releases chemicals that propagate pain message.
• Action potential moves along an afferent fiber to the spinal cord.

Na^+ K^+
Na^+ K^+
Na^+ Na^+
Na^+
Na^+

Noxious stimuli

CLINICAL JUDGMENT QUESTIONS

This test is for you to check your own mastery of the content. Answers are provided in Appendix A.

1. A 30-year-old woman reports having persistent, intense pain in her right arm related to trauma sustained from a car accident 5 months ago. She states that the slightest touch or clothing can exacerbate the pain. This report is suggestive of:

   a. Referred pain.
   b. Psychogenic pain.
   c. Complex regional pain I.
   d. Cutaneous pain.

2. You are caring for a 36-year-old male who presents to the emergency department with acute right lower quadrant abdominal pain rated at 10/10 on the numeric pain rating scale. The patient is tachycardic, tachypneic, grimacing, and curled in the fetal position. During the workup, the provider refuses to order any pain medication. You should:

   a. Advocate for the patient to receive pain medication. It will be easier to complete the workup if the patient is comfortable.
   b. Let the patient know that no pain medication can be given until the workup is complete, as the medication may mask symptoms.
   c. Recognize that the provider understands the need for the patient to feel the pain so he can adequately describe it.
   d. Call your supervisor to intervene. The patient should have pain medication ordered immediately.

3. A patient has osteoarthritis in her hips and knees. She can move around in her room this morning and has offered no complaints. When asked, she states that her pain is "bad this morning" and rates the pain at an 8 on a 0 to 10-point scale. The nurse suspects the patient:

   a. Is addicted to her pain medication and cannot obtain relief from small doses.
   b. Does not want to trouble anyone with her complaints.
   c. Is not in severe pain but would like pain medication.
   d. Has experienced pain for years and adapted to the chronic pain.

4. You are assessing the pain in a patient in the neonatal intensive care unit. J.K. is a female infant born at 34 weeks gestation who underwent surgery to correct esophageal atresia. When you admit the patient postoperatively, she is not actively crying, does not require oxygen to maintain an oxygen saturation above 98%, her HR and BP are increased from baseline though not significantly, she grimaces frequently, and she wakes frequently. Using the CRIES instrument on page 174 of the textbook, how would you rate the infant's pain?

   a. 2
   b. 3
   c. 6
   d. 1
   e. 4

5. When caring for a patient with advanced dementia, which of the following categories are included in the PAINAD Scale? **Select all that apply.**

   a. Breathing independent of vocalization
   b. Yelling
   c. Body language
   d. Consolability
   e. Activity
   f. Negative vocalization
   g. Positive vocalization
   h. Facial expression
   i. Face
   j. Vital signs

6. Mu-opioid receptors are located in the: **Select all that apply.**
   a. Small intestine
   b. Amygdala
   c. Hypothalamus
   d. Thalamus
   e. Insula
   f. Prefrontal cortex
   g. Spinal cord ventral horn
   h. Brainstem
   i. Spinal cord dorsal horn

7. Acute and chronic pain result in a variety of physiological changes. Mark the following as a result of acute pain or chronic pain.

Physiological Change	Acute Pain	Chronic Pain
Depression		
Nausea		
Fear		
Isolation		
Limited functioning		
Tachycardia		

Complete the following paragraph using the Options listed below:

8. Mu-opioid receptors found in the _____1_____ lead to respiratory depression while mu-receptors located in the dorsal horn are responsible for pain ___2___ and those located in the ventral tegmental area are responsible for _____3_____.

Options for 1	Options for 2	Options for 3
Brainstem	Transduction	Transduction
Dorsal horn	Modulation	Modulation
Medulla	Pleasure	Pleasure
Ventral tegmental area	Transmission	Transmission
Thalamus	Perception	Perception

9. Highlight the findings that would require follow-up.
   You are caring for a 62-year-old male who is receiving morphine to treat pain related to metastatic bone cancer. The patient also has chemotherapy-induced peripheral neuropathy. Vital signs: HR 124, regular; RR 30 bpm, shallow; BP 148/88, R arm, lying down. Complains of burning pain in bilateral feet, rated at 8/10.

SKILLS LABORATORY AND CLINICAL SETTING

The purpose of the clinical component is to practice pain assessment in the clinical setting and to achieve the following:

Clinical objectives

1. Assess pain in patients using objective and subjective indicators of pain.
2. Use the Brief Pain Inventory to assess pain in at least one patient.
3. Use the numeric pain scale (0 to 10) to assess pain in at least one patient.

Instructions

Use the Brief Pain Inventory, and numeric pain scale (0 to 10) to assess pain in at least one patient. If possible, use each tool on multiple patients to assure understanding of how to use each assessment tool. Discuss your findings with your laboratory faculty member and classmates.

Brief Pain Inventory

Date:___/___/___   Time: _____
Name:_____
        Last   First   Middle initial

1. Throughout our lives, most of us have had pain from time to time (such as minor headaches, sprains, and tooth-aches). Have you had pain other than these everyday kinds of pain today?
   1. Yes   2. No

2. On the diagram, shade in the areas where you feel pain. Put an X on the area that hurts the most.

Right   Left   Left   Right

3. Please rate your pain by circling the one number that best describes your pain at its **worst** in the past 24 hours.

   | 0 | 1 | 2 | 3 | 4 | 5 | 6 | 7 | 8 | 9 | 10 |
   No pain   Pain as bad as you can imagine

4. Please rate your pain by circling the one number that best describes your pain at its **least** in the past 24 hours.

   | 0 | 1 | 2 | 3 | 4 | 5 | 6 | 7 | 8 | 9 | 10 |
   No pain   Pain as bad as you can imagine

5. Please rate your pain by circling the one number that best describes your pain on the **average**.

   | 0 | 1 | 2 | 3 | 4 | 5 | 6 | 7 | 8 | 9 | 10 |
   No pain   Pain as bad as you can imagine

6. Please rate your pain by circling the one number that tells how much pain you have **right now**.

   | 0 | 1 | 2 | 3 | 4 | 5 | 6 | 7 | 8 | 9 | 10 |
   No pain   Pain as bad as you can imagine

7. What treatments or medications are you receiving for your pain?

   _____
   _____

8. In the past 24 hours, how much **relief** have pain treatments or medications provided? Please circle the one percentage that most shows how much relief you have received.

   | 0% | 10 | 20 | 30 | 40 | 50 | 60 | 70 | 80 | 90 | 100% |
   No relief   Complete relief

9. Circle the one number that describes how, during the past 24 hours, pain has **interfered** with your:

   A: General activity

   | 0 | 1 | 2 | 3 | 4 | 5 | 6 | 7 | 8 | 9 | 10 |
   Does not interfere   Completely interferes

   B: Mood

   | 0 | 1 | 2 | 3 | 4 | 5 | 6 | 7 | 8 | 9 | 10 |
   Does not interfere   Completely interferes

   C: Walking ability

   | 0 | 1 | 2 | 3 | 4 | 5 | 6 | 7 | 8 | 9 | 10 |
   Does not interfere   Completely interferes

   D: Normal work (includes both work outside the home and housework)

   | 0 | 1 | 2 | 3 | 4 | 5 | 6 | 7 | 8 | 9 | 10 |
   Does not interfere   Completely interferes

   E: Relations with other people

   | 0 | 1 | 2 | 3 | 4 | 5 | 6 | 7 | 8 | 9 | 10 |
   Does not interfere   Completely interferes

   F: Sleep

   | 0 | 1 | 2 | 3 | 4 | 5 | 6 | 7 | 8 | 9 | 10 |
   Does not interfere   Completely interferes

   G: Enjoyment of life

   | 0 | 1 | 2 | 3 | 4 | 5 | 6 | 7 | 8 | 9 | 10 |
   Does not interfere   Completely interferes

(Copyright © Charles S. Cleeland, 1991.)

NOTES

CHAPTER 12

Nutrition Assessment

PURPOSE

This chapter presents the components of nutritional assessment, including the assessment of dietary intake and nutritional status of individuals; identify the possible occurrence, nature, and extent of impaired nutritional status (ranging from undernutrition to overnutrition); and record the assessment accurately.

READING ASSIGNMENT

Jarvis: *Physical Examination and Health Assessment*, 9th ed., Chapter 12, pp. 181–198.

Suggested reading:
Graf, M. D., Karp, S. M., Lutenbacher, M., et al. (2021). Clinical strategies for addressing obesity in infants and toddler. *Nurse Pract, 46*(2), 28–34.

GLOSSARY

Study the following terms after completing the reading assignment. You should be able to cover the definition on the right and define the term out loud.

Android obesity .... excess body fat that is placed predominantly within the abdomen and upper body, as opposed to the hips and thighs.

Anthropometry .... measurement of the body (e.g., height, weight, circumferences, skinfold thickness).

Body mass index .... weight in kilograms divided by height in meters squared (W/H^2); value of 30 or more is indicative of obesity; value of less than 18.5 is indicative of undernutrition.

Diet history .... a detailed record of dietary intake obtainable from 24-hour recalls, food frequency questionnaires, food diaries, and similar sources.

Kwashiorkor .... primarily a protein deficiency characterized by edema, growth failure, and muscle wasting.

Malnutrition .... may mean any nutrition disorder but usually refers to long-term nutritional inadequacies or excesses.

Marasmic kwashiorkor .... combination of chronic energy deficit and chronic or acute protein deficiency.

Marasmus .... results from energy and protein deficiency, manifesting with significant loss of body weight, skeletal muscle, and adipose tissue mass but with serum protein concentrations relatively intact.

Nutritional monitoring .... assessment of dietary or nutritional status at intermittent times with the aim of detecting changes in the dietary or nutritional status of a population.

Nutrition screening .... a process used to identify individuals at nutritional risk or with nutritional problems.

Obesity .... excessive accumulation of body fat; usually defined as 20% above desirable weight or body mass index of 30.0 to 39.9.

Protein-calorie malnutrition (PCM) .... inadequate consumption of protein and energy, resulting in a gradual body wasting and increased susceptibility to infection.

Recommended dietary allowance (RDA) .... levels of intake of essential nutrients considered to be adequate to meet the nutritional needs of almost all healthy persons.

Sarcopenic obesity .... combined loss of muscle mass with weight gain occurring in old age.

Skinfold thickness .... double fold of skin and underlying subcutaneous tissue that is measured with skinfold calipers at various body sites.

Waist-to-hip ratio (WHR) .... waist or abdominal circumference divided by the hip or gluteal circumference; method for assessing fat distribution.

STUDY GUIDE

After completing the reading assignment, you should be able to answer the following questions in the spaces provided.

1. Define optimal nutritional status.

2. Describe the unique nutritional needs of various developmental periods throughout the life cycle.

3. Describe the role that cultural heritage and values may play in an individual's nutritional intake.

4. Describe four sources of error that may occur when using the 24-hour diet recall.

5. Describe the difference between monogenic and polygenic obesity.

6. Explain the clinical changes associated with each type of malnutrition:

Obesity _____

Marasmus _____

Kwashiorkor _____

Marasmus-kwashiorkor mix _____

CLINICAL JUDGMENT QUESTIONS

This test is for you to check your own mastery of the content. Answers are provided in Appendix A.

1. You are doing an initial history and physical on a patient who is new to the clinic. The patient recently immigrated to the United States and reports significant malnutrition in his home country. His current weight is 110 pounds, and he is 5′10″ (BMI 15.8). Upon assessment, you notice foamy plaques on the corneas and dry skin. Given his self-report and the assessment findings, you believe the patient may have:

   a. Vitamin A deficiency
   b. Vitamin B_6 deficiency
   c. Iron deficiency
   d. Riboflavin deficiency
   e. Niacin deficiency

2. Metabolic syndrome is diagnosed when patients have at least three of the biomarkers. Please identify which biomarkers are considered diagnostic for metabolic syndrome. **Select all that apply.**

   a. On medication for high triglycerides
   b. On medication for low LDL
   c. On medication for low HDL
   d. LDL >99 mg/dL
   e. HDL >50 mg/dL
   f. On medication for elevated glucose
   g. Fasting glucose ≥100 mg/dL
   h. Fasting glucose <100 mg/dL
   i. HDL <40 mg/dL in men
   j. Systolic blood pressure ≥135 mm Hg
   k. Waist circumference >35 inches in men
   l. Waist circumference ≥40 inches in men
   m. On medication for hypertension

3. While it is important to confirm food restrictions with your patient, you know that the following foods are often not eaten by Muslims. **Select all that apply.**

   a. Pork and pork products
   b. All meat
   c. Alcohol
   d. Shellfish
   e. Coffee
   f. Pungent spices
   g. Hot beverages
   h. Leavened bread

4. Underline the findings below that are concerning for the following patient.

You are caring for a 9-year-old female who is being seen in the clinic today for a well-child visit. A.L. reports that she has a good appetite and enjoys a variety of food. Her parents confirm access to fresh fruits and vegetables. They also confirm adequate resources to provide nutritious meals. A.L. is 54 inches tall and weighs 93 pounds. Vital signs: HR 85, RR 20, BP 110/80. Her BMI is 22.4, which puts her in the 96th percentile. Her total cholesterol is 165 mg/dL, her LDL is 99 mg/dL, and her HDL is 35 mg/dL. Her fasting glucose was 101 mg/dL.

5. Based on the information in question 4:

    a. A.L. has pediatric metabolic syndrome. This puts her at a higher risk for cardiovascular disease and early mortality. She should be immediately treated for hypertension, high cholesterol, and obesity.
    b. A.L. has concerning laboratory and assessment findings. Counseling to promote lifestyle modifications and close monitoring are necessary. Due to age, A.L. should not be diagnosed with PMetS.
    c. A.L. has three of the biomarkers that are indicative of pediatric metabolic syndrome. She should be diagnosed with PMetS. She will need follow-up and medication therapy to avoid long-term consequences of PMetS.
    d. A.L. is a growing child. While her findings are not within normal limits, they are not concerning until she is at least 16 years old. The health care team will continue to monitor for any changes.

6. Fill in the blanks using the terms: marasmus, kwashiorkor, marasmus/kwashiorkor mix, common obesity, monogenic obesity.

    _____ is caused by inadequate protein intake, while _____ is caused by diets high in calories but deficient in protein. A patient with _____ often has an emaciated appearance due to prolonged inadequate intake of protein and calories due to starvation.

7. For each sign of malnutrition, mark which deficiency or deficiencies is the potential cause.

Sign of malnutrition	Vitamin A	Vitamin B6	Vitamin D	Thiamine	Calcium
Rickets					
Peripheral neuropathy					
Pale conjunctiva					
Bitot spots					
Osteomalacia					
Dry skin					

8. In the following patient scenario, underline the assessment findings that place the person at risk for metabolic syndrome.

    K.L. is a 52-year-old female who comes to the clinic today for her annual checkup. During the history, she reports no recent changes to diet and has no acute concerns. Her current medications include simvastatin (for high cholesterol), metformin (oral hypoglycemic), calcium supplement, fish oil supplement, and a multivitamin. Weight 205 pounds. Height 5′4″. BMI 35.2. WC 41 inches. Vital signs: HR 89, RR 20, BP 138/90. Lungs are clear to auscultation. Mild edema bilateral lower extremities. All lab values are within normal limits.

9. Given the information in question 8, K.L. should:

    a. Be diagnosed with MetS. She is on medication for cholesterol and glucose. Her BP is high and her waist circumference is ≥40 inches.
    b. Be diagnosed with MetS. Her BP, BMI, and waist circumference are all indicative of metabolic syndrome in an adult.
    c. Be counseled on lifestyle modification. Her BP and BMI are high, but her lab values are all within normal limits, so she is at a low risk.
    d. Be counseled on lifestyle modification. By reducing her weight and waist circumference, she can avoid the diagnosis of MetS.

10. J.H. is in the clinic for his 6-month checkup. He is an 89-year-old widower who lost his wife 8 months ago. He has two children who live approximately 8 hours away. He lives alone and no longer drives. He has lost 10 pounds in the previous 6 months but denies trying to lose weight. Select all appropriate questions related to J.H.'s nutritional status.

    a. Do you currently wear dentures? If yes, do they fit appropriately?
    b. Who do you eat with for meals?
    c. What did you eat for dinner last night?
    d. Can you tell me everything you ate in the last 24 hours including drinks?
    e. Do you go grocery shopping yourself? If not, who buys your groceries?
    f. Is your income adequate to purchase food?
    g. What medications do you take? I only need to know about prescription medications.

SKILLS LABORATORY AND CLINICAL SETTING

The purpose of the clinical component is to practice the steps of the assessment on a peer in the skills laboratory and to achieve the following:

Clinical Objectives

1. Identify persons at risk of developing malnutrition.
2. Develop an appreciation for cultural influences on nutritional status.
3. Use anthropometric measures and laboratory data to assess the nutritional status of an individual.
4. Use nutritional assessment in the provision of health care.
5. Record the assessment findings accurately.

Instructions

1. Gather nutritional assessment forms and anthropometric equipment. Practice the steps of the *Malnutrition Screening Tool* on a peer in the skills laboratory.
2. Review the questions in the *Mini Nutritional Assessment* with an aging adult. Persons identified as being at risk (MNA score 0 to 11 points) should undergo a more comprehensive assessment.

MALNUTRITION SCREENING TOOL (MST)	
Have you lost weight recently without trying?	
No	0
Unsure	2
If yes, how much weight (kilograms) have you lost?	
1–5	1
6–10	2
11–15	3
>15	4
Unsure	2
Have you been eating poorly because of a decreased appetite?	
No	0
Yes	1
Total	
Score of 2 or more = patient at risk for malnutrition	

Mini Nutritional Assessment
MNA®

Nestlé
NutritionInstitute

Last name:		First name:		
Sex:	Age:	Weight, kg:	Height, cm:	Date:

Complete the screen by filling in the boxes with the appropriate numbers. Total the numbers for the final screening score.

Screening

A Has food intake declined over the past 3 months due to loss of appetite, digestive problems, chewing or swallowing difficulties?
0 = severe decrease in food intake
1 = moderate decrease in food intake
2 = no decrease in food intake ☐

B Weight loss during the last 3 months
0 = weight loss greater than 3 kg (6.6 lbs)
1 = does not know
2 = weight loss between 1 and 3 kg (2.2 and 6.6 lbs)
3 = no weight loss ☐

C Mobility
0 = bed or chair bound
1 = able to get out of bed / chair but does not go out
2 = goes out ☐

D Has suffered psychological stress or acute disease in the past 3 months?
0 = yes   2 = no ☐

E Neuropsychological problems
0 = severe dementia or depression
1 = mild dementia
2 = no psychological problems ☐

F1 Body Mass Index (BMI) (weight in kg) / (height in m)^2
0 = BMI less than 19
1 = BMI 19 to less than 21
2 = BMI 21 to less than 23
3 = BMI 23 or greater ☐

IF BMI IS NOT AVAILABLE, REPLACE QUESTION F1 WITH QUESTION F2.
DO NOT ANSWER QUESTION F2 IF QUESTION F1 IS ALREADY COMPLETED.

F2 Calf circumference (CC) in cm
0 = CC less than 31
3 = CC 31 or greater ☐

Screening score (max. 14 points)

12 - 14 points: Normal nutritional status
8 - 11 points: At risk of malnutrition
0 - 7 points: Malnourished ☐☐

References
1. Vellas B, Villars H, Abellan G, *et al.* Overview of the MNA® - Its History and Challenges. *J Nutr Health Aging.* 2006;**10**:456-465.
2. Rubenstein LZ, Harker JO, Salva A, Guigoz Y, Vellas B. Screening for Undernutrition in Geriatric Practice: Developing the Short-Form Mini Nutritional Assessment (MNA-SF). *J. Geront.* 2001; **56A**: M366-377
3. Guigoz Y. The Mini-Nutritional Assessment (MNA®) Review of the Literature - What does it tell us? *J Nutr Health Aging.* 2006; **10**:466-487.
4. Kaiser MJ, Bauer JM, Ramsch C, et al. Validation of the Mini Nutritional Assessment Short-Form (MNA®-SF): A practical tool for identification of nutritional status. *J Nutr Health Aging.* 2009; **13**:782-788.
® Société des Produits Nestlé, S.A., Vevey, Switzerland, Trademark Owners © Nestlé, 1994, Revision 2009. N67200 12/99 10M
For more information: www.mna-elderly.com

CHAPTER 13

Skin, Hair, and Nails

PURPOSE

This chapter presents the structure and function of the skin and its appendages, explains the rationale for and methods of inspection and palpation of the skin, and records the assessment accurately.

READING ASSIGNMENT

Jarvis: *Physical Examination and Health Assessment*, 9th ed., Chapter 13, pp. 199–250.

Suggested readings:
Feutz, K., Shirey, D. (2022). Measles: Moving toward eradication. *Nurse Pract 47*(5), 14–21.
Solazzo, A. L., Geller, A. C., Hay, J. L., et al. (2020). Indoor ultraviolet tanning among U.S. adolescents and young adults: Results from a prospective study of early onset and persistence. *J Adolesc Health*, *67*(4), 609–611. doi:10.1016/j.jadohealth.2020.03.027.

GLOSSARY

Study the following terms after completing the reading assignment. You should be able to cover the definition on the right and define the term out loud.

Alopecia .... baldness; hair loss

Annular .... circular shape to skin lesion

Bulla .... elevated cavity containing free fluid larger than 1 cm in diameter

Confluent .... skin lesions that run together

Crust .... thick, dried-out exudate left on the skin when vesicles or pustules burst or dry up

Cyanosis .... dusky blue color to skin or mucous membranes, as a result of an increased amount of nonoxygenated hemoglobin

Erosion .... scooped-out, shallow depression in the skin

Erythema .... intense redness of the skin due to excess blood in dilated superficial capillaries, as in fever or inflammation

Excoriation .... self-inflicted abrasion on skin due to scratching

Fissure .... linear crack in skin extending into dermis

Furuncle .... boil; suppurative inflammatory skin lesion due to infected hair follicle

Hemangioma .... skin lesion due to benign proliferation of blood vessels in the dermis

Iris .... target shape of skin lesion

Jaundice .... yellow color to skin, palate, and sclera due to excess bilirubin in the blood

Keloid .... hypertrophic scar, elevated beyond the site of original injury

Lichenification .... tightly packed set of papules that thickens skin; caused by prolonged, intense scratching

Lipoma .... benign fatty tumor, composed of mature fat cells

Maceration .... softening of tissue by soaking in liquid

Macule .... flat skin lesion with only a color change

Nevus .... mole; circumscribed skin lesion due to excess melanocytes

Nodule .... elevated skin lesion larger than 1 cm in diameter

Pallor .... excessively pale, whitish-pink color to lightly pigmented skin

Papule .... palpable skin lesion smaller than 1 cm in diameter

Plaque .... skin lesion in which papules coalesce or come together

Pruritus .... itching

Purpura .... red-purple skin lesion due to blood in tissues from breaks in blood vessels

Pustule .... elevated cavity containing thick, turbid fluid

Scale .... compact desiccated flakes of skin from shedding of dead skin cells

Telangiectasia .... skin lesion due to permanently enlarged and dilated blood vessels that are visible

Ulcer .... sloughing of necrotic inflammatory tissue that causes a deep depression in skin, extending into dermis

Vesicle .... elevated cavity containing free fluid up to 1 cm in diameter

Wheal .... raised red skin lesion due to interstitial fluid

Zosteriform .... linear shape of skin lesion along a nerve route

STUDY GUIDE

After completing the reading assignment, you should be able to answer the following questions in the spaces provided.

1. List the 3 layers associated with the skin, and describe the contents of each layer.

2. Differentiate among sebaceous, eccrine, and apocrine glands.

3. List at least 5 functions of the skin.

4. Describe the appearance of pallor, erythema, cyanosis, and jaundice in both light-skinned and dark-skinned persons. State common causes of each.

5. List causes of changes in skin temperature, texture, moisture, mobility, and turgor.

6. The white linear markings that are normally visible through the nail and on the pink nail bed are termed _____.

7. Describe the following findings that are common variations on the infant's skin:

Mongolian spot _____

Café au lait spot _____

Erythema toxicum _____

Cutis marmorata _____

Physiologic jaundice _____

Milia _____

8. Describe the following findings that are common variations on the aging adult's skin:

Lentigines _____

Seborrheic keratosis _____

Actinic keratosis _____

Acrochordons (skin tags) _____

Sebaceous hyperplasia _____

9. Differentiate among these purpuric lesions: petechiae, bruise, hematoma.

10. Differentiate among the appearance of the skin rash in light and dark skin of 3 childhood illnesses: measles (rubeola), German measles (rubella), chickenpox (varicella).

11. List and describe the 4 stages of pressure injury development.

12. Define and give an example of the following Primary skin lesions: macule, papule, plaque, nodule, tumor, wheal, vesicle, and pustule.

13. Define and give an example of these Secondary lesions: crust, scale, fissure, erosion, and ulcer.

Fill in the labels indicated on the following illustrations:

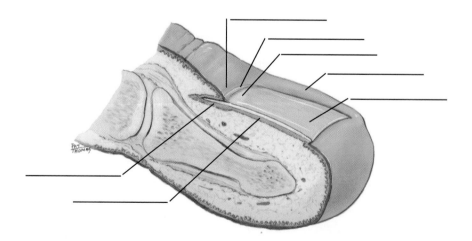

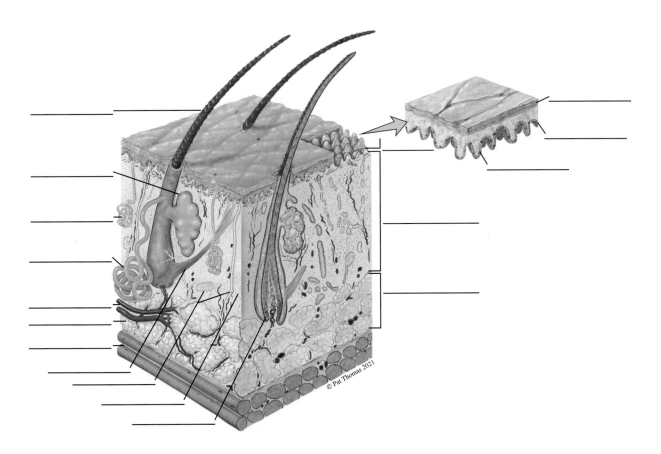

© Pat Thomas 2021

CRITICAL THINKING ACTIVITIES

1. Read the article by Solazzo et al., listed on the first page of this chapter. You encounter a 17-year-old adolescent at your clinic for a sports physical. Compose what you would say in response to the history of using a tanning bed in the gym twice per week. During which part of the examination would you give your response? Try your response out on your lab partner. Ask for feedback concerning facts, avoiding scolding.

2. You are caring for an 18-year-old male who has paraplegia (complete sensory and motor loss of both legs) following a motorcycle accident 2 weeks prior. He has learned to use a straight catheter to empty the bladder. As you talk, he does not maintain eye contact but responds appropriately in short answers. He has not learned to use a wheelchair independently but is lifted into a chair 3 times per day for 1 hour. He refuses breakfast; for lunch and dinner, he eats about half the food offered on his tray.

    Study the Braden Scale at www.bradenscale.com. How would you rate the risk of your patient developing a pressure injury? On what part(s) of his body?

CLINICAL JUDGMENT QUESTIONS

This test is for you to check your own mastery of the content. Answers are provided in Appendix A.

1. You are conducting a class for new graduates on skin assessment. Which statement is true regarding the epidermis?

    a. The epidermis consists mostly of connective tissue or collagen.
    b. The epidermis contains the blood vessels.
    c. The epidermal cells are continually lost and replaced with new cells.
    d. A "paper cut" stimulates nerve cells in the epidermis.

2. You are preparing to care for a 63-year-old Black man with a history of heart attack who now presents with heart failure. What is the best technique to assess for cyanosis?

    a. Palpate the skin for increased heat.
    b. Inspect the hard palate of the mouth.
    c. Inspect the feet for an ashen gray look.
    d. Inspect the nail beds for a dusky pale color.

3. You are taking a history for a 25-year-old woman with a rash on her upper chest and neck. Which question would give you further information on the woman's rash?

    a. How much alcohol would you say you drink each week?
    b. Have you tried a new food or medicine?
    c. Have you recently started oral contraceptives?
    d. With which racial-ethnic group do you identify?

4. You are caring for a 48-year-old with a history of chronic alcohol abuse and liver disease. Which site is the best technique to assess for early jaundice?

    a. Sclera and hard palate.
    b. Nail beds.
    c. Lips.
    d. Visible skin surfaces.

5. You are assessing the skin of a 57-year-old during a clinic appointment. Which technique is the best to assess for increased skin temperature?

    a. A grasping with your fingertips of both the hands.
    b. Laying the palmar surface of your hands on the abdomen.
    c. Placing the ventral surface of your hands on the person's shins and feet.
    d. Laying the dorsal surface of your hands on the person's neck.

6. You are assessing the general skin color of a darkly pigmented person. You would expect which finding?

    a. Lighter pigmentation on the palms of the hands.
    b. A reddened color of the lips.
    c. Patchy pigmentation on the dorsal surface of the hands.
    d. Small flat macules of browner pigment melanin on the chest.

7. You are in the ED when a 70-year-old woman is brought by ambulance after falling in her assisted living space and then not being found for 14 hours. Vital signs are stable. Imaging shows no broken bones. She is alert and oriented. One of your assessment findings is that the skin on her upper chest "tents" after you lift it. This finding is consistent with:

   a. Edema.
   b. Dehydration.
   c. Dry skin (xerosis) of aging.
   d. A normal finding for her age and upper chest.

8. During your skin assessment of a 65-year-old White landscape worker, you notice a raised, thickened area of increased pigmentation of 1.5 cm that looks dark brown and greasy. What is your next most appropriate action?

   a. Interpret this as seborrheic keratosis and move on with the examination.
   b. Notify the physician.
   c. Inquire about recent exposure to toxic outdoor plants.
   d. Inquire about recent exposure to deer ticks.

9. A 78-year-old retired physical examination teacher comes to your clinic for a routine assessment. The teacher asks about small, round, flat, evenly brown macules on the backs of the hands. After assessing the area, what is your best response?

   a. "These are the result of sun exposure and do not require treatment."
   b. "These are related to sun exposure and may become cancerous."
   c. "These are skin tags that occur with older age and do not require treatment."
   d. "I'm glad you brought this to my attention. I will refer you for a biopsy."

10. A 50-year-old is admitted to your medical surgical unit with chronic obstructive lung disease (emphysema). Signs are: alert and oriented, on low-flow oxygen, with BP 156/78 mm Hg, HR 88 bpm and regular, respirations 20 per minute and unlabored. During initial assessment, you observe a rounded appearance of the nail beds to their base in all 10 fingers. Your next most appropriate action is to:

    a. Notify the physician.
    b. Increase the oxygen flow.
    c. Note this is an expected finding for this person and move on.
    d. Take his vital signs again.

11. During a routine assessment of a 35-year-old, you notice the makings in the nail beds of the photo below. These linear streaks are appropriately recorded as:

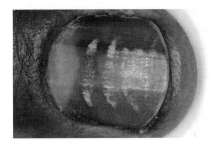

    a. Increased linear pigmentation.
    b. Leukonychia striata.
    c. Melanoma of the nail matrix.
    d. Splinter hemorrhages.

12. A 3-day-old infant has had healthy assessments since birth. On this 3rd day, you notice a yellowing of the skin, sclera, and mucous membranes. Your next most appropriate action is:

    a. Ask the breast-feeding mom to avoid carotene-rich foods.
    b. Notify the physician that this may be hemolytic disease of the newborn.
    c. Record this as physiologic jaundice and proceed with the assessment.
    d. Perform deep palpation on the abdomen to elicit possible pain associated with biliary tract obstruction.

13. During a sports physical for a 14-year-old adolescent, you observe many papules, pustules, nodules, and "blackheads" covering the cheeks and jaw on the face. Which of these statements would be your most appropriate one?

    a. "Have you heard any other kids say anything about your acne?"
    b. "You have severe acne; it is at its peak and will get better in a year."
    c. "How do you feel about the acne on your face?"
    d. "Would you say your acne has made you feel depressed?"

14. You are collecting a health history on a 52-year-old woman. Vital signs and weight are within normal range. At one point, she reports, "the last few weeks, I have had sudden drenching sweating through my shirt." How would you proceed with data collection?

    a. "Can you tell me the date of your last menstrual period?"
    b. "Do you have chest pain at this time?"
    c. "Would you say you are depressed?"
    d. "What was your activity level at these times?"

15. A 74-year-old woman presents with a history of intense itching and a raised red linear rash on one side of her upper back. You know that these findings are consistent with: **Select all that apply**.

    a. A bacterial skin infection.
    b. Herpes zoster infection (shingles).
    c. Poison ivy contact.
    d. History of childhood chicken pox infection.

16. A father brings his 18-month-old infant to your clinic because of a red blotchy rash on the face and neck. Father reports cough, runny nose, and "doesn't want to eat or drink much." Vital signs are 39°C (102.4°F), HR 120 bpm, respirations 24/min. Infant looks sick and miserable. What are the best techniques to continue with the assessment? **Select all that apply**.

    a. Check for immunization history for the infant.
    b. Ask if any other children at home or daycare with the same rash?
    c. Inspect infant's inner cheeks for blue-white "pearls" on the mucosa.
    d. Check nailbeds for capillary refill.

Match column A to column B; items in column B may be used more than once.

Column A: Descriptor

17. _____ Basal cell layer
18. _____ Aids protection by cushioning
19. _____ Collagen
20. _____ Adipose tissue
21. _____ Uniformly thin
22. _____ Stratum corneum
23. _____ Elastic tissue

Column B: Skin Layer

a. Epidermis
b. Dermis
c. Subcutaneous layer

Column A: Descriptor Column

24. _____ Pallor
25. _____ Erythema
26. _____ Cyanosis
27. _____ Jaundice

B: Color Change

a. Intense redness of the skin due to excess blood in the dilated superficial capillaries
b. Bluish mottled color that signifies decreased perfusion
c. Absence of red-pink tones from the oxygenated hemoglobin in blood
d. Increase in bilirubin in the blood causing a yellow color in the skin

Column A: Descriptor of Infant

28. _____ Tiny, punctate red macules and papules on the cheeks, trunk, chest, back, and buttocks
29. _____ Lower half of body turns red, upper half blanches
30. _____ Transient mottling on trunk and extremities
31. _____ Bluish color around the lips, hands, fingernails, feet, and toenails
32. _____ Large round or oval patch of light brown usually present at birth
33. _____ Yellowing of skin, sclera, and mucous membranes due to increased numbers of red blood cells hemolyzed after birth
34. _____ Yellow-orange color in light-skinned persons from large amounts of foods containing carotene

Column B: Skin Color Change

a. Harlequin
b. Erythema toxicum
c. Acrocyanosis
d. Physiologic jaundice
e. Carotenemia
f. Café au lait spot
g. Cutis marmorata

SKILLS LABORATORY AND CLINICAL SETTING

Usually, the clinical examination of the integumentary system is performed along with the examination of each particular body region. The purpose of practicing the steps of this examination separately is so that you begin to think of the skin and its appendages as a separate organ system and so that you learn the components of skin examination.

Clinical Objectives

1. Inspect and palpate the skin, noting its color, vascularity, edema, moisture, temperature, texture, thickness, mobility, turgor, and any lesions.
2. Inspect the fingernails, noting color, shape, and any lesions.
3. Inspect the hair, noting texture, distribution, and any lesions.
4. Record the history and physical examination findings accurately, reach an assessment of the health state, and develop a plan of care.

Instructions

Prepare the examination setting. Wash your hands. Practice the steps of the examination on a peer in the skills laboratory, giving appropriate instructions as you proceed. Choosing a peer from an ethnic background other than your own will further heighten your recognition of the range of normal skin tones. Record your findings using the regional write-up sheet that follows. The front of the page is intended as a worksheet; the back of the page is intended for your narrative summary recording using the SOAP format.

Note the student performance checklist that follows the regional write-up sheet. It lists the essential behaviors that you should display as an examiner, and it may be used by your clinical instructor to evaluate your clinical teaching of the skin self-examination.

REGIONAL WRITE-UP—SKIN, HAIR, AND NAILS

Date _____

Examiner _____

Patient _____ Age _____ Gender _____

Reason for visit _____

I. **Health History**

	No	Yes, explain
1. Any past skin disease?	_____	_____
2. Any change in skin color or pigmentation?	_____	_____
3. Any changes in a mole?	_____	_____
4. Excessive dryness or moisture?	_____	_____
5. Any skin itching?	_____	_____
6. Any excess bruising?	_____	_____
7. Any skin rash or lesions?	_____	_____
8. Taking any medications?	_____	_____
9. Any recent hair loss?	_____	_____
10. Any change in nails?	_____	_____
11. Any environmental hazards for skin?	_____	_____
12. How do you take care of your skin? Sunscreen?	_____	_____
13. What is your amount of sun exposure? Indoor tanning?	_____	_____

II. **Physical Examination**

A. **Inspect and palpate skin.**

Color_____

Pigmentation_____

Temperature_____

Moisture_____ Texture _____

Thickness_____ Any edema _____

Mobility and turgor _____

Vascularity and bruising _____

Any lesions (describe) _____

B. **Inspect and palpate hair.**

Color_____

Texture_____Distribution_____

Any lesions (describe) _____

C. **Inspect and palpate nails.**

Shape and contour _____

Consistency_____Distribution_____

Color_____

Capillary refill _____

D. **Teach skin self-examination.**

REGIONAL WRITE-UP—SKIN, HAIR, AND NAILS

Summarize your findings using the SOAP format.

Subjective (reason for seeking care, health history)

Objective (physical examination findings)

Record distribution of any rash or lesions below.

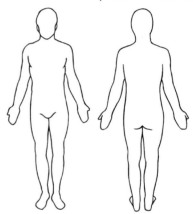

Assessment (assessment of problem, diagnosis)

Plan (diagnostic evaluation, follow-up care, teaching)

STUDENT COMPETENCY CHECKLIST

Teaching Skin Self-Examination (SSE)

	S	U	Comments
I. **Cognitive**			
A. Explain:			
1. why skin is examined.			
2. who should perform skin self-examination.			
3. frequency of skin examination.			
B. Define the ABCDE rule.			
C. Describe any equipment the patient may need.			
II. **Performance**			
A. Explain to the patient the need for SSE.			
B. Instruct the patient on the technique of SSE by:			
1. demonstrating the order and body positioning for inspecting skin.			
2. describing normal skin characteristics.			
3. describing abnormal findings to look for.			
C. Instruct the patient to report unusual findings to the provider.			

NOTES

Head, Face, Neck, and Regional Lymphatics

PURPOSE

This chapter presents the anatomy and function of structures in the head and neck, the methods of inspection and palpation of these structures, and the accurate recording of the assessment.

READING ASSIGNMENT

Jarvis: *Physical Examination and Health Assessment*, 9th ed., Chapter 14, pp. 251–280.

Suggested readings:
Rogers, J., & Spain, S. (2020). Understanding the most commonly billed diagnoses in primary care: Headache disorders. *Nurse Pract*, *45*(10), 41–47.

GLOSSARY

Study the following terms after completing the reading assignment. You should be able to cover the definition on the right and define the term out loud.

Bruit .... blowing, swooshing sound heard through the stethoscope over an area of abnormal blood flow

Dysphagia .... difficulty in swallowing

Goiter .... increase in size of thyroid gland that occurs with hyperthyroidism

Lymphadenopathy .... enlargement of the lymph nodes due to infection, allergy, or neoplasm

Macrocephalic .... an abnormally large head

Microcephalic .... an abnormally small head

Normocephalic .... a round, symmetric skull that is appropriately related to body size

Torticollis .... head tilt due to shortening or spasm of one sternomastoid muscle

Vertigo .... illusory sensation of either the room or one's own body spinning; not the same as dizziness

STUDY GUIDE

After completing the reading and media assignments, write or draw the answers in the spaces provided.

1. The major neck muscles are the _____.

2. Name the borders of two regions in the neck—the anterior triangle and the posterior triangle.

3. List facial structures that should appear symmetric when inspecting the head.

4. Describe the characteristics of lymph nodes often associated with:

   Acute infection _____

   Chronic inflammation _____

   Cancer _____

5. Differentiate *caput succedaneum* from *cephalhematoma* in the newborn infant.

6. Describe the tonic neck reflex in the infant.

7. Describe the characteristics of normal cervical lymph nodes during childhood.

8. List the condition(s) associated with parotid gland enlargement.

9. Describe the facial characteristics that occur with Down syndrome.

10. Contrast the facial characteristics of hyperthyroidism versus hypothyroidism.

Fill in the labels indicated on the following illustrations.

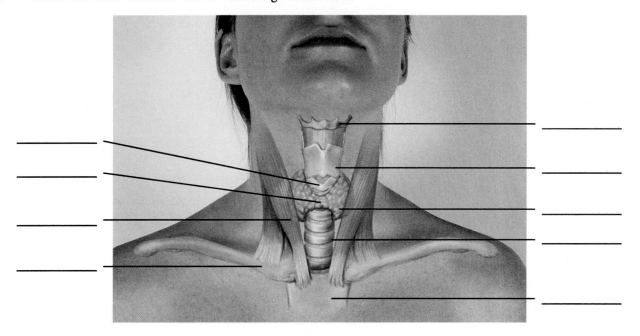

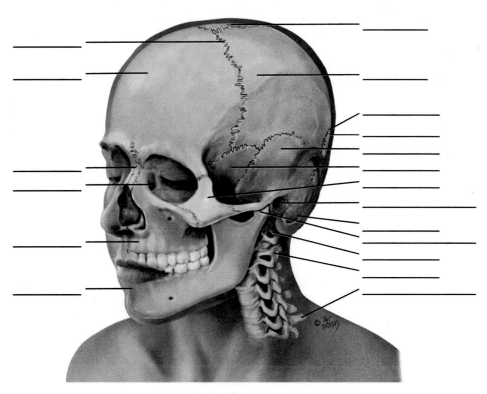

(© Pat Thomas, 2018.)

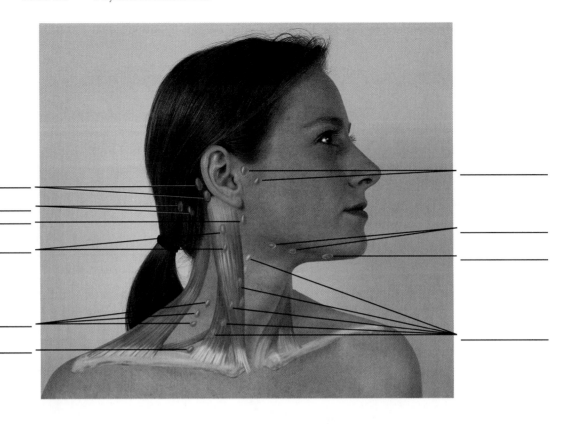

CLINICAL JUDGMENT QUESTIONS

This test is to check your own mastery of the content. Find the Answers in Appendix A.

1. You are assessing the oral structures in a 58-year-old man with a 40-year history of smoking cigarettes. You will search for the sublingual glands at which location?

   a. In the cheeks, over the mandible, anterior to the ear.
   b. Beneath the mandible at the angle of the jaw.
   c. In the floor of the mouth under the side of the tongue.
   d. Above the temporalis muscle, anterior to the ear.

2. During physical examination, a 30-year-old man shows a bulging blood vessel that runs diagonally across the sternomastoid muscle. You are aware that this is the:

   a. Temporal artery.
   b. Carotid artery.
   c. External jugular vein.
   d. Internal jugular vein.

3. You stand behind a 28-year-old pregnant woman to palpate the thyroid gland. You search for the isthmus of the thyroid gland just below the:

   a. Mandible.
   b. Cricoid cartilage.
   c. Hyoid cartilage.
   d. Thyroid cartilage.

4. You are taking a health history for a 35-year-old woman who reports having had cluster headaches in the past. Which findings would you expect for cluster headaches?

   a. They may be triggered by alcohol, pain, or perfume.
   b. Their usual occurrence is two per month, each lasting 1 to 3 days.
   c. They are described as throbbing.
   d. They tend to be supraorbital, retro-orbital, or frontotemporal.

5. You are inspecting the face of a 20-year-old woman who reports, "I woke up this morning and looked in the mirror and my face is flat! Help! I think I'm paralyzed!" Which action(s) would you direct? **Select all that apply.**

   a. Ask the woman to wrinkle the forehead.
   b. Ask her to show the teeth with lips pulled back.
   c. Palpate for pain using firm pressure under the maxillae (cheekbones).
   d. Inquire if she has experienced any drooling.

6. You are testing active range of motion (ROM) in a 79-year-old man. When turning his head to right and left, you observe he turns more at his shoulders than at his neck. What is your next most appropriate action?

   a. Palpate his shoulders for any pain or tenderness.
   b. Direct him to bend over and touch the toes for complete ROM of spine.
   c. Continue with the examination; this is a common finding in an older adult.
   d. Refer him to an orthopedic specialist.

7. As you palpate the anterior fontanel on a 6-month-old infant, you note it feels about 2 cm wide and dips inward. Your next most appropriate action is to:

   a. Inspect for cranial asymmetry due to early closure of fontanel.
   b. Suspect dehydration and inquire about number of wet diapers.
   c. Auscultate over the fontanel for a systolic bruit.
   d. Move on with the examination; these data are expected.

8. The thyroid gland is enlarged bilaterally in the neck of a 50-year-old woman; which maneuver would be your next most appropriate?

   a. Check for deviation of the trachea.
   b. Continue with the examination; this is an expected finding in a menopausal woman.
   c. Listen for a murmur over the aortic area causing thyroid enlargement.
   d. Listen for a bruit over the thyroid lobes indicating increased blood flow.

9. A 22-year-old adult comes to your clinic for an employment physical examination. As you palpate the cervical lymph nodes, which characteristics would be healthy and expected?

   a. Mobile, soft, nontender
   b. Large, clumped, tender
   c. Matted, fixed, hard
   d. One isolated enlargement, fixed, nontender

10. You assess a newborn infant 3 hours after birth and note a soft, fluctuant swelling just over one cranial bone. The parents report a difficult head presentation delivery. What is (are) your next action(s)? **Select all that apply.**

    a. Inform the parents that this will go away on its own over the next few weeks.
    b. Request an order for blood results to screen for possible jaundice.
    c. Suspect increased intracranial pressure and request a referral.
    d. Inspect the infant's face for sunsetting eyes.

11. A 20-year-old man suffers a blow to his head from another player's leg during a soccer game. You assess him 6 hours later, and he reports a moderate headache and nausea, vomiting one time, and blurred vision while reading his phone screen. He had no loss of consciousness after the injury. There are no further assessment abnormalities. Your most appropriate advice is:

    a. Bed rest for 24 hours, no reading, screen watching, or other brain work activity.
    b. Rest with only slow walking for next 24 hours.
    c. Remain at home for 24 hours, mild stretching allowed.
    d. No return to game play for 24 hours; otherwise perform usual activity.

12. You suspect an infant's head is of abnormal size and can use which procedure to verify these findings?

    a. Palpation.
    b. Measuring tape.
    c. Observing for symmetry of facial features.
    d. Noting absence of the tonic neck reflex.

For questions 13–22, match column B to column A.

Column A: Lymph Nodes

13. _____ Preauricular

14. _____ Posterior auricular

15. _____ Occipital

16. _____ Submental

17. _____ Submandibular

18. _____ Jugulodigastric

19. _____ Superficial cervical

20. _____ Deep cervical

21. _____ Posterior cervical

22. _____ Supraclavicular

Column B: Location

a. Above and behind the clavicle

b. Deep under the sternomastoid muscle

c. In front of the ear

d. In the posterior triangle along the edge of the trapezius muscle

e. Superficial to the mastoid process

f. At the base of the skull

g. Halfway between the angle and the tip of the mandible

h. Behind the tip of the mandible

i. Under the angle of the mandible

j. Overlying the sternomastoid muscle

CRITICAL THINKING ACTIVITIES

Headache (HA) disorders are common neurologic disorders but are not fully assessed, diagnosed, or treated. Consider your own personal and clinical experience with HA. Review data on HA in Chapter 14 in Jarvis 9th ed., Table 14-1, and in the suggested reading by Rogers and Spain (2020) listed on p. 251. Discuss these points:
- List non-medication interventions for tension-type HA and migraine HA. Discuss your own experiences with these interventions.
- List triggers for tension-type, migraine, and cluster HA. Then practice your patient teaching to present these points in the clinical area.
- Discuss lifestyle modifications that may aid in the care of the person with chronic HA.
- Discuss Red Flag HAs that command immediate referral.

SKILLS LABORATORY AND CLINICAL SETTINGS

The purpose of the clinical component is to practice the steps of the head, face, and neck examination on a peer in the skills laboratory and to achieve the following objectives.

Clinical Objectives

1. Collect a health history related to pertinent signs and symptoms of the head and neck.
2. Inspect and palpate the skull, noting size, contour, lumps, or tenderness.
3. Inspect the face, noting facial expression, symmetry, skin characteristics, or lesions.
4. Inspect and palpate the neck for symmetry, range of motion, and integrity of lymph nodes, trachea, and thyroid gland.
5. Record the findings systematically, reach an assessment of the health state, and develop a plan of care.

Instructions

Prepare the examination setting. Wash your hands. Practice the steps of the examination on a peer in the skills laboratory, giving appropriate instructions as you proceed. Record your findings using the regional write-up sheet that follows. The front of the page is intended as a worksheet; the back of the page is intended for your narrative summary recording using the SOAP format.

REGIONAL WRITE-UP—HEAD, FACE, AND NECK

Date _____

Examiner _____

Patient _____ Age _____ Gender _____

Reason for visit _____

I. Health History

	No	Yes, explain
1. Any unusually frequent or severe **headaches**?		
2. Any **head injury**?		
3. Experienced any **dizziness**?		
4. Any neck **pain**?		
5. Any **lumps** or **swelling** in head or neck?		
6. Any surgery on head or neck?		

II. Physical Examination

A. **Inspect and palpate the skull.**
General size and contour _____
Deformities, lumps, tenderness _____
Temporal artery _____
Temporomandibular joint _____

B. **Inspect the face.**
Facial expression _____
Symmetry of structures _____
Involuntary movements _____
Edema _____
Masses or lesions _____
Color and texture of skin _____

C. **Inspect the neck.**
Symmetry _____
Range of motion, active _____
Test strength of cervical muscles. _____
Abnormal pulsations _____
Enlargement of thyroid _____
Enlargement of lymph and salivary glands _____

D. **Palpate the lymph nodes.**
Exact location _____
Size and shape _____
Presence or absence of tenderness _____
Freely movable, adherent to deeper structures, or matted together _____
Presence of surrounding inflammation _____
Texture (hard, soft, firm) _____

E. **Palpate the trachea.** _____

F. **Palpate the thyroid gland.** _____

G. **Auscultate the thyroid gland (if enlarged).** _____

REGIONAL WRITE-UP—HEAD, FACE, AND NECK

Summarize your findings using the SOAP format.

Subjective (reason for seeking care, health history)

Objective (physical examination findings)

Assessment (assessment of health state or problem, diagnosis)

Plan (diagnostic evaluation, follow-up care, patient teaching)

PURPOSE

This chapter presents the structure and function of the external and internal components of the eyes, the methods of examination of vision, external eye, and ocular fundus, and the accurate recording of the assessment.

READING ASSIGNMENT

Jarvis: *Physical Examination and Health Assessment*, 9th ed., Chapter 15, pp. 281–322.

Suggested readings:
Carlson, C., Howe, T., Pedersen, C., & Yoder, L. (2020). Caring for visually impaired patients in the hospital. *Am J Nurs, 120*(5), 48–55.

GLOSSARY

Study the following terms after completing the reading assignment. You should be able to cover the definition on the right and define the term out loud.

Accommodation .... adaptation of the eye for near vision by increasing the curvature of the lens

Anisocoria .... unequal pupil size

Arcus senilis .... gray-white arc or circle around the limbus of the iris that is common with aging

Argyll Robertson pupil .... pupil does not react to light; does constrict with accommodation

Astigmatism .... refractive error of vision due to differences in curvature in refractive surfaces of the eye (cornea and lens)

A-V crossing .... crossing paths of an artery and vein in the ocular fundus

Bitemporal hemianopsia .... loss of both temporal visual fields

Blepharitis .... inflammation of the glands and eyelash follicles along the margin of the eyelids

Cataract .... opacity of the lens of the eye that develops slowly with aging and gradually obstructs vision

Chalazion .... infection or retention cyst of a meibomian gland, showing as a beady nodule on the eyelid

Conjunctivitis .... infection of the conjunctiva, "pinkeye"

Cotton wool area .... abnormal soft exudates visible as gray-white areas on the ocular fundus

Cup-to-disc ratio .... ratio of the width of the physiologic cup to the width of the optic disc, normally half or less

Diopter .... unit of strength of the lens settings on the ophthalmoscope that changes focus on the eye structures

Diplopia .... double vision

Drusen .... benign deposits on the ocular fundus that show as round yellow dots and occur commonly with aging

Ectropion .... lower eyelid loose and rolling outward

Entropion .... lower eyelid rolling inward

Exophthalmos .... protruding eyeballs

Fovea .... area of keenest vision at the center of the macula on the ocular fundus

Glaucoma .... a group of eye diseases characterized by an increased intraocular pressure

Hordeolum .... (stye) red, painful pustule that is a localized infection of hair follicle at eyelid margin

Lid lag .... abnormal white rim of sclera visible between the upper eyelid and the iris when a person moves the eyes downward

Macula .... round darker area of the ocular fundus that mediates vision only from the central visual field

Microaneurysm .... abnormal finding of round red dots on the ocular fundus that are localized dilations of small vessels

Miosis .... constricted pupils

Mydriasis .... dilated pupils

Myopia .... nearsighted; refractive error in which near vision is better than far vision

Nystagmus .... involuntary, rapid, rhythmic movement of the eyeball

Optic atrophy .... pallor of the optic disc due to partial or complete death of optic nerve

Optic disc .... area of ocular fundus in which blood vessels exit and enter

Papilledema .... stasis of blood flow out of the ocular fundus; sign of increased intracranial pressure

Presbyopia .... decrease in power of accommodation that occurs with aging

Pterygium .... triangular opaque tissue on the nasal side of the conjunctiva that grows toward the center of the cornea

Ptosis .... drooping of upper eyelid over the iris and possibly covering the pupil

Red reflex .... red glow that appears to fill the person's pupil when first visualized through the ophthalmoscope

Strabismus .... (squint, crossed eye) disparity of the eye axes

Xanthelasma .... soft, raised yellow plaques occurring on the skin at the inner corners of the eyes

STUDY GUIDE

After completing the reading assignment and the media assignment, write or draw the answers in the spaces provided.

1. Name the 6 sets of extraocular muscles and the cranial nerve that innervates each one.

2. Name and describe the 3 concentric coats of the eyeball.

3. Name the functions of the ciliary body, the pupil, and the iris.

4. Describe the anterior chamber, the posterior chamber, and the vitreous body.

5. Describe how an image formed on the retina compares with its actual appearance in the outside world.

6. Describe the lacrimal system.

7. Define pupillary light reflex, fixation, and accommodation.

8. Concerning the pupillary light reflex. Describe and contrast a direct light reflex with a consensual light reflex.

9. Identify the common age-related changes in the eye.

10. Discuss the most common causes of decreased visual function in older adults.

11. Explain the statement: normal visual acuity is 20/20.

12. Describe the method of testing for presbyopia.

13. To test for accommodation, the person focuses on a distant object and then shifts the gaze to a near object about 6 inches away. At a near distance, you would expect the pupils to _____ (dilate/constrict) and the axes of the eyes to _____.

14. Concerning malalignment of the eye axes, contrast *phoria* with *tropia.*

15. Describe abnormal findings of tissue color that are possible on the conjunctiva and sclera, and describe their significance.

16. Describe the method of everting the upper eyelid for examination.

17. Contrast *pinguecula* with *pterygium.*

18. Contrast the use of the negative diopter or red lens settings with the positive diopter or black lens settings on the ophthalmoscope.

19. Explain the rationale for testing for strabismus during early childhood.

20. Describe these findings and explain their significance: epicanthal fold; pseudostrabismus; ophthalmia neonatorum; Brushfield spots.

21. Describe the following 4 types of red eye, and explain their significance:

a. Conjunctivitis:

b. Subconjunctival hemorrhage:

c. Iritis:

d. Acute glaucoma:

Fill in the labels indicated on the following illustrations.

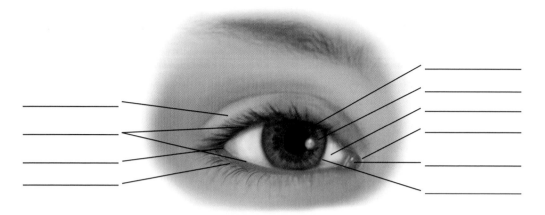

(© Pat Thomas, 2006.)

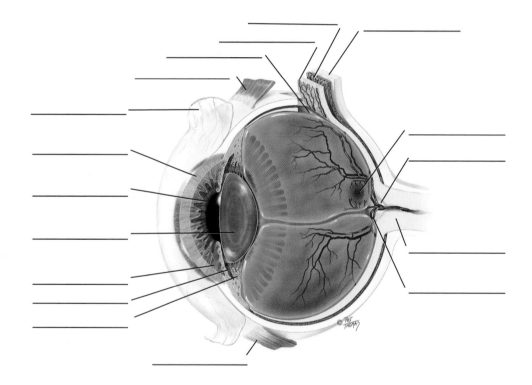

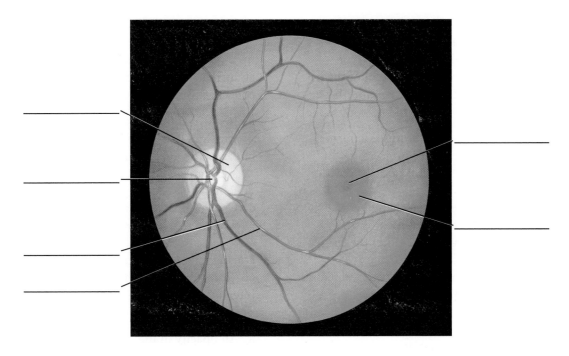

CLINICAL JUDGMENT QUESTIONS

This test is for you to check your own mastery of the content. Answers are provided in Appendix A.

1. During history collection, a 78-year-old retired female gardener reports blurry vision existing for about 5 to 6 years. Her husband says the woman's pupils look "milky." What would be your most appropriate response(s) to this statement? **Select all that apply.**

   a. "Does your blurry vision affect your daily activities?"
   b. Continue with the health history; this is an expected visual response to aging.
   c. "Do objects appear out of focus?"
   d. "I am going to refer you to our Emergency Department now, so that a specialist will check your eyes."

2. You are testing vision using the Snellen alphabet chart. A 14-year-old girl has a result of 20/40 Right eye and 20/50-1 Left eye. You observe her pausing and hesitant about some of the letters. Your next best action would be to:

   a. Move her 10 feet closer to the Snellen chart and retest.
   b. Assess her near vision using a handheld vision screener.
   c. Alert the girl and her parent for the need to refer to an eye specialist.
   d. Continue with the exam; this is a common finding during teenage growth spurt.

3. A 44-year-old man presents to your outpatient clinic for an examination for a bus driving job. During the Diagnostic Positions Test, you observe a back-and-forth movement of the iris when he looks to the extreme side. Your best action would be to:

a. Proceed with the exam, as this is a normal finding.
b. Inquire about the amount of daily alcohol drinking.
c. Ask about dizziness when changing positions, as this eye movement is associated with inflammation of the semicircular canals in the ears.
d. Refer to a physician, as this eye movement is associated with multiple sclerosis.

4. You are inspecting the conjunctiva and sclera of a 53-year-old Black woman. Which of the findings below are abnormal and worthy of referral? **Select all that apply.**

a. Overall reddening of the blood vessels on sclera of one eye but clearer near the iris.
b. A gray-blue or muddy color of the sclera.
c. An even yellow color of both sclera, extending up to the iris.
d. A small brown macule on the sclera that the person says has always been there.

5. You plan to assess the pupillary light reflex on a hospitalized 20-year-old soccer player suspected of concussion. Your correct action(s) would be to: **Select all that apply.**

a. Ask the person to stare into the distance behind you.
b. Advance your penlight in from the front to test both pupil responses.
c. Use a pupil gauge to assess the findings in millimeters.
d. Refer unequal pupil response to the physician.

6. During a screening examination, you inspect the ocular fundus using the ophthalmoscope on a 21-year-old woman who reports no abnormal symptoms during the history collection. Your best action would be to:

a. Remove your own glasses and approach the woman's left eye with your left eye.
b. Leave the light on in the examining room and remove glasses from the woman.
c. Remove glasses and set the diopter setting a 0.
d. Use the smaller white light and instruct the woman to focus on the ophthalmoscope.

7. During the ophthalmoscope examination of a 66-year-old woman, the red reflex is interrupted and appears with a black center. This finding is associated with:

a. An opacity in the cornea or lens.
b. A pathologic disease in the optic tract.
c. Tortuous and crossing blood vessels in the ocular fundus
d. Constricted pupils.

8. During the ophthalmoscopic examination, the mechanism causing the red reflex is:

a. Petechial hemorrhages in the sclera.
b. Diabetic retinopathy.
c. Light reflecting from the retina.
d. Blood in the vitreous humor.

9. You are assessing infants during screening examinations in a pediatric outpatient clinic. You are alert for the following attending behaviors that suggest the infant can receive visual images and indeed *see*. **Select all that apply.**

a. At 2 to 4 weeks of age, the infant can fixate on an object (bright toy).
b. At 6 weeks of age, the infant can make some visual response to your face.
c. At 6 to 10 months of age, the infant can fixate at a toy and follow it as you move it in all directions.
d. At 12 months of age, the infant refuses to reopen eyes for about 20 seconds after exposure to your bright penlight.

10. You are assessing the vision of a 4-year-old child. Which of the following responses are abnormal and indicate referral to an eye specialist? **Select all that apply.**

    a. Unable to read letters on the Snellen alphabet chart.
    b. During the Corneal Light Reflex, the reflected light in the left eye is off center but the reflected light in the right eye is centered on the pupil.
    c. During the Cover test, one eye jumps in gaze following removal of the opaque card.
    d. The child has an extra fold of skin at the epicanthus of both eyes.

11. You are assessing the eyes and vision at a retirement center for adults aged 65 years and older. Which of the following responses are abnormal and indicate referral to an eye specialist? **Select all that apply.**

    a. The tissue of the upper eyelid is relaxed and rests close to the upper eyelashes.
    b. Bulging exists on the tissue of the lower eyelids.
    c. An opaque wedge-shaped tissue is present on the sclera and continues over the cornea.
    d. A gray-white circle is present around the cornea on the iris.
    e. Yellow papules are present on the upper lids near the inner canthus.
    f. Pupils are small with a resting size of 2 mm.
    g. During the ophthalmoscope exam, a black spot is present in the red reflex.

12. A 19-year-old man presents to the university health center holding a tissue pressed to his eye. A yellow raised pustule exists at the upper eyelid margin. It has a small red area around it and is extremely painful. The sclera are white and vision is normal. Which of the following are your appropriate actions? **Select all that apply.**

    a. Inspect the other eye for a similar lesion.
    b. Request prescriptions for antibiotic drops/ ointment.
    c. Instruct the man this will resolve on its own and no treatment is necessary.
    d. Instruct the man to avoid touching both eyes with the same tissue.
    e. Refer the man to the Emergency Department of the hospital.

13. A 25-year-old woman has been blind in her left eye since birth. What response would you expect in her pupils when the right eye is illuminated by a penlight beam?

    a. No response in both pupils.
    b. Both pupils constrict.
    c. Right pupil constricts, left has no response.
    d. Left pupil constricts, right has no response.

14. Which of the following eye disorders prompt urgent referral to an Emergency Department? **Select all that apply.**

    a. Sudden acute loss of vision in one eye.
    b. Obvious trauma to the eyeball.
    c. Unequal resting pupil size of 1 or 2 mm; both constrict to light.
    d. Diagnosis of herpes zoster infection (shingles) on the face.
    e. One unequal pupil that is dilated, distorted in shape, with redness around iris.

CRITICAL THINKING ACTIVITIES

Work with a partner in the lab, but try to pair with someone you do not know well. One person is blind-folded. Each person should guide the other on a campus walk with the following requirements:

1. Go through two different sets of doors.
2. Go up *and* down a set of stairs.
3. Drink at a water fountain.

Walk into buildings with which you are less familiar; this highlights a vision deficit in an unfamiliar environment. Be the blindfolded partner for 7 to 10 minutes and then switch roles. Back in the lab, discuss the following:

1. Frustration levels.
2. How did it feel to be led?
3. How did it feel to lead?
4. What worked? What failed to work?
5. What actions developed your trust in the partner who was leading?
6. How did you handle the doorways? The stairs? The drinking fountain?
7. Did you talk to anyone else on campus? Did you feel self-conscious, as if others were looking at you?
8. What is your takeaway for applying this exercise to your low-vision patients?

SKILLS LABORATORY AND CLINICAL SETTING

The purpose of the clinical component is to practice the steps of the examination on a peer in the skills laboratory. Note that the first practice session usually takes a long time because there are so many separate steps. Be aware that success with the use of the ophthalmoscope is hard to achieve during the first practice session. Make sure you are holding the instrument correctly, and practice focusing on various objects around the room before you try to look at a person's fundus. When you do examine a peer's eye, make sure to offer occasional rest times. It is very tiring for the "patient" to have the ophthalmoscope light shining in their eye. During the first practice session, aim to find the red reflex and a retinal vessel or two; if you can locate the optic disc, so much the better.

Clinical Objectives

1. Collect a health history related to pertinent signs and symptoms of the eye system.
2. Demonstrate and explain the assessment of visual acuity, visual fields, external eye structures, and ocular fundus.
3. Record the history and physical examination findings accurately, reach an assessment of the health state, and develop a plan of care.

Instructions

Prepare the examination setting. Wash your hands. Practice the steps of the examination on a peer in the skills laboratory, giving appropriate instructions as you proceed. Record your findings using the regional write-up sheet that follows. The front of the page is intended as a worksheet; the back of the page is intended for your narrative summary recording using the SOAP format.

REGIONAL WRITE-UP—EYES

Date _____

Examiner _____

Patient _____ Age _____ Gender _____

Reason for visit _____

I. Health History

	No	Yes, explain
1. Any **difficulty seeing** or blurring?	_____	_____
2. Any eye **pain**?	_____	_____
3. Any history of **crossed eyes**?	_____	_____
4. Any **redness** or **swelling** in the eyes?	_____	_____
5. Any **watering** or **tearing**?	_____	_____
6. Any **injury** or **surgery** to the eye?	_____	_____
7. Ever tested for **glaucoma**?	_____	_____
8. Wear **glasses** or **contact lenses**?	_____	_____
9. Ever had vision tested?	_____	_____
10. Taking any medications?	_____	_____

II. Physical Examination

A. **Test visual acuity**.
   Snellen eye chart _____
   Pocket vision screener for near vision _____

B. **Test visual fields**.
   Confrontation test _____

C. **Inspect extraocular muscle function**.
   Corneal light reflex _____
   Diagnostic positions test _____

D. **Inspect external eye structures**.
   General _____
   Eyebrows _____
   Eyelids and lashes _____
   Eyeballs _____
   Conjunctiva and sclera _____
   Lacrimal gland, puncta _____

E. **Inspect anterior eyeball structures**.
   Cornea _____
   Iris _____
   Pupil size _____
   Pupil direct and consensual light reflex _____
   Accommodation _____

F. **Inspect ocular fundus**.
   Optic disc _____
   Vessels _____
   General background of fundus _____
   Macula _____

REGIONAL WRITE-UP—EYES

Summarize your findings using the SOAP format.

Subjective (reason for seeking care, health history)

Objective (physical examination findings)

Record findings on diagram below.

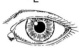

Assessment (assessment of problem, diagnosis)

Plan (diagnostic evaluation, follow-up care, teaching)

PURPOSE

This chapter reviews the structure and function of the ears, the methods of examination of hearing, external ear structures, and the tympanic membrane using the otoscope, and how to record the assessment accurately.

READING ASSIGNMENT

Jarvis: *Physical Examination and Health Assessment*, 9th ed., Chapter 16, pp. 323–350.

Suggested reading:
Tiefel, N. L. (2020). A review of the management of sudden sensorineural hearing loss. *Nurse Pract, 45*(12), 43–48.

GLOSSARY

Study the following terms after completing the reading assignment. You should be able to cover the definition on the right and define the term out loud.

Annulus... outer fibrous rim encircling the eardrum

Atresia... congenital absence or closure of ear canal

Cerumen................................... yellow waxy material that lubricates and protects the ear canal

Cochlea................................... inner ear structure containing the central hearing apparatus

Eustachian tube......................... connects the middle ear with the nasopharynx and allows the passage of air

Helix... superior posterior free rim of the pinna

Incus... "anvil"; middle of the 3 ossicles of the middle ear

Malleus... "hammer"; outermost of the 3 ossicles of the middle ear

Mastoid... bony prominence of the skull located just behind the ear

Organ of Corti........................... sensory organ of hearing

Otalgia... pain in the ear

Otitis externa............................. inflammation of the outer ear and ear canal

Otitis media................................ inflammation of the middle ear and tympanic membrane

Otorrhea..discharge from the ear

Pars flaccida ....small, slack, superior section of the tympanic membrane

Pars tensa...................................thick, taut, central-inferior section of the tympanic membrane

Pinna...auricle, or outer ear

Stapes ...."stirrup"; innermost of the 3 ossicles of the middle ear

Tinnitus ....ringing in the ears

Tympanic membrane.................."eardrum"; thin, translucent, oval membrane that stretches across the ear canal and separates the middle ear from the outer ear

Umbo...knob of the malleus that shows through the tympanic membrane

Vertigo..a spinning, twirling sensation

STUDY GUIDE

After completing the reading assignment and the media assignment, write or draw the answers in the spaces provided.

1. List the 3 functions of the middle ear.

2. Contrast 2 pathways of hearing.

3. Differentiate among the types of hearing loss and give examples.

4. Relate the anatomic differences that place the infant at a greater risk for middle ear infections.

5. Describe the whispered voice test of hearing acuity.

6. Explain the positioning of normal ear alignment in the child.

7. Define otosclerosis and presbycusis.

8. Contrast the motions used to straighten the ear canal when using the otoscope with an infant versus an adult.

9. Describe the appearance of these nodules that could be present on the external ear: Darwin tubercle, sebaceous cyst, tophi, chondrodermatitis, keloid, and carcinoma.

10. Describe the appearance of these conditions that could appear in the ear canal: osteoma, exostosis, furuncle, polyp, and foreign body.

11. List the disease state suggested by the following descriptions of the appearance of the eardrum: yellow-amber color, pearly gray color, air-fluid level, distorted light reflex, red color, dense white areas, oval dark areas, black or white dots on drum, and blue drum.

Fill in the labels indicated on the following illustrations.

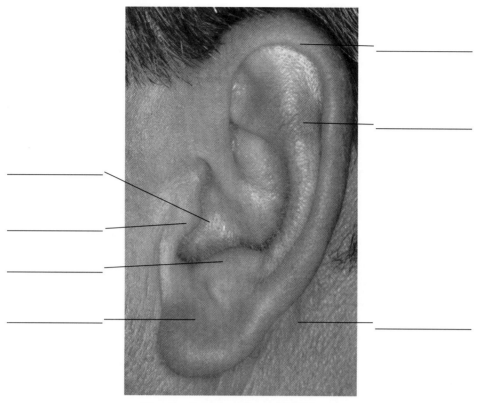

(Courtesy Lemmi and Lemmi, 2011.)

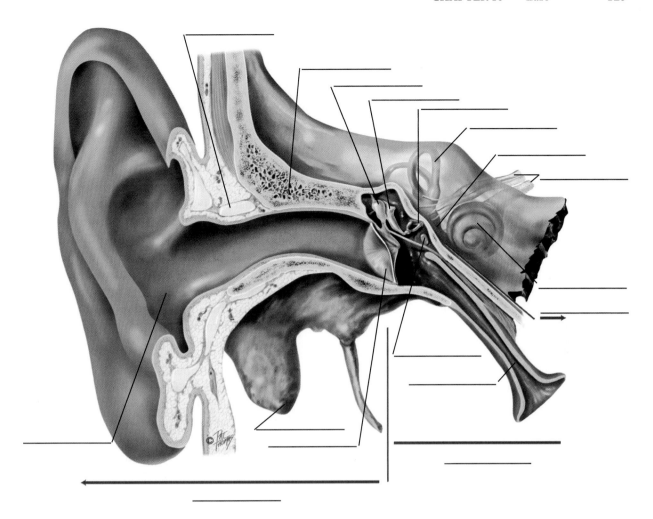

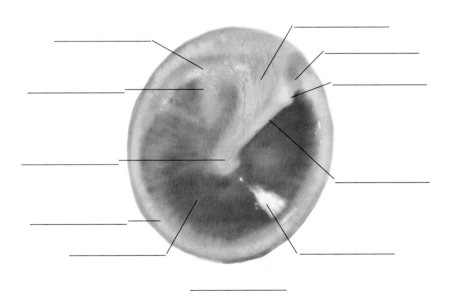

CLINICAL JUDGMENT QUESTIONS

This test is for you to check your own mastery of the content. Answers are provided in Appendix A.

1. During history collection, the mother of a 5-year-old boy tells you that he has discharge from one ear. What would be your most appropriate response(s) to this statement? **Select all that apply.**

   a. "Is your child allergic to any drugs?"
   b. "Does it look like pus, or is it bloody?"
   c. "Any odor to the discharge?"
   d. "Does your child feel dizzy?"

2. You inspect a 45-year-old woman's ear canal using the otoscope. The tympanic membrane is pearly gray and slightly concave. Your next action should be to:

   a. Assume acute otitis media and refer to physician.
   b. Assume scarring of the drum and refer to audiologist.
   c. Proceed with the exam as this is an expected finding.
   d. Assess the ear canal again in 20 minutes after testing the hearing.

3. You are assessing hearing acuity using the whispered voice test on a 74-year-old woman. She is able to repeat 2 of the 6 numbers/letters you present. Your next action should be to:

   a. Consider a high-tone hearing sensorineural loss and refer for audiology.
   b. Assume this is an expected response to aging and proceed with the exam.
   c. Inspect the ear canal for foreign bodies.
   d. Inquire if the woman experienced recent head trauma.

4. You are preparing to examine a person's ear with the otoscope. Your correct action would be to palpate which areas for tenderness?

   a. Helix, external auditory meatus, and lobule.
   b. Mastoid process, tympanic membrane, and malleus.
   c. Pinna, pars flaccida, and antitragus.
   d. Pinna, tragus, and mastoid process.

5. You prepare to examine a child's ear who is younger than 3 years old. Your correct action would be to:

   a. Pull the pinna up and back.
   b. Pull the pinna down.
   c. Hold the pinna gently but firmly in its normal position.
   d. Tilt the child's head slightly toward you, the examiner.

6. The patient's history and the assessment of the Weber and Rinne tuning fork tests suggest a 45-year-old man has a conductive hearing loss. You proceed knowing that the common cause of conductive hearing loss is:

   a. Impacted cerumen.
   b. Acute rheumatic fever.
   c. A stroke (CVA).
   d. Otitis externa.

7. You assess a person's tympanic membrane and the findings suggest an infection of acute otitis media. Which of the following findings support this?

   a. Absent light reflex, bluish drum, oval dark areas.
   b. Absent light reflex, reddened drum, bulging drum.
   c. Oval dark areas on drum.
   d. Absent light reflex, air fluid level, and bubbles behind drum.

8. A 64-year-old woman states she has no problems hearing and is able to repeat all 6 numbers/letters presented on the whispered voice test. During otoscopy, her eardrum looks more white and more opaque than you have seen in a younger adult. Your next appropriate response would be to:

   a. Ask her if she feels "isolated" in family groups.
   b. Consider conductive hearing loss and refer her to an audiologist.
   c. Proceed with the exam, as this is a common finding in aging.
   d. Ask if she has been hit on the side of her head in the past.

9. The mother of an 18-month-old is concerned because her son has had 3 ear infections in the past year. He attends daycare and takes a pacifier at bedtime. He has not had a pneumococcal vaccine. What would be your most appropriate response?

   a. "We need to check your son's immune system to see why he is having so many ear infections."
   b. "Ear infections are common in infants and toddlers because they tend to have more cerumen in their external ear."
   c. "At 18 months, the child's Eustachian tube is shorter and wider than an adult's, so infections in the throat can extend up to the ear."
   d. "This suggests nerve damage in the inner ear and we will refer you to a specialist in ear-nose-throat disorders."

10. When examining the ears and hearing of a 45-year-old Black woman, you notice a 2-cm nodule on the back of the lobule. Skin color is consistent with the woman's usual pigment. Nodule is soft, painless, and not ulcerated. How would you proceed?

    a. Inquire about amount of sun exposure and refer for biopsy.
    b. Inquire if the woman has the joint/cartilage disease of gout.
    c. Assess for enlarged tender lymph nodes.
    d. Explain that the nodule is likely the overgrowth of scar tissue.

11. A 38-year-old woman enters your clinic concerned with roaring/ringing in her ears that is driving her "crazy." What is your best response to this concern?

    a. "How would you say the ringing in your ears affects your ability to do your usual activities?"
    b. "Are you allergic to any drugs that you know of?"
    c. "How do you clean your ears?"
    d. "Are you exposed to chronic loud noises in your work or your hobby?"

12. A woman has had hearing screening by an audiologist through her community center. The results suggest a sensorineural hearing loss in one ear. During your assessment, your best approach is to:

    a. Speak loudly so she can hear your questions.
    b. Look for a source of obstruction using the otoscope.
    c. Ask the woman what medications she is taking.
    d. Assess the tympanic membrane for the source of infection.

13. You assess a 25-year-old man and note the pinna is tender, is red-blue in color, and has small clear vesicles. What is the most appropriate question?

    a. "Have you been out in the cold for a long time recently?"
    b. "Any recent trauma to your ear?"
    c. "Any change in your usual hearing?"
    d. "Do you have drainage from your ear?"

SKILLS LABORATORY AND CLINICAL SETTING

The purpose of the clinical component is to practice the steps of the ear examination on a peer in the skills laboratory or on a patient in the clinical setting. The use of the otoscope is somewhat easier than the use of the ophthalmoscope. However, you still must be sure that you are holding the instrument correctly. Holding the otoscope in an upside-down position seems awkward at first, but it is important to make sure the otoscope tip does not cause pain to the delicate parts of the ear canal. Have someone correct your positioning before you insert the instrument.

Clinical Objectives

1. Collect a health history related to the pertinent signs and symptoms of the ear system.
2. Describe the appearance of the normal outer ear and external ear canal.
3. Describe and demonstrate the correct technique of an otoscopic examination.
4. Describe and perform tests for hearing acuity.
5. Systematically describe the normal tympanic membrane, including position, color, and landmarks.
6. Record the history and physical examination findings accurately, reach an assessment about the health state, and develop a plan of care.

Instructions

Prepare the examination setting and gather your equipment. Make certain that the otoscope light is bright and that the batteries are freshly charged. Wash your hands. Practice the steps of the examination on a peer in the skills laboratory, giving appropriate instructions as you proceed. Record your findings using the regional write-up sheet that follows. The front of the page is intended as a worksheet; the back of the page is intended for your narrative summary recording using the SOAP format.

REGIONAL WRITE-UP—EARS

Date _____

Examiner _____

Patient _____ Age _____ Gender _____

Reason for Visit _____

I. Health History (subjective)

	No	Yes, explain
1. Any **earache** or ear pain?		
Trauma to head?		
2. Any ear **infections**?		
Now or in the past?		
3. Any **discharge** from ears?		
4. Any hearing loss now?		
5. Any **loud noises** at home or at work?		
6. Any **ringing** or **buzzing** in ears?		
Taking any medications?		
7. Ever felt **vertigo** (spinning)?		
8. How do you clean your ears?		
9. Use ear protection from loud noise or while swimming?		

II. Physical Examination (objective)
A. Inspect and palpate external ear.
Size and shape _____

Skin condition _____

Tenderness _____

External auditory meatus _____
B. Inspect using the otoscope.
External canal _____

Tympanic membrane _____

Color and characteristics _____

Position _____

Integrity of membrane _____
C. Test hearing acuity.
Whispered voice test _____

REGIONAL WRITE-UP—EARS

Summarize your findings using the SOAP format.

Subjective (reason for seeking care, health history)

Objective (physical examination findings)

Record findings on diagram below.

R   L

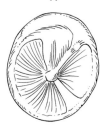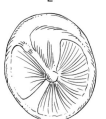

Assessment (assessment of health state or problem, diagnosis)

Plan (diagnostic evaluation, follow-up care, patient teaching)

Nose, Mouth, and Throat

PURPOSE

This chapter presents the structure and function of the nose, mouth, and throat; the methods of inspection and palpation of these structures; and the accurate recording of the assessment.

READING ASSIGNMENT

Jarvis: *Physical Examination and Health Assessment*, 9th ed., Chapter 17, pp. 351–382.

Suggested reading:
DiSilvio, B., Baqdunes, M., et al. (2021). Smoking addiction and strategies for cessation. *Crit Care Nurs Q*, *44*(1), 33–48. Read this, then practice Critical Thinking Activities, p. 137.
Rogers, J., Eastland, T. (2021). Acute Pharyngitis. *Nurse Pract*, *46*(5), 48–54.

GLOSSARY

Study the following terms after completing the reading assignment. You should be able to cover the definition on the right and define the term out loud.

Aphthous ulcers .... "canker sores"; small, painful, round ulcers in the oral mucosa of unknown cause

Buccal .... pertaining to the cheek

Candidiasis .... (moniliasis) white, cheesy, curd-like patch on buccal mucosa due to superficial fungal infection

Caries .... decay in the teeth

Cheilitis .... red, scaling, shallow, painful fissures at corners of mouth

Choanal atresia .... closure of nasal cavity due to congenital septum between nasal cavity and pharynx

Crypts .... indentations on surface of tonsils

Epistaxis .... nosebleed, usually from anterior septum

Epulis .... nontender, fibrous nodule of the gum

Fordyce granules .... small, isolated, white or yellow papules on oral mucosa

Gingivitis .... red, swollen gum margins that bleed easily

Herpes simplex .... "cold sores"; clear vesicles with red base that evolve into pustules, usually at lip-skin junction

Koplik spots .... small, blue-white spots with red halo over oral mucosa; early sign of measles

Leukoplakia .... chalky white, thick, raised patch on sides of tongue; precancerous

Malocclusion .... upper or lower dental arches out of alignment

Papillae .... rough, bumpy elevations on dorsal surface of tongue

Parotid glands .... pair of salivary glands in the cheeks in front of the ears

Pharyngitis .... inflammation of the throat

Plaque .... soft, whitish debris on teeth

Polyp .... smooth, pale gray nodules in the nasal cavity due to chronic allergic rhinitis

Rhinitis .... red, swollen inflammation of nasal mucosa

Thrush .... oral candidiasis in the newborn

Turbinate .... one of 3 bony projections into nasal cavity

Uvula .... free projection hanging down from the middle of the soft palate

STUDY GUIDE

After completing the reading assignment and the media assignment, write or draw the answers in the spaces provided.

1. Name the functions of the nose.

2. Describe the size and components of the nasal cavity.

3. List the 4 sets of paranasal sinuses, and describe their function.

4. List the 3 pairs of salivary glands, including their location and the locations of their duct openings.

5. After tooth loss in the middle or older adult, describe the consequences of chewing with the remaining maloccluded teeth.

6. Describe the appearance of a deviated nasal septum and a perforated septum.

7. Describe the appearance of a torus palatinus, and explain its significance.

8. Contrast the physical appearance and clinical significance of the following: leukoedema, candidiasis, leukoplakia, and Fordyce granules.

9. List the 4-point grading scale for the size of tonsils.

10. Describe the appearance and clinical significance of these findings in the infant: sucking tubercle, Epstein pearls, and Bednar aphthae.

11. Contrast the appearance of nasal turbinates versus nasal polyps.

12. Describe the appearance and clinical significance of these findings on the tongue: ankyloglossia, fissured tongue, geographic tongue, black hairy tongue, macroglossia.

13. In the space below, sketch a cleft palate and a bifid uvula.

Fill in the labels indicated on the following illustrations.

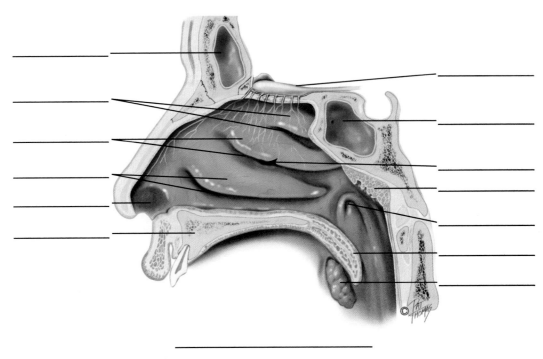

(© Pat Thomas, 2006)

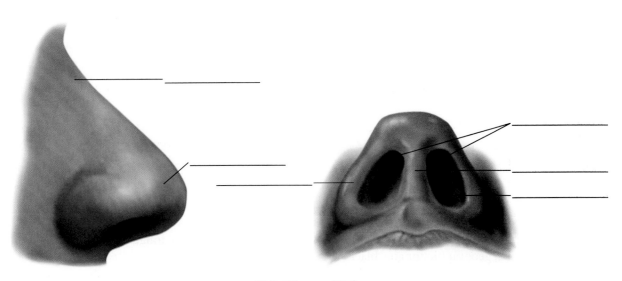

(© Pat Thomas, 2006)

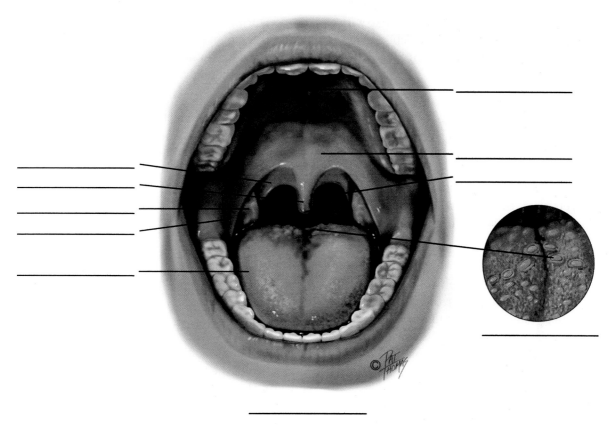

(© Pat Thomas, 2006)

CLINICAL JUDGMENT QUESTIONS

This test is for you to check your own mastery of the content. Find the answers in Appendix A.

1. A 30-year-old man enters your Emergency Department with profuse bleeding from the nose. He reports no prescription medicine, no street drugs, and no chronic conditions. You proceed with your intervention, knowing that 80% to 90% of nose bleeds occur in which site?

   a. The turbinates.
   b. The columellae.
   c. Kiesselbach plexus.
   d. The meatus.

2. For the man with the nosebleed in Question 1, your next action(s) would be to: **Select all that apply.**

   a. Don gloves and compress the lower third of the nose.
   b. Ask the man to sit and lean forward.
   c. Measure the body temperature for signs of fever.
   d. Alert about a decreased sense of smell following this episode.

3. A 39-year-old woman enters your clinic with symptoms of acute sinusitis. Which sinuses can you assess through examination?

   a. Ethmoid and sphenoid.
   b. Frontal and ethmoid.
   c. Maxillary and sphenoid.
   d. Frontal and maxillary.

4. During history collection, a 35-year-old man tells you that he takes oral antibiotics whenever he gets a sore throat because "I can't afford to lose any time at work." Your most appropriate response is:

   a. "Please bring me your bottle of antibiotics so I can check the label."
   b. "You do not need a throat culture as long as you already have the antibiotics."
   c. "Most sore throats are caused by viruses that do not respond to antibiotics."
   d. "A streptococcal sore throat is more likely to occur when you don't have a fever."

5. During history collection, a 70-year-old woman reports dry mouth. You are aware that the most frequent cause of this is:

   a. The aging process.
   b. Related to medications she may be taking.
   c. The use of dentures.
   d. Related to a diminished sense of smell.

6. During an inspection of a patient's nares, you observe a deviated septum. What is your next most appropriate action?

   a. Request a consultation with an EarNose-Throat specialist.
   b. Proceed with the examination; this is not significant unless airflow is obstructed.
   c. Teach the person what to do if a nosebleed should occur.
   d. Explore further because polyps frequently accompany a deviated septum.

7. During the examination of a 45-year-old Black man recently immigrated from Nigeria, you note a dark melanotic line along the pink gingival margin. Your next action should be to:

   a. Ask about any food or vitamin deficiency in the man's country of origin.
   b. Inquire about tobacco use in any form.
   c. Request a physician consult for a possible tissue biopsy.
   d. Proceed with the exam; this is a normal finding.

8. A 45-year-old woman has a 23-year history of smoking over one pack of cigarettes per day. During the oral exam, you inspect knowing that malignancies are most likely to develop: **Select all that apply.**

   a. On the soft palate.
   b. On the tongue.
   c. In the buccal cheek mucosa.
   d. In the mucosal "gutter" under the tongue.

9. A 16-year-old boy has fever and a sore throat. You grade his tonsils as 3+ because the tonsils are:

   a. Visible.
   b. Halfway between the tonsillar pillars and uvula.
   c. Touching the uvula.
   d. Touching each other.

10. During oral exam, you note a small pink papule on the buccal mucosa opposite to the person's upper 2nd molar. Your next action should be to:

    a. Proceed with the exam; this is the opening of Stenson duct.
    b. Search for accompanying Koplik spots.
    c. Inquire about level of alcohol drinking.
    d. Inquire about teeth grinding during the night.

11. During examination of the nose in a person with chronic allergies, you note a protruding nodule. You can distinguish a nasal polyp from the nasal turbinates by the following sign(s): **Select all that apply.**

    a. The polyp is highly vascular.
    b. The polyp is movable.
    c. The polyp is pale gray in color.
    d. The polyp is nontender.

12. You note small, round, white, shiny papules on the hard palate and gums of a 2-month-old infant. You are aware that these signify:

    a. Aphthous areas or ulcers that are the result of sucking.
    b. Teeth buds are beginning to appear.
    c. A normal finding called *Epstein pearls.*
    d. The presence of a monilial or yeast infection.

13. When assessing the tongue, your best technique includes:

    a. Palpating the U-shaped area under the tongue.
    b. Checking tongue color for cyanosis.
    c. Using a tongue blade to elevate the tongue while placing a finger under the jaw.
    d. Asking the person to say "ahhh" and note the tongue rise in the midline.

14. You are assessing a 79-year-old woman in a residential facility. Which of the following would most likely be present?

    a. Hypertrophy of the gums.
    b. An increased production of saliva.
    c. Decreased ability to identify odors.
    d. Finer and less prominent nasal hair.

CRITICAL THINKING ACTIVITIES

Review the strategies, Ask, Advise, Access, Assist, Arrange, for smoking cessation in the DiSilvio article and in Jarvis: *Physical Examination and Health Assessment,* 9th ed., p. 367–370 and Fig. 17.25. Plan teaching in your own words, and role-play with a peer in the laboratory setting. Take turns being the "smoker" and the counselor.

How would you alter your teaching strategy for the adolescent or adult who reports vaping?

SKILLS LABORATORY AND CLINICAL SETTING

The purpose of the clinical component is to practice the steps of the examination on a peer in the skills laboratory or on a patient in the clinical setting and to achieve the following:

Clinical Objectives

1. Inspect the external nose.
2. Demonstrate use of the otoscope and nasal attachment to inspect the structures of the nasal cavity.
3. Demonstrate knowledge of infection control practices during inspection and palpation of structures of the mouth and pharynx.
4. Record the history and physical examination findings accurately, reach an assessment of the health state, and develop a plan of care.

Instructions

Prepare the examination setting, and gather your equipment: gloves, penlight, otoscope with broad nasal speculum, tongue blade, cotton gauze pad.

Wash your hands. Practice the steps of the examination on a peer in the skills laboratory, giving appropriate instructions as you proceed. Record your findings using the regional write-up sheet that follows. The front of the page is intended as a worksheet; the back of the page is intended for your narrative summary recording using the SOAP format.

REGIONAL WRITE-UP—NOSE, MOUTH, AND THROAT

Date _____

Examiner _____

Patient _____ Age _____ Gender _____

Reason for visit _____

I. Health History

	No	Yes, explain
A. Nose		
1. Any nasal **discharge**?	_____	_____
2. Unusually frequent or severe colds?	_____	_____
3. Any **sinus pain** or sinusitis?	_____	_____
4. Any **trauma** or injury to nose?	_____	_____
5. Any **nosebleeds**? How often?	_____	_____
6. Any **allergies** or hay fever?	_____	_____
7. Any change in sense of smell?	_____	_____
B. Mouth and throat	_____	_____
1. Any **sores** in mouth, tongue?	_____	_____
2. Any **sore throat**? How often?	_____	_____
3. Any bleeding gums? Any toothache?	_____	_____
4. Any **hoarseness**, voice change?	_____	_____
5. Any difficulty in **swallowing**?	_____	_____
6. Any change in sense of taste?	_____	_____
7. Do you smoke? How much per day?	_____	_____
8. Drink alcohol? How many times per week? Drinks per occasion?	_____	_____
9. Use of nasal sprays? Use of nose for illicit drugs?	_____	_____
10. Tell me about usual dental care.	_____	_____

II. Physical Examination

A. **Inspect and palpate the nose.**

Symmetry _____

Deformity, asymmetry, inflammation _____

Test patency of each nostril _____

Using a nasal speculum, note:

   Color of nasal mucosa _____

   Discharge, foreign body _____

   Septum: deviation, perforation, bleeding _____

   Turbinates: color, swelling, exudate, polyps _____

B. **Palpate the sinus area.**

Frontal _____ Maxillary _____

C. **Inspect the mouth.**

Lips _____

Teeth and gums _____

Buccal mucosa _____

Palate and uvula _____

Tonsils (grade) _____ Tongue _____

D. **Inspect the throat.**

Tonsils: condition and grade _____

Pharyngeal wall _____

Any breath odor _____

REGIONAL WRITE-UP—NOSE, MOUTH, AND THROAT

Summarize your findings using the SOAP format.

Subjective (reason for seeking care, health history)

Objective (physical examination findings)   Record findings on the diagram below.

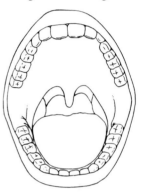

Assessment (assessment of health state or problem, diagnosis)

Plan (diagnostic evaluation, follow-up care, patient teaching)

Breasts, Axillae, and Regional Lymphatics

PURPOSE

This chapter presents the structure and function of the breast, the rationale and methods of examination of the breast, the accurate recording of the assessment, and the techniques of breast self-examination.

READING ASSIGNMENT

Jarvis: *Physical Examination and Health Assessment*, 9th ed., Chapter 18, pp. 383–408.

Suggested readings:

Freudenheim, J. L. (2020). Alcohol's effects on breast cancer in women. *Alcohol Res Curr Rev, 40*(2), 1–12. https://doi.org/10.35946/arcr.v40.2.11

Yurdaisik, I. (2020). Analysis of the most viewed first 50 videos on YouTube about breast cancer. *BioMed Res Int*, 1–7. https://doi.org/10.1155/2020/2750148

GLOSSARY

Study the following terms after completing the reading assignment. You should be able to cover the definition on the right and define the term out loud.

Alveoli .... smallest structures in the mammary gland

Areola .... darkened area surrounding the nipple

Colostrum .... thin, yellow fluid, precursor of milk, secreted for a few days after birth

Cooper ligaments .... suspensory ligaments; fibrous bands extending from the inner breast surface to the chest wall muscles

Fibroadenoma .... benign breast mass

Galactorrhea .... persistent white discharge of milk between nursing sessions or after weaning

Gynecomastia .... excessive breast development in the male

Intraductal papilloma .... serosanguineous nipple discharge

Inverted .... nipples that are depressed or invaginated

Lactiferous .... conveying milk

Mastalgia .... pain in breast

Mastitis .... inflammation of the breast

Montgomery glands .... sebaceous glands in the areola that secrete protective lipid during lactation; also called *tubercles of Montgomery*

Paget disease .... intraductal carcinoma in the breast

Peau d'orange .... orange peel appearance of breast due to edema

Retraction .... dimple or pucker on the skin

Striae .... atrophic pink, purple, or white linear streaks on the breasts, associated with pregnancy, excessive weight gain, or rapid growth during adolescence

Supernumerary nipple .... minute extra nipple along the embryonic milk line

Tail of Spence .... extension of breast tissue into the axilla

Thelarche .... beginning of prepubertal breast development

STUDY GUIDE

After completing the reading assignment and the media assignment, write or draw the answers in the spaces provided.

1. Identify appropriate history questions to ask regarding the breast examination.

2. Describe the anatomy of the breast.

3. Correlate changes in the female breast with normal developmental stages.

4. Describe the components of the breast examination.

5. List points to include in teaching breast self-examination.

6. Explain the significance of a supernumerary nipple or breast.

7. Differentiate between the female and male examination procedures and findings.

8. Discuss pathologic changes that may occur in the breast:

Benign breast disease _____

Abscess _____

Acute mastitis _____

Fibroadenoma _____

Cancer _____

Paget disease _____

9. List and describe the characteristics to consider when a mass is noted in the breast.

10. Define gynecomastia.

11. Describe screening mammography and clinical breast examination (CBE) for the diagnosis of breast lesions.

12. List the added risk factors that increase the usual risk for breast cancer.

Fill in the labels on the following diagrams.

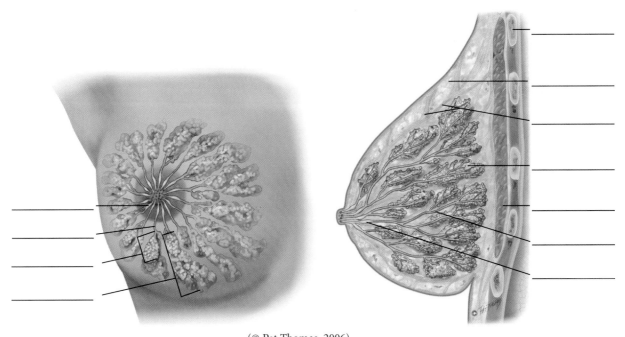

(© Pat Thomas, 2006)

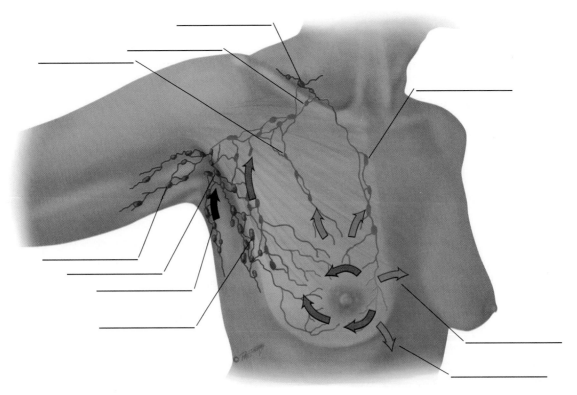

(© Pat Thomas, 2006)

CLINICAL JUDGMENT QUESTIONS

This test is for you to check your own mastery of the content. Answers are provided in Appendix A.

1. You are presenting the internal anatomy of the breast for a community health care clinic. Which of the following are accurate points to include? **Select all that apply.**

   a. The bulk of the breast is mainly pectoralis muscle tissue.
   b. The fibrous connective tissue extends from inside the breast skin surface toward the chest wall muscles.
   c. The breast tissue slopes upward into the axilla.
   d. Most lymphatic drainage of the breast flows inward to deeper chest lymph ducts.

2. A 13-year-old girl presents to your clinic for a school physical examination. She asks you why her breasts "don't match" in size. What is your best response?

   a. "One breast may temporarily grow faster than the other during development."
   b. "In these cases, I usually ask another examiner to come in and double check."
   c. "It is a sign that you will have small cystic lumps in one side; these are common."
   d. "This may show a temporary hormonal imbalance. We will check again in 6 months."

3. When teaching the breast self-examination, you would inform the woman that the best time to conduct breast self-examination is:

   a. At the onset of the menstrual period.
   b. On the 14th day of the menstrual cycle.
   c. On the 4th to 7th days of the cycle.
   d. Just before the menstrual period.

4. You are providing health promotion for a 50-year-old woman. What is the current recommendation for women aged 45 to 54 years of age for screening mammography?

   a. Opportunity to begin mammograms at age 55.
   b. Mammogram now and every 2 years.
   c. Annual mammogram.
   d. Only baseline examination needed unless the woman has symptoms.

5. You are inspecting an adult woman's breasts for retraction signs. Her best position is:

   a. Lying supine with arms at the sides.
   b. Leaning forward with hands outstretched.
   c. Sitting with hands pushing onto hips.
   d. Lying supine with one arm elevated over her head.

6. The bimanual technique is your preferred approach for a woman:

   a. Who is pregnant.
   b. Who is having the first breast examination by a health care provider.
   c. With large pendulous breasts.
   d. Who has felt a change in the breast during self-examination.

7. During the examination of a 70-year-old man, you note gynecomastia. You next best action is to:

   a. Request a breast biopsy.
   b. Request a mammogram.
   c. Review the medications for drugs that have gynecomastia as a side effect.
   d. Proceed with the examination; this is a normal part of the aging process.

8. A 57-year-old woman presents to your clinic for a health checkup, having deferred any health care visits for 1.5 years. During a breast examination, you palpate a 2-cm firm mass with irregular edges. What is your next best action?

   a. Request a breast biopsy.
   b. Request a mammogram.
   c. Review her medication list for drugs that cause breast lumps.
   d. Proceed with the examination; this is a common finding in a menopausal woman.

9. You are teaching a 34-year-old woman who is 2 months pregnant what common breast changes to expect. You would include: **Select all that apply.**

   a. The areolae become darker brown.
   b. Nipple retraction.
   c. Able to express breast milk after 2 months.
   d. Blue vascular pattern over both breasts.

10. You have examined the following women during one shift. Which ones should you refer for further evaluation? **Select all that apply.**

    a. A 28-year-old with multiple distinct nodules palpated in each breast.
    b. A 48-year-old who has a 6-month history of reddened and sore left nipple and areolar area.
    c. A 22-year-old with asymmetric breasts and inversion of nipples since adolescence.
    d. A 64-year-old with an ulcerated area at the tip of the right nipple; no masses, tenderness, or enlarged lymph nodes present.

11. You are examining a 10-year-old girl for a sports physical. What is the first physical change associated with puberty in girls? **Select all that apply.**

    a. Breasts enlarge and areolae enlarge over breasts.
    b. A small mound of breast tissue develops under the nipple.
    c. Height spurt.
    d. Pubic hair development.

12. During the examination of a 30-year-old woman, she asks about "the large mole" below her left breast. After inspecting a 1-cm circular brown area with a central bump, what is your best response?

    a. "I think you should be examined by a dermatologist."
    b. "This is a common finding of an extra, undeveloped nipple."
    c. "These are Montgomery glands, which are common."
    d. "Is there a possibility that you are pregnant?"

13. You visit the home of a 35-year-old mother with her first baby. She is 4 days postpartum. She has a tender thickening in one breast with the overlying skin reddened and tender. She has fatigue but no fever. What teaching would you give? **Select all that apply.**

    a. "Nurse the baby on the affected side first at each nursing."
    b. "Nurse the baby frequently to keep the breast as empty as possible."
    c. "This condition is common when you and the baby are both learning to nurse."
    d. "I will request an antibiotic for you that will not harm the baby."

CRITICAL THINKING ACTIVITIES

Perform a review of 3 to 4 YouTube™ videos about breast cancer. First read the Yurdaisik article on this analysis cited in this chapter's opening. This author states that YouTube™ is commonly used by patients who have new diagnoses of breast cancer, yet the videos do not include accurate information about diagnosis, screening, or follow-up. For the YouTube™ videos you choose: What is the overall quality? What is the proportion of anecdotal information, i.e., one personal case presentation? What is the proportion of scientifically accurate content? Discuss your findings in your laboratory group or in your class.

SKILLS LABORATORY AND CLINICAL SETTING

The purpose of the clinical component is to practice the steps of the assessment on a peer in the skills laboratory and to achieve the following.

Clinical Objectives

1. Demonstrate knowledge of the symptoms related to the breasts and axillae by obtaining a health history.
2. Perform inspection and palpation of the breasts with the woman in sitting and supine positions, using proper technique and providing appropriate draping.
3. Teach breast self-examination to a woman, or list the points to include in teaching breast self-examination.
4. Record the history and physical examination findings accurately, reach an assessment of the health state, and develop a plan of care.

Instructions

Gather the health history of a peer or a woman in the clinical area. Gather any equipment (small pillow, centimeter ruler, handout on breast self-examination). Then practice the steps of the breast examination. Record your findings on the regional write-up sheet that follows. The front of the page is intended as a worksheet; the back of the page is intended for your narrative summary recording using the SOAP format.

   Note the student performance checklist that follows the regional write-up sheet. It lists the essential behaviors you should display as an examiner, and it may be used by your clinical instructor to evaluate your clinical teaching of breast self-examination.

Using a computer or electronic device, enter www.cancer.gov/bcrisktool/default/aspx. This Breast Cancer Risk Assessment is an interactive tool to help estimate a woman's risk of developing breast cancer. It has been updated for Black women and for Asian and Pacific Islander women. The model does not apply to women with a history of breast cancer or chest irradiation or women younger than 35 years. Practice using the tool in your laboratory setting. The screen should look like this:

Before using the tool, please note the following:

> The Breast Cancer Risk Assessment Tool was designed for use by health professionals. If you are not a health professional, you are encouraged to discuss the results and your personal risk of breast cancer with your doctor.

> Although the tool may accurately estimate a woman's risk of developing breast cancer, these risk estimates do not allow one to say precisely which woman will develop breast cancer. In fact, the distribution of risk estimates for women who develop breast cancer overlaps the estimates of risk for women who do not.

> The tool should not be used to calculate breast cancer risk for women who have already had a diagnosis of breast cancer, lobular carcinoma in situ (LCIS), or ductal carcinoma in situ (DCIS).

> The BCRA risk calculator may be updated periodically as new data or research becomes available.

> Although the tool has been used with success in clinics for women with strong family histories of breast cancer, more specific methods of estimating risk are appropriate for women known to have breast cancer–producing mutations in the BRCA1 or BRCA2 genes.

> Other factors may also affect risk and are not accounted for by the tool. These factors include previous radiation therapy to the chest for the treatment of Hodgkin lymphoma or women who have recently immigrated to the United States from certain regions of Asia where breast cancer risk is low. Further, the tool may not be appropriate for women living outside the United States. The tool's risk calculations assume that a woman is screened for breast cancer as in the general U.S. population. A woman who does not have mammograms will have a somewhat lower chance of a diagnosis of breast cancer.

www.cancer.gov/bcrisktool/default.aspx

Risk Tool

(Click a question number for a brief explanation, or read all explanations.)

1. Does the woman have a medical history of any breast cancer or of ductal carcinoma in situ (DCIS) or lobular carcinoma in situ (LCIS) or has she received previous radiation therapy to the chest for treatment of Hodgkin lymphoma?   [Select ⬍]

2. Does the woman have a mutation in either the *BRCA1* or *BRCA2* gene, or a diagnosis of a genetic syndrome that may be associated with elevated risk of breast cancer?   [Select ⬍]

3. What is the woman's age?
   This tool only calculates risk for women 35 years of age or older.   [Select ⬍]

4. What was the woman's age at the time of her first menstrual period?   [Select ⬍]

5. What was the woman's age at the time of her first live birth of a child?   [Select ⬍]

6. How many of the woman's first-degree relatives - mother, sisters, daughters - have had breast cancer?   [Select ⬍]

7. Has the woman ever had a breast biopsy?   [Select ⬍]

   7a. How many breast biopsies (positive or negative) has the woman had?   [Select ⬍]

   7b. Has the woman had at least one breast biopsy with atypical hyperplasia?   [Select ⬍]

8. What is the woman's race/ethnicity?   [Select ⬍]

   8a. What is the sub race/ethnicity?   [Select ⬍]

   [Calculate Risk >]

REGIONAL WRITE-UP—BREASTS AND AXILLAE

Date _____

Examiner _____

Patient _____ Age _____ Gender _____

Reason for Visit _____

I. Health History

	No	Yes, explain
1. Any **pain** or tenderness in breasts?		
2. Any **lump** or thickening in breasts?		
3. Any **discharge** from nipples?		
4. Any **rash** on breasts?		
5. Any **swelling** in the breasts?		
6. Any **trauma**, injury, or radiation to breasts?		
7. Any **history** of breast disease?		
8. Ever had **surgery** on breasts?		
9. List medications:		
10. Ever been taught breast self-examination?		
11. Ever had mammography? When?		

12. Past health:
   a. Age at menses _____   b. Age at first birth _____
   c. Age at menopause _____   d. Ever take hormone therapy? _____
   e. Usual number of alcoholic drinks/week _____

II. Physical Examination
A. Inspection
   1. Breast symmetry _____
   Skin color and condition _____
   Lesions _____
   Rash or edema _____
   2. Areolae and nipples
   Direction _____
   Discharge _____
   3. Response to arm movement _____
   4. Axillae _____

B. Palpation
   1. Breast texture _____
   Masses _____
   Tenderness _____
   2. Areolae and nipples
   Masses _____
   Discharge _____
   3. Axillae and lymph nodes
   Size _____   Shape _____
   Consistency _____   Mobility _____
   Discrete or matted _____   Tenderness _____

C. Teach breast self-examination

REGIONAL WRITE-UP—BREASTS AND AXILLAE

Summarize your findings using the SOAP format.

Subjective (reason for seeking care, health history)

Objective (physical examination findings)   Record findings on diagram below.

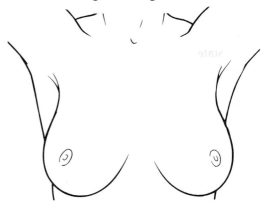

Assessment (assessment of health state or problem, diagnosis)

Plan (diagnostic evaluation, follow-up care, teaching)

STUDENT COMPETENCY CHECKLIST

Teaching Breast Self-Examination (BSE)

	S	U	Comments
A. Cognitive			
1. Explain the following:			
a. Why breasts are examined			
(1) in the shower.			
(2) before a mirror.			
(3) supine with pillow under side of breast being examined.			
b. Who should do breast examination			
c. Frequency options of breast examination			
d. Best time of the month to do breast examination and rationale			
2. State the area of breast where most lumps are found.			
3. Give two reasons why a person may not report significant findings to the health care provider.			
B. Performance			
1. Explains to woman the need for BSE			
2. Instructs woman on technique of BSE by:			
a. inspecting and bilaterally comparing breasts in front of mirror.			
b. noting new or unusual rash or redness on the skin and areola.			
c. palpating breast in a systemic manner, using pads of three fingers and with the woman's arm raised overhead.			
d. palpating tail of Spence and axilla.			
e. gently compressing nipples.			
3. Instructs woman to report unusual findings to the health professional at once			
4. Asks woman to do return demonstration			

NOTES

Thorax and Lungs

PURPOSE

This chapter presents the structure and function of the thorax and lungs, methods of examination of the respiratory system, normal lung sounds, characteristics of adventitious lung sounds, and accurate recording of the assessment.

READING ASSIGNMENT

Jarvis: *Physical Examination and Health Assessment*, 9th ed., Chapter 19, pp. 409–454.

Suggested readings:
Cook, L. K., & Wulf, J. A. (2020). Community-acquired pneumonia: A review of current diagnostic criteria and management. *Am J Nurs*, *120*(12), 34–42.
Acosta, R. A. H., Garrigos, Z. E., Marcelin, J. R., & Vijayvargiya, P. (2022). COVID-19 pathogenesis and clinical manifestations. *Infect Dis Clin N Am*, *36*(2), 231–249.

GLOSSARY

Study the following terms after completing the reading assignment. You should be able to cover the definition on the right and define the term out loud.

Alveoli ....functional units of the lung; the thin-walled chambers surrounded by networks of capillaries that are the site of respiratory exchange of carbon dioxide and oxygen

Angle of Louis ....manubriosternal angle, the articulation of the manubrium and body of the sternum, continuous with the second rib

Apnea ....cessation of breathing

Asthma ....an abnormal respiratory condition associated with allergic hypersensitivity to certain inhaled allergens, characterized by inflammation, bronchospasm, wheezing, and dyspnea

Atelectasis ....an abnormal respiratory condition characterized by collapsed, shrunken, deflated sections of alveoli

Bradypnea ....slow breathing, fewer than 10 breaths per minute, regular rate

Bronchiole .... one of the smaller respiratory passageways into which the segmental bronchi divide

Bronchitis .... inflammation of the bronchi with partial obstruction of bronchi due to excessive mucus secretion

Bronchophony .... the spoken voice sound heard through the stethoscope, which sounds soft, muffled, and indistinct over normal lung tissue

Bronchovesicular .... the normal breath sound heard over major bronchi, characterized by a moderate pitch and an equal duration of inspiration and expiration

Carina .... ridge of cartilage located inside the trachea where it bifurcates into the right and left mainstem bronchi

Chronic obstructive
pulmonary disease (COPD) .... a functional category of abnormal respiratory conditions characterized by airflow obstruction (e.g., emphysema, chronic bronchitis)

Cilia .... millions of hairlike cells lining the tracheobronchial tree

Consolidation .... the solidification of portions of lung tissue as it fills up with infectious exudate, as in pneumonia

Crackles .... abnormal, discontinuous, adventitious lung sounds heard on inspiration

Crepitus .... coarse, crackling sensation palpable over the skin when air abnormally escapes from the lung and enters the subcutaneous tissue

Dead space .... passageways that transport air but are not available for gaseous exchange (e.g., trachea, bronchi)

Dyspnea .... difficult, labored breathing

Emphysema .... type of chronic obstructive pulmonary disease characterized by enlargement of the alveoli distal to terminal bronchioles

Fissure .... the narrow crack dividing the lobes of the lungs

Fremitus .... a palpable vibration from the spoken voice felt over the chest wall

Friction rub .... a coarse, grating, adventitious lung sound heard when the pleurae are inflamed

Hypercapnia .... (also termed hypercarbia) increased levels of carbon dioxide in the blood

Hyperventilation .... increased rate and depth of breathing

Hypoxemia .... decreased level of oxygen in the blood

Intercostal space .... space between the ribs

Kussmaul respiration .... type of hyperventilation that occurs with diabetic ketoacidosis

Orthopnea .... difficulty breathing when supine

Paroxysmal nocturnal
dyspnea .... sudden awakening from sleeping, with shortness of breath

Percussion .... striking over the chest wall with short, sharp blows of the fingers to determine the size and density of the underlying organ

Pleural effusion .... abnormal fluid collection between the layers of the pleura

Stridor .... high-pitched inspiratory crowing sound caused by upper airway obstruction, louder over the neck than the chest wall

Tachypnea .... rapid, shallow breathing; more than 24 breaths per minute

Vesicular .... refers to soft, low-pitched, normal breath sounds heard over peripheral lung fields

Wheeze .... high-pitched, musical, squeaking adventitious lung sound; also used with low-pitched (sonorous) adventitious sounds

Xiphoid process .... sword-shaped lower tip of the sternum

STUDY GUIDE

After completing the reading assignment and the media assignment, write or draw your answers in the spaces provided.

1. Describe the most important points about the health history for the respiratory system.

2. A patient reports a history of cigarette smoking that includes smoking 2 packs per day (ppd) from 1990 to 2012, then 1 ppd from 2013 until quitting in 2022. Calculate the number of pack years smoked.

3. Describe the pleura and its function.

4. List the structures that compose the respiratory dead space.

5. Summarize the mechanics of respiration.

6. List the elements included in the inspection of the respiratory system.

7. List and describe common thoracic deformities.

8. Define 2 types of adventitious breath sounds.

9. The sternal angle is also called _____. Why is it a useful landmark?

10. How many degrees is the normal costal angle? _____

11. When comparing the anteroposterior diameter of the chest with the transverse diameter, what is the expected ratio? What is the significance of this?

12. What is the tripod position?

13. List 3 factors that affect the normal intensity of the tactile fremitus.

    1. _____

    2. _____

    3. _____

14. During percussion, which sound would you expect to predominate over normal lung tissue?

15. List 6 factors that can cause extraneous noise during auscultation.

    1. _____

    2. _____

    3. _____

    4. _____

    5. _____

    6. _____

16. Describe the 3 types of normal breath sounds.

Name	Location	Description

Fill in the labels indicated on the following illustration.

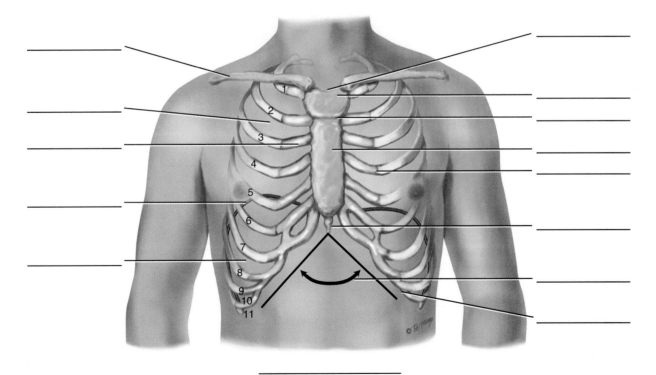

(© Pat Thomas, 2010.)

Study the lobes of the lungs and label their landmarks on the following two illustrations.

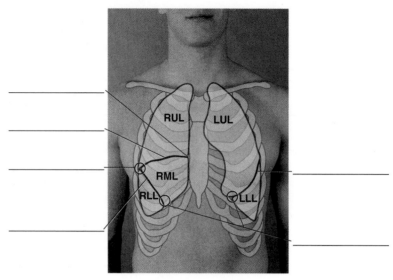

(© Pat Thomas, 2010.)

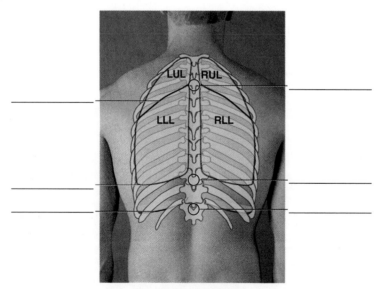

(© Pat Thomas, 2010.)

Label the normal location of the three types of breath sounds on the posterior and anterior chest walls.

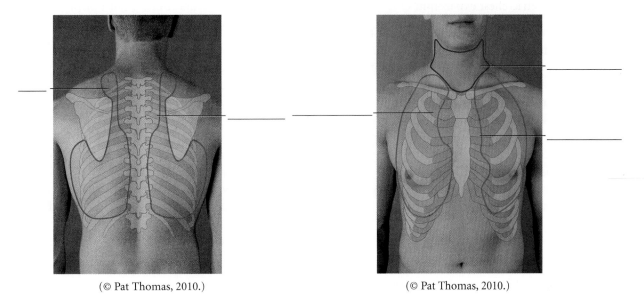

(© Pat Thomas, 2010.) (© Pat Thomas, 2010.)

CLINICAL JUDGMENT QUESTIONS

This test is for you to check your own mastery of the content. Answers are provided in Appendix A.

1. You are examining a hospitalized woman who is on bedrest and has difficulty turning. Which is your best approach to completing the inspection, palpation, and auscultation of the thorax?

   a. Inspect, palpate, and auscultate the anterior and lateral thorax only, omitting the posterior thorax to optimize patient comfort.
   b. Find an assistant to help you turn the woman side to side, and perform the complete assessment while comparing bilaterally as much as possible.
   c. Have the woman turn as best as she can, omitting assessment of areas of the thorax that are not accessible.
   d. Omit inspection of the posterior thorax and push down the mattress to move your hand and stethoscope endpiece under the woman while palpating and auscultating.

2. You are taking a health history on a 44-year-old man who reports use of cigarettes. You calculate a 24-pack year history of smoking, and learn that he has never attempted to quit before. What is your best statement to facilitate a discussion of quitting smoking?
   a. "Smoking is deadly; you really need to stop as soon as possible."
   b. "Do you have any family members who have died because of smoking-related illnesses?"
   c. "Here is a list of resources for when you are ready to quit smoking."
   d. "Are you interested in exploring options to help you quit smoking?"

3. A patient reports dry cough, shortness of breath with activity, and orthopnea. You auscultate fine inspiratory crackles over the bilateral posterior lung bases. What is your next best action?

   a. Request pulmonary function studies to check for emphysema.
   b. Request an x-ray image to check for lobar pneumonia.
   c. Auscultate for absent breath sounds to check for pneumothorax.
   d. Report to provider; these findings are consistent with heart failure.

4. Which of the following assessments best confirms symmetric chest expansion?

   a. Place hands on the posterolateral chest wall with thumbs at the level of T9 or T10.
   b. Inspect the shape and configuration of the chest wall.
   c. Compare bilateral auscultatory points for the presence of any adventitious sounds.
   d. Percuss the posterior chest.

5. You are auscultating breath sounds on a 70-year-old man who states he feels dizzy. Which is your next best action?

   a. Quickly move through the remaining auscultatory points.
   b. Stop the exam and record that the patient could not tolerate auscultation portion.
   c. Ask the patient to hold his breath for 10 seconds, then continue with auscultation.
   d. Allow the patient to take a break, then resume auscultation while monitoring for any worsening dizziness.

6. Which assessment finding is most likely to be immediately life-threatening?

   a. Bronchial breath sounds over a peripheral lung field.
   b. Stridor.
   c. Absent breath sounds over one lung lobe.
   d. Soft high-pitched expiratory wheezing with forced expiration.

7. After examining a patient, you note: fever, increased respiratory rate, chest expansion decreased on the left side, dull to percussion over the left lower lobe, and breath sounds louder with fine crackles over the left lower lobe. These findings are consistent with:

   a. Acute bronchitis.
   b. Asthma.
   c. Pleural effusion.
   d. Lobar pneumonia.

8. On auscultating a patient, you note a coarse, low-pitched sound during both inspiration and expiration. This patient reports pain with breathing. These findings are consistent with:

   a. Fine crackles.
   b. Wheezes.
   c. Atelectatic crackles.
   d. Pleural friction rub.

9. You are examining a patient and count a respiratory rate of 30 breaths per minute. There are no adventitious sounds, but you do note that the breath sounds are decreased and the patient's breathing seems shallow. Which term best describes this breathing pattern?

   a. Hyperventilation.
   b. Hypoventilation.
   c. Tachypnea.
   d. Cheyne-Stokes respirations.

10. You are examining a patient with respiratory distress. Which of the following assessments would best determine if that patient has acute hypoxemia?

   a. Inspect the nailbeds for presence of clubbing.
   b. Palpate for areas of decreased tactile fremitus.
   c. Auscultate for presence of any adventitious breath sounds.
   d. Inspect the nailbeds and mucous membranes for presence of cyanosis.

For questions 15–19, match column B to column A.

Column A: Lung Borders

11. _____ Apex
12. _____ Base
13. _____ Lateral left
14. _____ Lateral right
15. _____ Posterior apex

Column B: Location

a. Rests on the diaphragm
b. C7
c. Sixth rib, midclavicular line
d. Fifth intercostal
e. 3 to 4 cm above the inner third of the clavicles

For questions 20–25, match column B to column A.

Column A: Configurations of the Thorax

16. _____ Normal chest
17. _____ Barrel chest
18. _____ Pectus excavatum
19. _____ Pectus carinatum
20. _____ Scoliosis
21. _____ Kyphosis

Column B: Description

a. Anteroposterior = transverse diameter
b. Exaggerated posterior curvature of thoracic spine
c. Lateral S-shaped curvature of the thoracic and lumbar spines
d. Sunken sternum and adjacent cartilages
e. Elliptic shape with an anteroposterior to transverse diameter in the ratio of 1:2
f. Forward protrusion of the sternum with ribs sloping back at either side

22. You are admitting a patient with shortness of breath and hypoxia to a respiratory care unit. For each assessment finding, indicate whether the finding is associated with left-sided pneumothorax or pneumonia. Each row must have at least one response but may have more than one response selected.

Assessment finding	Left-sided pneumothorax	Left-sided pneumonia
Dullness to percussion on the left side		
Decreased breath sounds on the left side		
Coarse crackles on the left side		
Decreased tactile fremitus on the left side		
Lag in expansion on the left side		

23. A patient with an extensive smoking history reports a productive cough of at least 3 months' duration for each of the last 2 years. Based on the patient's history, select the best condition and an appropriate physical assessment finding to complete the sentence.

This history suggests _____, and a likely assessment finding would be _____.

Condition	Assessment Finding
A. acute bronchitis	A. fever
B. heart failure	B. pink, frothy sputum
C. chronic bronchitis	C. localized dullness to percussion
D. lobar pneumonia	D. expiratory wheezes

CRITICAL THINKING ACTIVITIES

Spend 10 to 15 minutes with the lung sounds simulator in your Skills Laboratory. Or use various websites on the Internet to access audio recordings of healthy lung sounds, as well as adventitious sounds, at various locations over the lungs. One Internet source is https://www.easyauscultation.com/lung-sounds

SKILLS LABORATORY AND CLINICAL SETTING

The purpose of the clinical component is to practice the regional examination on a peer in the skills laboratory or on a patient in the clinical setting and to achieve the following:

Clinical Objectives

1. Demonstrate knowledge of the symptoms related to the respiratory system by obtaining a regional health history from a peer or patient.
2. Correctly locate anatomic landmarks on the thorax of a peer.
3. Using a grease pencil and, with the peer's permission, draw lobes or landmarks of the lungs on the peer's thorax.
4. Demonstrate correct techniques for inspection, palpation, percussion, and auscultation of the respiratory system.
5. Demonstrate the technique for estimation of diaphragmatic excursion.
6. Record the history and physical examination findings accurately, reach an assessment of the health state, and develop a plan of care.

Instructions

Gather your equipment. Wash your hands. Clean the stethoscope endpiece with an alcohol wipe. Practice the steps of the examination of the thorax and lungs on a peer or on a patient in the clinical area. Record your findings using the regional write-up sheet. The front of the sheet is intended as a worksheet; the back of the sheet is intended for a narrative summary using the SOAP format.

REGIONAL WRITE-UP—THORAX AND LUNGS

Date _____

Examiner _____

Patient _____ Age _____ Gender _____

Reason for Visit _____

I. Health History

	No	Yes, explain

1. Do you have a **cough?**

2. Any shortness of **breath?**

3. Any **chest pain** with breathing?

4. Any **past history** of lung diseases?

5. Ever **smoke** cigarettes? What age did you start at?

   How many per day? For how long? Ever tried to quit?

6. Any living or work conditions that affect your breathing?

7. Last TB skin test, chest radiography, flu vaccine?

II. Physical Examination

A. Inspection
1. Thoracic cage _____ Any deformity? _____
2. Respiratory rate and pattern _____ Use accessory muscles? _____
3. Skin and nails _____
4. Person's position _____
5. Person's facial expression _____
6. Level of consciousness _____

B. Palpation
1. Confirm symmetric chest expansion _____
2. Tactile fremitus _____
3. Skin temperature and moisture _____
4. Detect any lumps, masses, tenderness _____
5. Trachea _____

C. Percussion
1. Determine percussion note that predominates over lung fields _____

D. Auscultation
1. Listen: posterior, lateral, anterior _____
2. Any abnormal breath sounds? _____
   If so, perform bronchophony _____
   Whispered pectoriloquy _____,
   Egophony _____
3. Any adventitious sounds? _____

REGIONAL WRITE-UP—THORAX AND LUNGS

Summarize your findings using the SOAP format.

Subjective (reason for seeking care, health history)

Objective (physical examination findings)   Use the drawing to record your findings.

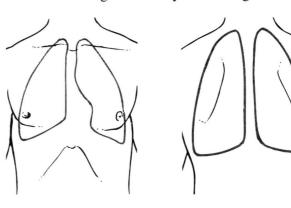

Assessment (assessment of health state or problem, diagnosis)

Plan (diagnostic evaluation, follow-up care, teaching)

Heart and Neck Vessels

PURPOSE

This chapter reviews the structure and function of the heart, valves, and great vessels; the cardiac cycle; heart sounds; the rationale and methods of examination of the heart; and how to accurately record the assessment. At the end of this chapter, you should be able to perform a complete assessment of the heart and neck vessels.

READING ASSIGNMENT

Jarvis: *Physical Examination and Health Assessment,* 9th ed., Chapter 20, pp. 455–504.

Suggested readings:
Rogers, J. R. (2020). Understanding the most commonly billed diagnoses in primary care: Hypertension. *Nurse Pract*, *45*(6), 50–55.
Rogers, J. R., & Baker, M. (2020). Understanding the most commonly billed diagnoses in primary care: Atherosclerotic cardiovascular disease. *Nurse Pract*, *45*(7), 35–41.

GLOSSARY

Study the following terms after completing the reading assignment. You should be able to cover the definition on the right and define the term out loud.

Angina pectoris .... acute chest pain that occurs when the myocardial demand exceeds its oxygen supply

Aortic regurgitation .... (aortic insufficiency) an incompetent aortic valve that allows backward flow of blood into the left ventricle during diastole

Aortic stenosis .... calcification of aortic valve cusps that restricts forward flow of blood during systole

Aortic valve .... the left semilunar valve separating the left ventricle and the aorta

Apex of the heart .... tip of the heart pointing down toward the 5th left intercostal space

Apical impulse .... point of maximal impulse (PMI); pulsation created as the left ventricle rotates against the chest wall during systole, normally at the 5th left intercostal space in the midclavicular line

Base of the heart .... broader area of the heart's outline located at the 3rd right and left intercostal spaces

Bell (of the stethoscope) .... cup-shaped endpiece used for soft, low-pitched heart sounds

Bradycardia .... slow heart rate, less than 50 beats per minute in the adult

Clubbing .... bulbous enlargement of distal phalanges of fingers and toes that occurs with chronic cyanotic heart and lung conditions

Coarctation of aorta .... severe narrowing of the descending aorta, a congenital heart defect

Cor pulmonale .... right ventricular hypertrophy and heart failure due to pulmonary hypertension

Cyanosis .... dusky blue discoloration of the skin and mucous membranes due to excessive amount of deoxygenated hemoglobin in the blood

Diaphragm (of the stethoscope) .... flat endpiece of the stethoscope used for hearing relatively high-pitched heart sounds

Diastole .... the heart's filling phase

Dyspnea .... difficult, labored breathing

Edema .... swelling of legs or dependent body part due to increased interstitial fluid

Erb's point .... traditional auscultatory area in the 3rd left intercostal space

First heart sound (S$_1$) .... occurs with closure of the atrioventricular valves signaling the beginning of systole

Fourth heart sound (S$_4$) .... S$_4$ gallop, atrial gallop; very soft, low-pitched ventricular filling sound that occurs in late diastole

Gallop rhythm .... the addition of a 3rd or a 4th heart sound; makes the rhythm sound like the cadence of a galloping horse

Inching .... technique of moving the stethoscope incrementally across the precordium through the auscultatory areas while listening to the heart sounds

Left ventricular hypertrophy (LVH) .... increase in thickness of the myocardial wall that occurs when the heart pumps against chronic outflow obstruction (e.g., aortic stenosis)

Midclavicular line (MCL) .... imaginary vertical line bisecting the middle of the clavicle in each hemithorax

Mitral regurgitation .... mitral insufficiency; incompetent mitral valve allows regurgitation of blood back into left atrium during systole

Mitral stenosis .... calcified mitral valve impedes forward flow of blood into left ventricle during diastole

Mitral valve .... left atrioventricular valve separating the left atrium and ventricle

Palpitation .... uncomfortable awareness of rapid or irregular heart rate

Paradoxical splitting .... Opposite of a normal split S$_2$, so that the split is heard in expiration, and in inspiration, the sounds fuse into one sound

Pericardial friction rub .... high-pitched, scratchy extracardiac sound heard when the precordium is inflamed

Physiologic splitting .... normal variation in S$_2$ heard as two separate components during inspiration

Precordium .... area of the chest wall overlying the heart and great vessels

Pulmonic regurgitation .... pulmonic insufficiency; backflow of blood through incompetent pulmonic valve into the right ventricle

Pulmonic stenosis .... calcification of pulmonic valve that restricts forward flow of blood during systole

Pulmonic valve .... right semilunar valve separating the right ventricle and pulmonary artery

Second heart sound (S_2) .... occurs with closure of the semilunar valves, aortic and pulmonic; signals the end of systole

Summation gallop .... abnormal mid-diastolic heart sound heard when both the pathologic S_3 and S_4 are present

Syncope .... temporary loss of consciousness due to decreased cerebral blood flow (fainting); caused by ventricular asystole, pronounced bradycardia, or ventricular fibrillation

Systole .... the heart's pumping phase

Tachycardia .... rapid heart rate, greater than 95 beats per minute in adults

Third heart sound (S_3) .... soft, low-pitched ventricular filling sound that occurs in early diastole (S_3 gallop) and may be an early sign of heart failure

Thrill .... palpable vibration on the chest wall accompanying severe heart murmur

Tricuspid valve .... right atrioventricular valve separating the right atrium and ventricle

STUDY GUIDE

After completing the reading assignment and the media assignment, write or draw the answers in the spaces provided.

1. Define apical impulse and describe its normal location, size, and duration.

   Which of these *abnormal* conditions may affect the location of the apical impulse?

2. Explain the mechanism producing normal first and second heart sounds.

3. Describe the effect of respiration on the heart sounds.

4. Describe the characteristics of the **first heart sound** and its intensity at the apex of the heart and at the base.

5. Describe the characteristics of the **second heart sound** and its intensity at the apex of the heart and at the base.

6. Explain the physiologic mechanism for the normal splitting of S_2 in the pulmonic valve area.

7. Define the **third heart sound.** When in the cardiac cycle does it occur? Describe its intensity, quality, location in which it is heard, and the method of auscultation.

8. Differentiate a physiologic S_3 from a pathologic S_3.

9. Define the **fourth heart sound.** When in the cardiac cycle does it occur? Describe its intensity, quality, location in which it is heard, and the method of auscultation.

10. Explain the position of the valves during the cardiac cycle in diastole, isometric contraction, systole, and isometric relaxation.

11. Define venous pressure and jugular venous pulse.

12. Differentiate between carotid artery pulsation and jugular vein pulsation.

13. List the major risk factors for heart disease and stroke as identified in this text.

14. Define bruit, and discuss what it indicates.

15. State 4 guidelines to distinguish S_1 from S_2.

    1. _____

    2. _____

    3. _____

    4. _____

16. Define pulse deficit and discuss what it indicates.

17. Define preload and afterload.

18. List the characteristics to explore when you hear a murmur, including the grading scale of murmurs.

19. Discuss the characteristics of an innocent or functional murmur.

Fill in the labels indicated on the following illustrations.

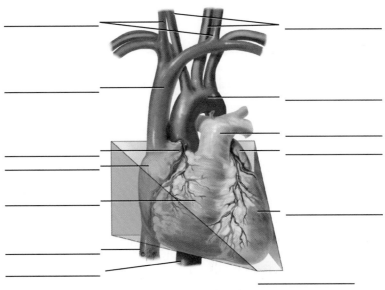

(© Pat Thomas, 2006.)

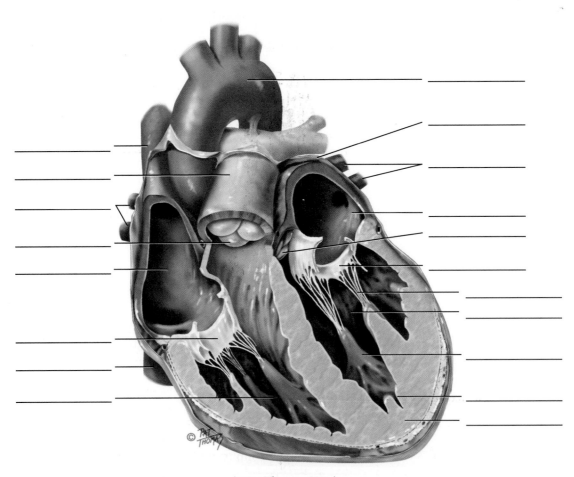

(© Pat Thomas, 2010.)

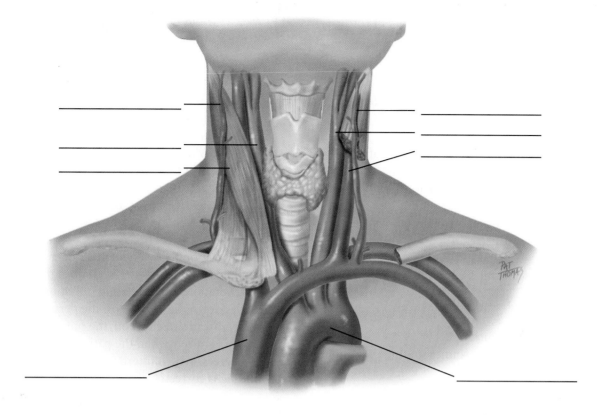

(© Pat Thomas, 2010.)

CLINICAL JUDGMENT QUESTIONS

This test is for you to check your own mastery of the content. Answers are provided in Appendix A.

1. The precordium is:

   a. A synonym for mediastinum.
   b. The area on the chest where the apical impulse is felt.
   c. The area on the anterior chest overlying the heart and great vessels.
   d. A synonym for the area where the superior and inferior venae cavae return unoxygenated venous blood to the right side of the heart.

2. Select the best description of the tricuspid valve.

   a. Left semilunar valve.
   b. Right atrioventricular valve.
   c. Left atrioventricular valve.
   d. Right semilunar valve.

3. The function of the pulmonic valve is to:

   a. Divide the left atrium and left ventricle.
   b. Guard the opening between the right atrium and right ventricle.
   c. Protect the orifice between the right ventricle and pulmonary artery.
   d. Guard the entrance to the aorta from the left ventricle.

4. Atrial systole occurs:

   a. During ventricular systole.
   b. During ventricular diastole.
   c. Concurrently with ventricular systole.
   d. Independently of ventricular function.

5. The second heart sound is the result of:

   a. Opening of the mitral and tricuspid valves.
   b. Closing of the mitral and tricuspid valves.
   c. Opening of the aortic and pulmonic valves.
   d. Closing of the aortic and pulmonic valves.

6. A 74-year-old woman has a history of coronary artery disease. Which 3 signs and symptoms lead you to suspect the woman may have heart failure? **Select all that apply.**

    a. Reports 2-month history of orthopnea, sleeping on 3 pillows because "it is easier to breathe"
    b. Reports burning epigastric pain after eating
    c. 2+ bilateral pretibial edema
    d. S3 gallop
    e. Clear, adventitious breath sounds
    f. Warm, flushed skin

7. When auscultating the heart, your first step is to:

    a. Identify S_1 and S_2.
    b. Listen for S_3 and S_4.
    c. Listen for murmurs.
    d. Identify all four sounds on the first round.

8. A murmur is heard after S_1 and before S_2. This murmur would be classified as:

    a. Diastolic (possibly benign).
    b. Diastolic (always pathologic).
    c. Systolic (possibly benign).
    d. Systolic (always pathologic).

9. When assessing the carotid artery, you will palpate:

    a. Bilaterally at the same time while standing behind the patient.
    b. Medial to the sternomastoid muscle, one side at a time.
    c. For a bruit while asking the patient to hold their breath briefly.
    d. For unilateral distention while turning the patient's head to one side.

10. For a patient experiencing orthopnea, which physical assessment findings would be most relevant? **Select all that apply.**

    a. Right-sided carotid bruit.
    b. Elevated jugular venous pressure.
    c. Presence of a split S_2 toward the end of every expiration.
    d. Presence of an S_3 heart sounds in both supine and sitting positions.

11. A 62-year-old man complains of chest pain. You ask him to describe the chest pain. Which statement would cause you to consider an ischemic cardiovascular cause?

    a. "The pain is much worse when I take a deep breath, and I keep coughing too."
    b. "It feels sharp and stabbing, but it's a bit better when I lean forward."
    c. "This pain is burning; I notice it more after I eat and my mouth tastes terrible."
    d. "My chest feels tight and heavy, but it does go away when I rest for a few minutes."

12. After positioning a patient at 45 degrees and shining a light across the neck from the right side, you note an undulating pulsation that moves down the neck when the person takes a deep breath. In addition, the pulsation disappears entirely when the patient sits up to 90 degrees. Which interpretation of this finding is correct?

    a. This is the carotid pulse, and the finding is normal.
    b. This is the carotid pulse, and the finding may suggest carotid stenosis.
    c. This is the jugular venous pulse, and the finding is normal.
    d. This is the jugular venous pulse, and the finding may suggest hypovolemia.

13. While auscultating a patient's heart rate and rhythm, you note it sounds irregular. What additional assessments would help you determine the cause? **Select all that apply.**

    a. Note if there is any pattern to the irregularity.
    b. Note if the rate varies with inspiration and expiration.
    c. Carefully listen to the bilateral carotid arteries.
    d. Auscultate the apical beat while palpating the radial pulse, and note any difference in rate.

14. You are auscultating heart sounds and hear a click early in systole at the 2nd right interspace and the apex. There is also a systolic murmur. Which question to the patient demonstrates you understand the significance of your auscultation findings?

    a. "Have you been told you have a mitral valve replacement?"
    b. "Have you been told you have aortic stenosis?"
    c. "Have you been told you have mitral valve prolapse?"
    d. "Have you been told you have heart failure?"

15. You are interviewing a 14-year-old adolescent who has just started playing soccer and has been complaining of cramping leg pain during practice. The teen is very concerned that something is wrong. What should be your next action?

    a. Tell the teen it's probably dehydration, and encourage intake of more fluids and electrolytes.
    b. Talk to the attending provider about obtaining further tests to assess for any atherosclerotic disease in the legs.
    c. Tell the teen that growing pains are normal, and that you will follow up for improvement at the next visit.
    d. Assess arm versus leg blood pressures, bilateral femoral pulse amplitude, and for presence of any murmurs.

For questions 17–22, match column B to Column A.

Column A

16. _____ Tough, fibrous, double-walled sac that surrounds and protects the heart
17. _____ Thin layer of endothelial tissue that lines the inner surface of the heart chambers and valves
18. _____ Reservoir for holding blood
19. _____ Ensures smooth, friction-free movement of the heart muscle
20. _____ Muscular pumping chamber
21. _____ Muscular wall of the heart

Column B

a. Pericardial fluid
b. Ventricle
c. Endocardium
d. Myocardium
e. Pericardium
f. Atrium

22. Fill in the blanks.

    S_1 is best heard at the _____ of the heart, whereas S_2 is loudest at the _____ of the heart. S_1 coincides with the pulse in the _____ and coincides with the _____ wave if the patient is on an ECG monitor.

23. You are auscultating a patient's precordium to rule out a pericardial friction rub. Select one stethoscope feature, one patient position, and one patient instruction to complete the sentence.

    Listen with the _____ of the stethoscope, with the patient _____, and instruct the patient to _____.

Stethoscope feature	Patient position	Patient instruction
A. bell	A. sitting up and leaning forward	A. breathe out and hold
B. diaphragm	B. turned on the left side	B. breathe normally

CRITICAL THINKING ACTIVITIES

Calculate the 10-year risk for atherosclerotic cardiovascular disease (ASCVD).

First try these online calculators yourself, and then interview a man older than 40 years and a woman older than 40 years, perhaps members of your family. Consider the multiple traditional cardiovascular risk factors for asymptomatic adults without a clinical history of cardiovascular disease. Obtain a global risk score using the tools given below, and then develop a teaching plan individualized for the risk score of your interviewee.

- American College of Cardiology and American Heart Association ASCVD Risk Estimator
  - https://tools.acc.org/ldl/ascvd_risk_estimator/index.html#!/calulate/estimator/
  - https://tools.acc.org/ascvd-risk-estimator-plus/#!/calculate/estimate/

SKILLS LABORATORY AND CLINICAL SETTING

The purpose of the clinical component is to practice the regional examination on a peer in the skills laboratory or on a patient in the clinical setting to achieve the following.

Clinical Objectives

1. Demonstrate knowledge of cardiovascular symptoms by obtaining a regional health history from a peer or patient.
2. Correctly locate anatomic landmarks on the chest wall of a peer.
3. Using a grease pencil and with the peer's permission, outline the borders of the heart and label auscultatory areas on a peer's chest wall.
4. Demonstrate correct technique for inspection and palpation of the neck vessels.
5. Demonstrate correct techniques for inspection, palpation, and auscultation of the precordium.
6. Record the history and physical examination findings accurately, reach an assessment of the health state, and develop a plan of care.

Instructions

Gather your equipment. Wash your hands. Clean the stethoscope endpiece with an alcohol wipe. Practice the steps of the examination of the cardiovascular system on a peer or on a patient in the clinical area. Record your findings using the regional write-up sheet that follows. The front of the page is intended as a worksheet; the back of the page is intended for your narrative recording using the SOAP format.

REGIONAL WRITE-UP—CARDIOVASCULAR SYSTEM

Date _____

Examiner _____

Patient _____ Age _____ Gender _____

Reason for visit _____

I. Health History

	No	Yes, explain
1. Any **chest pain** or tightness?		
2. Any **shortness of breath**?		
3. Do you use more than one pillow to sleep?		
4. Do you have a **cough**?		
5. Do you seem to **tire easily**?		
6. Facial skin ever turns blue or ashen?		
7. Any **swelling** of feet or legs?		
8. Awaken at night to urinate?		
9. Any past history of heart disease?		
10. Any family history of heart disease?		
11. Any change in usual daily activities?		
12. Current medications?		
13. Smoking? How many per day? Alcohol use? Number of drinks per day?		

14. Assess cardiac risk factors: diabetes, hypertension, smoking, high cholesterol, obesity, sedentary lifestyle, age _____

II. Physical Examination

A. Carotid arteries

Palpate R _____ L _____
(absent, weak, moderate, bounding)

B. Jugular venous system

External jugular veins (circle one): < collapsed supine / meniscus visible at _____ bed elevated

Internal jugular venous pulsations: < not visible / visible at _____ bed elevated

C. Precordium—inspect and palpate.

1. Skin color and condition _____
2. Chest wall pulsations _____
3. Heave or lift _____
4. Apical impulse in the _____ at _____
   Size _____

D. Auscultation

1. Identify the anatomic areas where you will listen.
2. Rate and rhythm _____
3. Identify S_1 and S_2 in diagram at right and note any variation.
   Fill in any murmur below:

   S_1 S_2 S S_2

   S_1 _____

   S_2 _____

4. Listen in systole and diastole:
Extra heart sounds _____
Systolic murmur _____
Diastolic murmur _____

REGIONAL WRITE-UP—CARDIOVASCULAR SYSTEM

Summarize your findings using the SOAP format.

Subjective (reason for seeking care, health history)

Objective (physical examination findings)   Record findings using diagram.

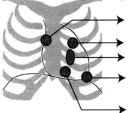

Assessment (assessment of the health state or problem, diagnosis)

Plan (diagnostic evaluation, follow-up care, patient teaching)

NOTES

Peripheral Vascular System and Lymphatic System

PURPOSE

This chapter presents the structure and function of the peripheral vascular system and the lymphatic system; the location of the peripheral pulse sites; the rationale and methods of examination of the peripheral vascular and lymphatic systems; and how to accurately record the assessment. At the end of this chapter, you should be able to perform a complete assessment of the peripheral vascular and lymphatic systems.

READING ASSIGNMENT

Jarvis: *Physical Examination and Health Assessment*, 9th ed., Chapter 21, pp. 502–532.

Suggested readings:
Kohlman-Trigoboff, D. (2021). Healthcare inequity in PAD. *J Vasc Nurs, 39*(3), 54–56.
Kohlman-Trigoboff, D. (2019) Update: Diagnosis and management of peripheral arterial disease. *J Nurse Pract, 15*(1), 87–95.

GLOSSARY

Study the following terms after completing the reading assignment. You should be able to cover the definition on the right and define the term out loud.

Allen test .... test that determines the patency of the radial and ulnar arteries by compressing one artery site and observing the return of skin color as evidence of patency of the other artery

Aneurysm .... defect or sac formed by dilation in artery wall due to atherosclerosis, trauma, or congenital defect

Arrhythmia .... variation from the heart's regular rhythm

Arteriosclerosis .... thickening and loss of elasticity of the arterial walls

Atherosclerosis .... plaques of fatty deposits formed in the inner layer (intima) of the arteries

Bradycardia .... slow heart rate, less than 50 beats per minute in the adult

Bruit .... blowing, swooshing sound heard through a stethoscope when an artery is partially occluded

Cyanosis .... dusky blue discoloration of the skin and mucous membranes due to excessive amount of deoxygenated hemoglobin in the blood

Diastole .... the heart's filling phase

Ischemia .... deficiency of arterial blood to a body part due to constriction or obstruction of a blood vessel

Lymph nodes .... small oval clumps of lymphatic tissue located at grouped intervals along lymphatic vessels

Lymphedema .... swelling of the extremity due to obstructed lymph channel, nonpitting

Pitting edema .... indentation left after the examiner depresses skin over swollen edematous tissue

Profile sign .... viewing the finger from the side to detect early clubbing

Pulse .... pressure wave created by each heartbeat, palpable at body sites where the artery lies close to the skin and over a bone

Pulsus alternans .... regular rhythm, but force of pulse varies with alternating beats of large and small amplitude

Pulsus bigeminus .... irregular rhythm; every other beat is premature; premature beats have weakened amplitude

Pulsus paradoxus .... beats have weaker amplitude with respiratory inspiration, stronger with expiration

Systole .... the heart's pumping phase

Tachycardia .... rapid heart rate, more than 95 beats per minute in the adult

Thrombophlebitis .... inflammation of the vein associated with thrombus formation

Ulcer .... open skin lesion extending into dermis, with sloughing of necrotic inflammatory tissue

Varicose veins .... dilated tortuous veins with incompetent valves

STUDY GUIDE

After completing the reading assignment and the media assignment, write or draw the answers in the spaces provided.

1. Describe the structure and function of arteries and veins.

2. List the pulse sites accessible to examination.

3. Describe the 3 mechanisms that help return venous blood to the heart.

4. Define the term *capacitance vessels* and explain its significance.

5. List the risk factors for venous stasis.

6. Describe the function of the lymphatic system.

7. Describe the function of the lymph nodes.

8. Name the related organs in the lymphatic system.

9. List the symptom areas to address during history-taking of the peripheral vascular system.

10. Fill in the grading scale for assessing the force of an arterial pulse: 0 _____; 1+ _____;
    2+ _____; 3+ _____

11. List the skin characteristics expected with arterial insufficiency to the lower legs.

12. Compare the characteristics of leg ulcers associated with arterial insufficiency with ulcers with venous insufficiency.

13. Fill in the description of the grading scale for pitting edema:

    1+ _____

    2+ _____

    3+ _____

    4+ _____

14. Describe the technique for using the Doppler ultrasonic probe to detect peripheral pulses.

15. Raynaud phenomenon has associated progressive tricolor changes of the skin from _____ to _____ and then to _____. State the mechanism for each of these color changes.

Fill in the labels indicated on the following arteries and name the pulse sites.

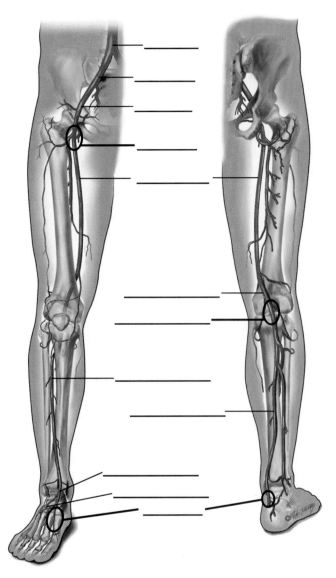

(@ Pat Thomas, 2010.)

CLINICAL JUDGMENT QUESTIONS

This test is for you to check your own mastery of the content. Answers are provided in Appendix A.

1. Which of the following organs aid the lymphatic system?

   a. Liver, lymph nodes, and stomach.
   b. Pancreas, small intestine, and thymus.
   c. Spleen, tonsils, and thymus.
   d. Pancreas, spleen, and tonsils.

2. Ms. T. has come for a prenatal visit. She reports dependent edema, varicosities in the legs, and hemorrhoids. What is your best response?

   a. "If these symptoms persist, we will perform an amniocentesis."
   b. "If these symptoms persist, we will discuss having you hospitalized."
   c. "The symptoms are caused by the pressure of the growing uterus on the veins. They are usual conditions of pregnancy."
   d. "At this time, the symptoms are a minor inconvenience. You should learn to accept them."

3. Inspection of a person's right hand reveals a red swollen area. To further assess for infection, you would palpate the:

   a. Cervical node.
   b. Axillary node.
   c. Epitrochlear node.
   d. Inguinal node.

4. To screen for deep vein thrombosis, you would:

   a. Measure the circumference of the ankle.
   b. Check the temperature with the palm of the hand.
   c. Compress the dorsalis pedis pulse, looking for blood return.
   d. Measure the widest point of the calf with a tape measure.

5. During the examination of the lower extremities, you are unable to palpate the popliteal pulse. Your next best action is to:

   a. Proceed with the examination. It is often impossible to palpate this pulse.
   b. Refer the patient to a vascular surgeon for further evaluation.
   c. Schedule the patient for a venogram.
   d. Schedule the patient for an arteriogram.

6. You assess a patient who has 4+ edema of the right leg. What is the best way to document this finding?

   a. Mild pitting, no perceptible swelling of the leg.
   b. Moderate pitting, indentation subsides rapidly.
   c. Deep pitting, leg looks swollen.
   d. Very deep pitting, indentation lasts a long time.

7. After raising a patient's legs 12 inches off the table for 30 seconds and then having the person sit up and dangle the legs, you note the color returned to both legs in 30 seconds. What should be your next action?

   a. Notify the provider of a potential acute arterial occlusion.
   b. Assess pulse amplitude and ask the patient about symptoms of claudication.
   c. Order a lower extremity venous ultrasound test.
   d. Proceed with the exam, as this is a normal finding.

8. A 54-year-old woman with five children has varicose veins of the lower extremities. Her most characteristic sign is:

   a. Reduced arterial circulation.
   b. Blanching, death-like appearance of the extremities on elevation.
   c. Loss of hair on feet and toes.
   d. Dilated, tortuous superficial bluish vessels.

9. Raynaud phenomenon occurs:

   a. When the patient's extremities are exposed to heat and compression.
   b. In hands and feet as a result of exposure to cold, vibration, and stress.

   c. After removal of lymph nodes or damage to lymph nodes and channels.
   d. As a result of leg cramps due to excessive walking or climbing stairs.

10. Match each patient to the expected pulse amplitude.

Patient	Pulse Amplitude
Patient with acute arterial occlusion of right leg. _____	i. 3+
Patient in septic shock with hypotension. _____	ii. 2+
Patient who just finished running on a treadmill. _____	iii. 1+
Patient in good health at pre-employment physical examination. _____	iv. 0

11. **Underline** the cues from the history and physical exam below that suggest lymphedema as the likely cause of the arm swelling.

You are assessing a woman with a history of breast cancer. She underwent a right mastectomy 2 months ago and is getting radiation therapy. She is concerned because her right arm is swollen and she thinks she may have a blood clot. Your examination reveals firm, non-pitting edema. Her arm pulses are 2+ bilaterally. Her skin is warm and there are no areas of redness or tenderness.

12. Complete the blanks using the options below.

You are caring for a patient who presented to the emergency department with right leg pain. She reports ____A____, and your physical exam reveals ____B____ in the right leg. You suspect the patient has ____C____, and your next action is to ____D____.

A – Subjective	B – Objective	C – Condition	D – Action
1. Gradual onset of pain over the last month	1. Warm intact skin, 2+ pulses, capillary refill <3 s.	1. Varicose veins	1. Contact the provider immediately
2. Dull, heavy pain after a long day	2. Warmth and redness over a tender, palpable calf vein	2. Acute arterial insufficiency	2. Document your findings carefully
3. Acute, sudden onset of very severe pain	3. Pallor, coolness, and pulselessness	3. Lymphedema	3. Teach the patient to avoid prolonged sitting

13. Match the finding to the most likely condition in each row.

Finding	Peripheral Artery Disease	Chronic Venous Insufficiency	Acute Deep Vein Thrombosis
Thin, shiny, hairless skin			
Thick skin with brown discoloration			
Red, warm skin			
Hair loss			
Bilateral diminished pulses			
Varicose veins			
Unilateral edema			

14. Complete the blanks using the options below.

A 62-year-old man presents with complaints of ___A___. You examine his legs and note ___B___. You are concerned that he may be experiencing ___C___.

A – Subjective	B – Objective	C – Condition
1. Claudication	1. Unilateral swelling and warmth	1. PAD
2. Pain in calf in multiple positions	2. Swelling of bilateral knee joints	2. Chronic venous insufficiency
3. Stumbling while walking and numb legs	3. Decreased reflexes, absent sensation to monofilament	3. Acute DVT

NOTES

CRITICAL THINKING ACTIVITIES

1. Calculate the Wells Score (see Jarvis: *Physical Examination and Health Assessment,* 9th ed., p. 21–18) for the following patient, then explain its significance: Your patient is a 48-year-old man who was in a motorcycle accident last month. He underwent general anesthesia for a splenectomy (due to internal bleeding), and his left foot through mid-calf is in a cast due to an ankle fracture. He is complaining that the cast has become tight in the last day. His left upper calf is tender to palpation along the venous system; the skin is of similar color and temperature to the right and there are no dilated vessels. While there is no visible swelling of the entire left leg, you measure a calf circumference of 33 cm on the right and 35 cm on the left; the left lower leg also has 1+ pitting edema while the right has none. He has no other past medical history.

2. Study the two photos following regarding foot and leg ulcers. The pathogenesis of these ulcers could be arterial (ischemic) dysfunction or venous (stasis) dysfunction. Choose which is which. To support your thinking, state the Subjective (history) symptoms and the Objective signs that would accompany these ulcers.

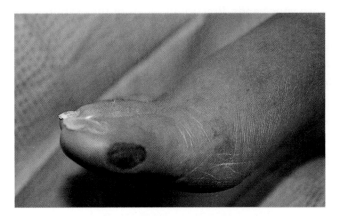

(From Dockery, G. L. (1997). *Cutaneous disorders of the lower extremity.* Philadelphia: Saunders.)

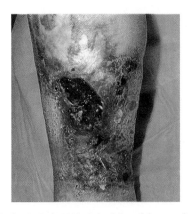

(From Lookingbill, D. P., & Marks, J. G. (1993). *Principles of dermatology* (2nd ed.). Philadelphia: Saunders.)

SKILLS LABORATORY AND CLINICAL SETTING

The purpose of the clinical component is to practice the regional examination on a peer in the skills laboratory or on a patient in the clinical setting to achieve the following.

Clinical Objectives

1. Demonstrate knowledge of the symptoms related to the peripheral vascular system by obtaining a regional health history from a peer or patient.
2. Demonstrate palpation of peripheral arterial pulses (brachial, radial, femoral, popliteal, posterior tibial, dorsalis pedis) by assessing amplitude and symmetry, noting any signs of arterial insufficiency.
3. Demonstrate inspection and palpation of peripheral veins by noting any signs of venous insufficiency.
4. Demonstrate palpation of the lymphatic system by identifying enlargement, clumping, or abnormal firmness of regional lymph nodes.
5. Demonstrate correct technique for performing the following additional tests when indicated: Allen test, Doppler ultrasonic stethoscope, computing the ankle-brachial index (ABI).
6. Record the history and physical examination findings accurately, reach an assessment of the health state, and develop a plan of care.

Instructions

Gather your equipment. Wash your hands. Practice the steps of the examination of the peripheral vascular system on a peer or on a patient in the clinical setting, giving appropriate instructions as you proceed. Record your findings using the regional write-up sheets that follow. The first part is intended as a worksheet; the last page is intended for your narrative summary recording using the SOAP format. Note that the peripheral examination and cardiovascular examination usually are practiced together.

REGIONAL WRITE-UP—PERIPHERAL VASCULAR SYSTEM

Date _____

Examiner _____

Patient _____ Age _____ Gender _____

Reason for Visit _____

I. Health History

	No	Yes, explain
1. Any leg **pain** (cramps)? Where?	_____	_____
2. Any **skin changes** in arms or legs?	_____	_____
3. Any sores or **lesions** in arms or legs?	_____	_____
4. Any **swelling** in the legs?	_____	_____
5. Any **swollen glands**? Where?	_____	_____
6. What medications are you taking?	_____	_____
7. Do you smoke cigarettes? How many per day? Ever tried to quit?	_____	_____

II. Physical Examination

A. Arms, Inspect:

Color of skin and nail beds _____

Symmetry _____

Lesions _____

Edema _____ Clubbing _____

Palpate

   Temperature _____ Texture _____

   Capillary refill _____

   Locate and grade pulses (record below)

   Check epitrochlear lymph nodes _____

   Modified Allen test (if indicated) _____

B. Legs, Inspect:

Color _____ Hair distribution _____

Venous pattern, varicosities _____

Swelling, edema _____ Atrophy _____

If so, measure calf circumference in centimeters: R _____ L _____

Skin lesions or ulcers _____

Palpate

   Temperature _____

   Calf tenderness _____

   Inguinal lymph nodes _____

   Locate and grade pulses (record below) _____

   Check pretibial edema (grade if present) _____

   Auscultate for bruit (if indicated) _____

REGIONAL WRITE-UP—PERIPHERAL VASCULAR SYSTEM

	Brachial	Radial	Femoral	Popliteal	Dorsalis pedis	P. tibial
R						
L						

0 = absent, 1+ = weak, 2+ = normal, 3+ = full, bounding

C. **Ankle-Brachial Index (ABI)**

Use Doppler ultrasonic probe and locate pulse sites: brachial, dorsalis pedis, and posterior tibial. Compute ABI. Optional: Visit https://ckdpcrisk.org/padrisk/ to calculate lifetime risk and prevalence of lower extremity PAD.

Ankle-Brachial Index Interpretation
Above 0.90: Normal or borderline
0.71 – 0.89: Mild PAD
0.41 – 0.70: Moderate PAD
0.00 – 0.40: Severe PAD

Right arm:
Systolic pressure ☐☐☐ mm Hg

Left arm:
Systolic pressure ☐☐☐ mm Hg

Right ankle:
Systolic pressure
Posterior tibial (PT) ☐☐☐ mm Hg
Dorsalis pedis (DP) ☐☐☐ mm Hg

Left ankle:
Systolic pressure
Posterior tibial (PT) ☐☐☐ mm Hg
Dorsalis pedis (DP) ☐☐☐ mm Hg

Right ABI equals ratio of:
Higher of the right ankle pressures (PT or DP) ☐☐☐ mm Hg
Higher arm pressure (right or left arm) ☐☐☐ mm Hg
= ☐.☐☐

Left ABI equals ratio of:
Higher of the left ankle pressures (PT or DP) ☐☐☐ mm Hg
Higher arm pressure (right or left arm) ☐☐☐ mm Hg
= ☐.☐☐

From AACN (2009). AACN Advanced Critical Care Nursing (ed. 1). Philadelphia: Saunders.

REGIONAL WRITE-UP—PERIPHERAL VASCULAR SYSTEM

Summarize your findings using the SOAP format.

Subjective (reason for seeking care, health history)

Objective (physical examination findings)

Record pulses on diagram below.

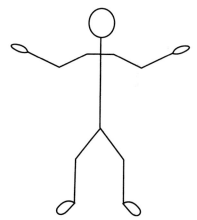

Assessment (assessment of health state or problem, diagnosis)

Plan (diagnostic evaluation, follow-up care, teaching)

NOTES

PURPOSE

This chapter presents the structure and function of the abdominal organs; the location of the abdominal organs; how to discriminate normal bowel sounds; the rationale and methods of examination of the abdomen; and how to accurately record the assessment. At the end of this chapter, you should be able to perform a complete assessment of the abdomen.

READING ASSIGNMENT

Jarvis: Physical Examination and Health Assessment, 9th ed., Chapter 22, pp. 533–572.

Suggested reading:
Rogers, J., & Schallmo, M. (2021). Understanding the most commonly billed diagnoses in primary care: Abdominal pain. *Nurse Pract, 46*(1), 13–20.

GLOSSARY

Study the following terms after completing the reading assignment. You should be able to cover the definition on the right and define the term out loud.

Aneurysm .... defect or sac formed by dilation in the artery wall due to atherosclerosis, trauma, or congenital defect

Anorexia .... loss of appetite for food

Ascites .... abnormal accumulation of serous fluid within the peritoneal cavity, associated with heart failure, portal hypertension, cirrhosis, hepatitis, pancreatitis, and cancer

Borborygmi .... loud, gurgling bowel sounds signaling increased motility or hyperperistalsis; occurs with early bowel obstruction, gastroenteritis, or diarrhea

Bruit .... blowing, swooshing sound heard through a stethoscope when an artery is partially occluded

Cecum .... first or proximal part of large intestine

Cholecystitis .... inflammation of the gallbladder

Costal margin .... lower border of the rib margin formed by medial edges of the 8th, 9th, and 10th ribs

Costovertebral angle (CVA) .... angle formed by the 12th rib and the vertebral column on the posterior thorax, overlying the kidney

Diastasis recti .... midline longitudinal ridge in the abdomen, a separation of abdominal rectus muscles

Dysphagia .... difficulty swallowing

Epigastrium .... the abdominal region between the costal margins

Hepatomegaly .... abnormal enlargement of liver

Hernia .... abnormal protrusion of bowel through weakening in the abdominal musculature

Inguinal ligament .... ligament extending from pubic bone to anterior superior iliac spine, forming lower border of abdomen

Linea alba .... midline tendinous seam joining the abdominal muscles

Paralytic ileus .... complete absence of peristaltic movement that may follow abdominal surgery or complete bowel obstruction

Peritoneal friction rub .... rough grating sound heard through the stethoscope over the site of peritoneal inflammation

Peritoneum .... double envelope of serous membrane that lines the abdominal wall and covers the surface of most abdominal organs

Peritonitis .... inflammation of peritoneum

Pyloric stenosis .... congenital narrowing of pyloric sphincter, forming outflow obstruction of stomach

Pyrosis .... heartburn; burning sensation in upper abdomen due to reflux of gastric acid

Rectus abdominis muscles ...... midline abdominal muscles extending from rib cage to pubic bone

Scaphoid .... abnormally sunken abdominal wall, as with malnutrition or in underweight individuals

Splenomegaly .... abnormal enlargement of spleen

Striae .... (lineae albicantes) silvery white or pink scar tissue formed by stretching of abdominal skin as with pregnancy or obesity

Suprapubic .... name of abdominal region just superior to pubic bone

Tympany .... high-pitched, musical, drum-like percussion note heard when percussing over the stomach and intestine

Umbilicus .... depression on the abdomen, marking the site of entry of umbilical cord

Viscera .... internal organs

STUDY GUIDE

After completing the reading assignment and the media assignment, write or draw the answers in the spaces provided.

1. Describe the proper positioning and preparation of the patient for the abdominal examination.

2. Discuss inspection of the abdomen, including the findings that you should note.

3. State the rationale for performing auscultation of the abdomen before palpation or percussion.

4. Describe the procedure for auscultation of bowel sounds.

5. Differentiate the following abdominal sounds: normal, hyperactive, and hypoactive bowel sounds; succession splash; bruit.

6. List the four conditions that may alter normal percussion notes heard over the abdomen.

7. Name the organs that are normally palpable in the abdomen.

8. Differentiate between light and deep palpation, and explain the purpose of each.

List 2 abnormalities that may be detected by light palpation and 2 that may be detected by deep palpation.

9. Contrast rigidity with voluntary guarding.

10. Contrast visceral pain and somatic (parietal) pain.

11. Describe rebound tenderness.

12. Distinguish abdominal wall masses from intraabdominal masses.

13. Describe the procedure and rationale for determining costovertebral angle (CVA) tenderness.

Fill in the labels indicated on the following illustrations.

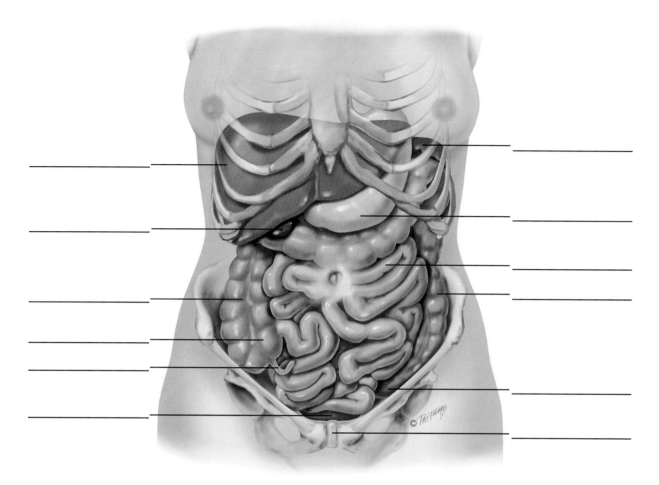

(@ Pat Thomas, 2010.)

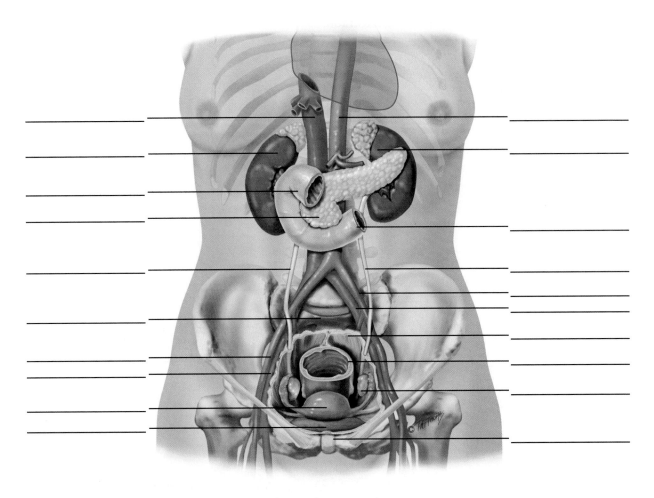

(@ Pat Thomas, 2006.)

CLINICAL JUDGMENT QUESTIONS

This test is for you to check your own mastery of the content. Answers are provided in Appendix A.

1. Select the sequence of techniques used during an examination of the abdomen.

   a. Percussion, inspection, palpation, auscultation.
   b. Inspection, palpation, percussion, auscultation.
   c. Inspection, auscultation, percussion, palpation.
   d. Auscultation, inspection, palpation, percussion.

2. You are auscultating a patient's abdomen and hear a soft, high-pitched, irregular gurgling sound over the right lower quadrant (RLQ). What is the next best action?

   a. Move on to percussion of the abdomen, as this is a normal finding.
   b. Continue auscultating the abdomen in all four quadrants, moving clockwise.
   c. Contact the practitioner or provider, as the patient may have a bowel obstruction.
   d. Continue listening to the RLQ for a full 5 minutes.

3. The absence of bowel sounds is established after listening for:

   a. 1 full minute.
   b. 3 full minutes.
   c. 5 full minutes.
   d. None of the above.

4. You are palpating the left lower quadrant, and the patient grimaces slightly and states the area is tender. What is your next best action?

   a. Contact the practitioner or provider; the patient may have appendicitis.
   b. Document the finding, which is normal, and move on with the exam.
   c. Explain to the patient that this is probably constipation.
   d. Contact the practitioner or provider; the patient may have cholecystitis.

5. You are auscultating the abdomen. Auscultation of the abdomen may reveal bruits in which arteries? **Select all that apply.**

   a. Carotid
   b. Pulmonic
   c. Aortic
   d. Radial
   e. Renal
   f. Iliac
   g. Femoral
   h. Popliteal
   i. Posterior tibial

6. A woman has pink-colored striae on the abdomen. What additional questions should you ask? **Select all that apply.**

   a. Tell me the date of your last menstrual period.
   b. Have you gained any weight recently?
   c. Have you recently been or is there a chance you could be pregnant?
   d. What caused these scars on your abdomen?

7. Auscultating the abdomen is begun in the RLQ because:

   a. Bowel sounds are always normally present here.
   b. Peristalsis through the descending colon is usually active.
   c. This is the location of the pyloric sphincter.
   d. Vascular sounds are best heard in this area.

8. A positive Blumberg sign indicates:

   a. Possible aortic aneurysm.
   b. Presence of renal artery stenosis.
   c. Enlarged, nodular liver.
   d. Peritoneal inflammation.

9. A positive Murphy sign is best described as:

   a. The pain felt when the examiner's hand is rapidly removed from an inflamed appendix.
   b. Pain felt when taking a deep breath when the examiner's fingers are on the approximate location of the inflamed gallbladder.
   c. A sharp pain felt by the patient when one hand of the examiner is used to thump the other at the costovertebral angle.
   d. This is not a reliable examination technique and is no longer recommended.

10. A patient complains of bloating, gas, and diarrhea after drinking milk or eating ice cream, and you suspect lactose intolerance. What is your best statement to the patient?

    a. "You probably should avoid all dairy products. Have you ever tried nondairy milks as an alternative?"
    b. "Consider taking an over-the-counter antacid to help manage these symptoms."
    c. "You many need to reduce the amount of lactose in your diet; I will talk to the physician about testing for lactose intolerance."
    d. "I think you should try low-lactose foods and probiotics for a while and see how your symptoms are affected."

11. A patient complains of a burning upper left abdominal pain that is worse on an empty stomach. What do you most suspect as the cause?

   a. Cholecystitis.
   b. Diverticulitis.
   c. Dysphagia.
   d. Gastric ulcers.

12. You are assessing the area of abdominal tenderness in the RLQ. Which finding supports involuntary guarding?

   a. The muscles contract, the area feels firm, and the patient grimaces during palpation; the muscles relax and the area feels soft when the patient is coaxed to exhale.
   b. The muscles contract, the area feels board-like, and the patient grimaces during palpation; the changes are not affected by exhalation and recur when the patient attempts to sit up.
   c. The pain is caused by your palpation of the opposite side; when you push in on the left lower quadrant, the patient reports pain in the RLQ when the pressure is released.
   d. The patient pushes your hands away when you attempt to palpate the area.

13. You are able to palpate the spleen in the lower quadrants. What is your best next action?

   a. Thoroughly palpate the borders to document a detailed description of its size and location.
   b. Proceed with the examination; this is a normal finding.
   c. Push into the spleen firmly while observing the facial expression for any signs of tenderness.
   d. Stop palpating the spleen and notify the practitioner or physician of possible enlarged spleen.

14. A 13-year-old girl comes to your clinic for a sports physical examination. She is lying flat on the table for assessment. As you inspect her abdomen you note occasional (1 to 2 times per minute) wavy rippling across her skin. What is your next best action?

   a. This is a normal finding for a young teen, proceed with the exam.
   b. Ask the girl about her last bowel movement.
   c. Inquire about the date of her last menstrual period.
   d. Avoid any palpation of the abdomen.

15. A 56-year-old woman arrives at your clinic with the following symptoms for the past 3 months: heartburn 30 minutes after eating, mouth tastes sour, some difficulty swallowing. You suspect the patient has GERD. Inspect the drawing and choose the area you anticipate her pain to occur.

   a. A
   b. B
   c. C
   d. D

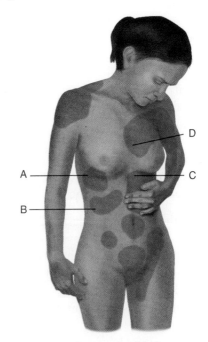

16. Underline the cues from his history and physical exam that suggest ascites as the likely cause of the abdominal distention.

   You are examining a patient with a distended abdomen. The patient has a history of cirrhosis and type 2 diabetes. The shape of the abdomen is protuberant with a single, uniform curve. The patient's flanks are bulging slightly, and the skin appears shiny and taut. The patient has no tenderness to palpation.

CRITICAL THINKING ACTIVITIES

Your patient is complaining of abdominal pain. Study Table 22.3, Common Sites of Referred Abdominal Pain, on p. 566 in Jarvis: *Physical Examination and Health Assessment,* 9th ed. Choose two conditions and list important subjective data to help determine what might be wrong with your patient.

SKILLS LABORATORY AND CLINICAL SETTING

The purpose of the clinical component is to practice the regional examination on a peer in the skills laboratory or on a patient in the clinical setting and to achieve the following.

Clinical Objectives

1. Demonstrate correct knowledge of the abdominal symptoms by obtaining a regional health history from a peer or patient.
2. Demonstrate correct inspection of the abdomen by inspection, auscultation, percussion, and palpation.
3. Demonstrate the correct technique of performing the following additional tests when indicated: fluid wave, rebound tenderness, and inspiratory arrest.
4. Record the history and physical examination findings accurately, reach an assessment of the health state, and develop a plan of care.

Instructions

Gather your equipment. Wash your hands. Assess the patient's comfort before starting. Practice the steps of the examination on a peer or on a patient in the clinical setting, giving appropriate instructions as you proceed. Record your findings using the regional write-up sheets that follow. The front of the page is intended as a worksheet; the back of the page is intended for your narrative summary recording using the SOAP format.

NOTES

REGIONAL WRITE-UP—ABDOMEN

Date _____

Examiner _____

Patient _____ Age _____ Gender _____

Reason for visit _____

I. Health History

	No	Yes, explain
1. Any change in **appetite?** Loss?	_____	_____
2. Any difficulty **swallowing?**	_____	_____
3. Any foods you **cannot tolerate?**	_____	_____
4. Any **abdominal pain?**	_____	_____
5. Any **nausea or vomiting?**	_____	_____
6. How often are **bowel movements?**	_____	_____
7. Any past history of **GI disease?**	_____	_____
8. What **medications** are you taking?	_____	_____

9. Tell me all food you ate in the last **24 hours**, starting with:
   Breakfast   snack   lunch   snack   dinner   snack

II. Physical Examination

A. Inspection

Contour of abdomen _____ General symmetry _____

Skin color and condition _____

Pulsation or movement _____

Umbilicus _____

State of hydration and nutrition _____

Person's facial expression and position in bed _____

B. Auscultation

Bowel sounds. _____

Note any vascular sounds. _____

C. Percussion

Percuss in all four quadrants. _____

If suspect ascites, test for fluid wave and shifting dullness. _____

D. Palpation

Light palpation in all four quadrants

Muscle wall _____ Tenderness _____

Enlarged organs _____

Masses _____

Deep palpation in all four quadrants

Masses _____

Contour of liver _____ Spleen _____

Kidneys _____ Aorta _____

Rebound tenderness _____

CVA tenderness _____

Jarvis, Carolyn and Eckhardt, Ann: PHYSICAL EXAMINATION & HEALTH ASSESSMENT:
Ninth Edition, Study Guide & Laboratory Manual. Copyright © 2024 by Elsevier Inc. All rights reserved.

REGIONAL WRITE-UP—ABDOMEN

Summarize your findings using the SOAP format.

Subjective (reason for seeking care, health history)

Objective (physical examination findings)

Record findings on diagram.

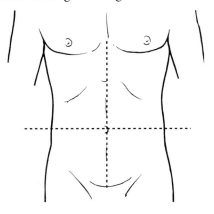

Assessment (assessment of health state or problem, diagnosis)

Plan (diagnostic evaluation, follow-up care, teaching)

Musculoskeletal System

PURPOSE

This chapter presents the structure and function of the various joints in the body, know their normal ranges of motion, position the patient comfortably during the examination, understand the rationale and methods of examination of the musculoskeletal system, assess functional ability, and accurately record the assessment. At the end of this chapter, you should be able to perform a complete assessment of the musculoskeletal system.

READING ASSIGNMENT

Jarvis: Physical Examination and Health Assessment, 9th ed., Chapter 23, pp. 573–628.

Suggested reading:
Niu, S., & Lim, F. (2020). The effects of smoking on bone health and healing. *Am J Nurs, 120*(7), 40–46.
Rogers, J., & Allen, J. (2021). Understanding the most commonly billed diagnoses in primary care: Generalized musculoskeletal pain. *Nurse Pract, 46*(3), 38–45.

GLOSSARY

Study the following terms after completing the reading assignment. You should be able to cover the definition on the right and define the term out loud.

Abduction .... moving a body part away from an axis or the median line

Adduction .... moving a body part toward the center or toward the median line

Ankylosis .... immobility, consolidation, and fixation of a joint because of disease, injury, or surgery; most often due to chronic rheumatoid arthritis

Ataxia .... inability to perform coordinated movements

Bursa .... enclosed sac filled with viscous fluid located in joint areas of potential friction

Circumduction .... moving the arm in a circle around the shoulder

Crepitation .... dry crackling sound or sensation due to grating of the ends of the damaged bone

Dorsal .... directed toward or located on the surface

Dupuytren contracture .... flexion contracture of the fingers due to chronic hyperplasia of the palmar fascia

Eversion .... moving the sole of the foot outward at the ankle

Extension .... straightening a limb at a joint

Flexion .... bending a limb at a joint

Ganglion .... round, cystic, nontender nodule overlying a tendon sheath or joint capsule, usually on the dorsum of wrist

Hallux valgus .... lateral or outward deviation of the great toe

Inversion .... moving the sole of the foot inward at the ankle

Kyphosis .... outward or convex curvature of the thoracic spine; hunchback

Ligament .... fibrous band running directly from one bone to another bone that strengthens the joint

Lordosis .... inward or concave curvature of the lumbar spine

Nucleus pulposus .... center of the intervertebral disc

Olecranon process .... bony projection of the ulna at the elbow

Patella .... kneecap

Plantar .... refers to the surface of the sole of the foot

Pronation .... turning the forearm so that the palm is down

Protraction .... moving a body part forward and parallel to the ground

Range of motion (ROM) .... extent of movement of a joint

Retraction .... moving a body part backward and parallel to the ground

Rheumatoid arthritis .... chronic systemic inflammatory disease of joints and surrounding connective tissue

Sciatica .... nerve pain along the course of the sciatic nerve that travels down from the back or thigh through the leg and into the foot

Scoliosis .... S-shaped curvature of the thoracic spine

Supination .... turning the forearm so that the palm is up

Talipes equinovarus .... (clubfoot) congenital deformity of the foot in which it is plantar flexed and inverted

Tendon .... strong fibrous cord that attaches a skeletal muscle to a bone

STUDY GUIDE

After completing the reading assignment, write or draw the answers in the spaces provided.

1. Differentiate synovial from nonsynovial joints.

2. List four signs that suggest acute inflammation in a joint.

3. Differentiate the following:

   Dislocation _____

   Subluxation _____

   Contracture _____

   Ankylosis _____

4. Differentiate testing of active range of motion versus passive range of motion.

5. Explain the method for measuring leg length.

6. Describe the Ortolani maneuver for checking an infant's hips.

7. When performing a functional assessment for an older adult, state the common adaptations that the older adult makes when attempting these maneuvers:

   Walking _____

   Climbing up stairs _____

   Walking downstairs _____

Picking up an object from the floor _____

Rising up from sitting in chair _____

Rising up from lying in bed _____

8. Draw and describe swan neck deformity and boutonnière deformity in rheumatoid arthritis.

9. Contrast Bouchard nodes with Heberden nodes in osteoarthritis.

Fill in the labels indicated on the following illustrations.

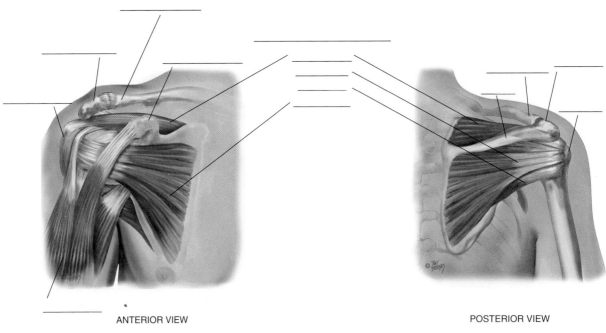

ANTERIOR VIEW   POSTERIOR VIEW

(© Pat Thomas, 2018.)

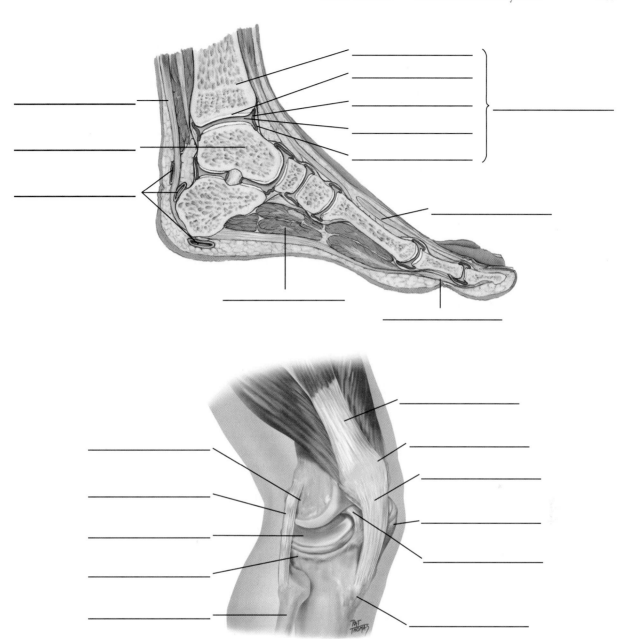

CLINICAL JUDGMENT QUESTIONS

This test is for you to check your own mastery of the content. Answers are provided in Appendix A.

1. You are caring for a 52-year-old woman with a 5-year history of rheumatoid arthritis. As you complete the musculoskeletal assessment, you identify the following assessment and history findings that are expected deviations with rheumatoid arthritis. **Select all that apply.**

   a. Symmetric joint involvement.
   b. Unilateral joint involvement.
   c. Lymphadenopathy.
   d. Increased appetite.
   e. Weight gain.
   f. Fatigue.
   g. Hard, bony protuberances.
   h. Ulnar drift.
   i. Bone spur.
   j. Anorexia.

2. Identify the appropriate order for the development of the normal spinal curvature from infancy to adulthood. Not all choices will be used.

   1. Posterior curve in lumbar region.
   2. C shaped curvature of spine.
   3. Lateral s-shaped curve develops.
   4. Anterior curve in lumbar region.
   5. Anterior curve in cervical neck region.
   6. Spinal curvature disappears.

3. You are providing osteoporosis education to a 67-year-old female who is at your clinic for her annual check-up. She has no chronic medical conditions, and her last bone mineral density was normal. The following is the most appropriate teaching for this patient.

   a. It is recommended that you have a DEXA scan to check for osteoporosis every 2 to 5 years. You'll want to continue to eat a healthy diet, exercise at least twice a week, and drink no more than one standard drink per day.

   b. It is recommended that you have a DEXA scan at least every 5 years. You should continue to eat the rainbow and maintain a healthy weight. Walking is the most appropriate exercise, and weightlifting should be avoided.
   c. Your last BMD was normal. Continue to maintain a healthy weight and avoid all alcohol. I'd like to check your vitamin D levels to ensure you are getting enough in your diet. Given your age, you should consume at least 1000 mg of calcium each day.
   d. Your last BMD was normal. It's important that you continue to eat a healthy diet and maintain a healthy weight. You should exercise at least five times each week and consider a combination of cardiovascular, balance, and strength training.

4. You are assessing a patient with a suspected rotator cuff tear. What assessment findings do you expect if the rotator cuff is torn? **Select all that apply.**

   a. Upright positioning.
   b. Hunched position.
   c. Limited adduction.
   d. Atrophy of shoulder girdle.
   e. Fluctuant to palpation.
   f. Limited abduction.
   g. Positive arm drop test.

For questions 5–18, match Column B to Column A.

Column A: Movement

5. _____ Flexion
6. _____ Extension
7. _____ Abduction
8. _____ Adduction
9. _____ Pronation
10. _____ Supination
11. _____ Circumduction
12. _____ Inversion
13. _____ Eversion
14. _____ Rotation
15. _____ Protraction
16. _____ Retraction
17. _____ Elevation
18. _____ Depression

Column B: Description

a. Turning the forearm so that the palm is up.
b. Bending a limb at a joint.
c. Lowering a body part.
d. Turning the forearm so that the palm is down.
e. Straightening a limb at a joint.
f. Raising a body part.
g. Moving a limb away from the midline of the body.
h. Moving a body part backward and parallel to the ground.
i. Moving a limb toward the midline of the body.
j. Moving the arm in a circle around the shoulder.
k. Moving the sole of the foot outward at the ankle.
l. Moving a body part forward and parallel to the ground.
m. Moving the sole of the foot inward at the ankle.
n. Moving the head around a central axis.

19. An 81-year-old woman has come for a health examination. As you complete the assessment, you notice several changes in the musculoskeletal system. Mark each change as expected or not expected with normal healthy aging.

Change in the Musculoskeletal System	Expected	Not expected
Boggy metacarpophalangeal joints		
Kyphosis		
Lordosis		
Flexion in hips		
Flexion in knees		
Osteoarthritis		

20. Identify which assessment findings are expected in each group. Some findings may be expected in multiple groups.

Assessment Finding	Infant	Toddler	Preschool/school age	Pregnant woman
Lordosis				
Varus position of feet/legs (flexible)				
Valgus position of feet/legs (flexible)				
Cervical flexion				

21. Underline the abnormal or concerning findings in the patient scenario below.

The client comes to the clinic with reports of bilateral swelling and pain in the DIP joints in her fingers. She also complains of fatigue and weight loss for the past year. VS: HR 86 bpm, regular, RR 18 bpm, unlabored, Temperature 100.5°F, BP 110/78. Upon physical examination, the DIP joints are tender and warm with a limited range of motion bilaterally. Full ROM in all other joints. Muscle strength—able to maintain flexion against resistance. Atrophy is noted in the interosseous muscles of the hands bilaterally.

22. Given the information in question 21, select the correct term to fill in each blank.

The client most likely has _____ which is a/an _____ typically involving _____ joints in the _____ and _____.

a. Rheumatoid arthritis.
b. Gouty arthritis.
c. knees.
d. hands.
e. inflammatory condition.
f. neck.
g. Osteoarthritis.
h. symmetric.
i. asymmetric.
j. noninflammatory condition.
k. feet.

23. Identify the correct order of steps in assessing a person for scoliosis. Not all steps will be used. Please number the steps correctly in the space provided.

Potential Steps	Appropriate steps
1. Position self in front of client so entire torso is visible.	
2. Note level of shoulders, scapulae, and iliac crests.	
3. Position self behind client so full spine is visible.	
4. Note level of shoulders, ribs, and superior iliac spine.	
5. Ask client to bend at the waist and reach for toes.	
6. Note the level of superior iliac spine while the patient is bent forward.	
7. Note level of shoulders, ribs, and iliac crests while they are bent forward.	

CRITICAL THINKING ACTIVITIES

The FRAX assessment tool is a computerized fracture risk algorithm developed by the World Health Organization and is available at *www.shef.ac.uk/FRAX*. To increase your experience and comfort with this tool, enter the website on your computer, click the calculation tool tab at the top of the page, and pick the correct regional version (e.g., U.S. Caucasian version).

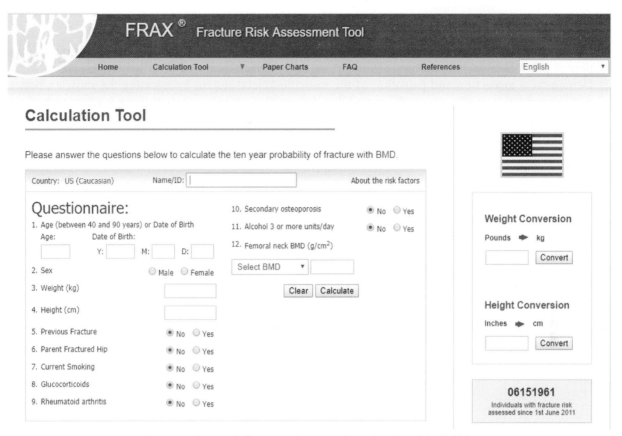

(© Centre for Metabolic Bone Diseases at the University of Sheffield.)

Enter the following data to determine fracture risk: C.M. is an 81-year-old white female, height: 5 feet 7 inches, weight: 124 lb. (Note: The tool includes a feature that converts height and weight to kg and cm; it will also calculate body mass index, shown in the red results box.) C.M. has no previous fractures, no smoking or glucocorticoid use, and alcohol use of 1 to 2 units per day. She has osteoporosis with a femoral neck T-score of –2.0. (Enter in field for question 12.)

The FRAX outcome gives you a 10-year absolute risk by percentages of hip fracture and major osteoporotic fracture. Write a teaching plan for C.M., including risk management and follow-up care. Present the plan to a peer, using simple, understandable layperson terms. If you have access to all the necessary patient data, complete a second FRAX assessment and conduct patient teaching for the client.

SKILLS LABORATORY AND CLINICAL SETTING

The purpose of the clinical component is to practice the regional musculoskeletal examination on a peer in the skills laboratory or on a patient in the clinical setting to achieve the following.

Clinical Objectives

1. Demonstrate knowledge of the musculoskeletal system by obtaining a regional health history from a peer or patient.
2. Demonstrate inspection and palpation of the musculoskeletal system by assessing the muscles, bones, and joints for size, symmetry, swelling, nodules, deformities, atrophy, and active range of motion.
3. Assess the person's ability to carry out functional activities of daily living.
4. Record the history and physical examination findings accurately, reach an assessment about the health state, and develop a plan of care.

Instructions

Gather your equipment. Wash your hands. Practice the steps of the examination on a peer or on a patient in the clinical setting, giving appropriate instructions as you proceed and maintaining the safety of the person during movement. Record your findings using the regional write-up sheet that follows. The first section is intended as a worksheet; the last page is intended for your narrative summary recording using the SOAP format.

REGIONAL WRITE-UP—MUSCULOSKELETAL SYSTEM

Date _____

Examiner _____

Patient _____ Age _____ Gender _____

Reason for visit _____

I. Health History

	No	Yes, explain
1. Any **pain** in the joints?	_____	_____
2. Any **stiffness** in the joints?	_____	_____
3. Any **swelling, heat, redness** in joints?	_____	_____
4. Any **limitation of movement**?	_____	_____
5. Any **muscle pain** or cramping?	_____	_____
6. Any **deformity** of bone or joint?	_____	_____
7. Any **accidents or trauma** to bones or joints?	_____	_____
8. Ever had **back pain**?	_____	_____
9. Any problems with **ADL:**	_____	_____
Bathing, toileting, dressing?	_____	_____
Grooming, eating, mobility?	_____	_____
Communicating?	_____	_____

II. Physical Examination
A. Cervical spine
1. Inspect size, contour _____ Deformity _____
2. Palpate for temperature _____ Pain _____
   Swelling or mass _____
3. Active range of motion
   Flexion _____ Extension _____
   Lateral bending right _____ Left _____
   Right rotation _____ Left _____

B. Shoulders
1. Inspect size, contour _____ Color, swelling _____
   Mass or deformity _____
2. Palpate for temperature _____ Pain _____
   Swelling or mass _____
3. Active range of motion
   Flexion _____ Extension _____
   Abduction _____ Adduction _____
   Internal rotation _____ External rotation _____

C. Elbows
1. Inspect for size, contour _____ Color, swelling _____
   Mass or deformity _____
2. Palpate for temperature _____ Pain _____
   Swelling or mass _____

3. Active range of motion
   Flexion _____ Extension _____
   Pronation _____ Supination _____

D. **Wrists and hands**
   1. Inspect for size, contour _____ Color, swelling _____
      Mass or deformity _____
   2. Palpate for temperature _____ Pain _____
      Swelling or mass _____
   3. Active range of motion
      Wrist extension _____ Flexion _____
      Finger extension _____ Flexion _____
      Ulnar deviation _____ Radial deviation _____
      Fingers spread _____ Make fist _____
      Touch thumb to each finger _____

E. **Hips**
   1. Inspect for size, contour _____ Color, swelling _____
      Mass or deformity _____
   2. Palpate for temperature _____ Pain _____
      Swelling or mass _____
   3. Active range of motion
      Extension _____ Flexion _____
      External rotation _____ Internal rotation _____
      Abduction _____ Adduction _____

F. **Knees**
   1. Inspect size, contour _____ Color, swelling _____
      Mass or deformity _____
   2. Palpate for temperature _____ Pain _____
      Swelling or mass _____
   3. Active range of motion
      Flexion _____ Extension _____
      Walk _____ Shallow knee bend _____

G. **Ankles and feet**
   1. Inspect for size, contour _____ Color, swelling _____
      Mass or deformity _____
   2. Palpate for temperature _____ Pain _____
      Swelling or mass _____
   3. Active range of motion
      Dorsiflexion _____ Plantar flexion _____
      Inversion _____ Eversion _____

H. **Spine**
1. Inspect for straight spinous processes. _____
   Equal horizontal positions for shoulders, scapulae, iliac crests, and gluteal folds _____
   Equal spaces between arms and lateral thorax _____
   Knees and feet align with trunk, point forward _____
   From side, note curvature: cervical, thoracic, lumbar _____
2. Palpate spinous processes.
3. Active range of motion
   Flexion _____ Extension _____
   Lateral bending right _____ Left _____
   Rotation right _____ Left _____

I. **Functional assessment (if indicated)**
Walk (with shoes on).
Climb up stairs.
Walk downstairs.
Pick up object from floor.
Rise up from sitting in chair.
Rise up from lying in bed.

REGIONAL WRITE-UP—MUSCULOSKELETAL SYSTEM

Subjective (reason for seeking care, health history)

Objective (physical examination findings)

Assessment (assessment of health state or problem, diagnosis)

Plan (diagnostic evaluation, follow-up care, patient teaching)

CHAPTER 24

Neurologic System

PURPOSE

This chapter presents the components of the neurologic system (the cranial nerves, cerebellar system, motor system, sensory system, and reflexes); the rationale and methods of examination of the neurologic system; and the accurate recording of the assessment. Together with the mental status assessment presented in Chapter 5, you should be able to perform a complete assessment of the neurologic system at the end of this chapter.

READING ASSIGNMENT

Jarvis: *Physical Examination and Health Assessment*, 9th ed., Chapter 24, pp. 629–684.

Suggested reading:
Washington, H. H., Glaser, K. R., & Ifejika, N. L. (2021). Acute Ischemic Strike: A review of updated guidelines, nursing assessment, and evidence-based treatment. *Am J Nurs, 121*(9), 26–32.

GLOSSARY

Study the following terms after completing the reading assignment. You should be able to cover the definition on the right and define the term out loud.

Agnosia .... loss of ability to recognize importance of sensory impressions

Agraphia .... loss of ability to express thoughts in writing

Amnesia .... loss of memory

Analgesia .... loss of pain sensation

Aphasia .... loss of power of expression by speech, writing, or signs; or loss of comprehension of spoken or written language

Apraxia .... loss of ability to perform purposeful movements in the absence of sensory or motor damage (e.g., inability to use objects correctly)

Ataxia .... inability to perform coordinated movements

Athetosis .... bizarre, slow, twisting, writhing movement resembling a snake or worm

Chorea .... sudden, rapid, jerky, purposeless movement involving limbs, trunk, or face

Clonus .... rapidly alternating involuntary contraction and relaxation of a muscle in response to sudden stretch

Coma .... state of profound unconsciousness from which a person cannot be aroused

Concussion .... collision or trauma causes violent shaking of brain, yielding behavioral changes but no changes on radiologic imaging

Decerebrate rigidity .... arms stiffly extended, adducted, internally rotated; legs stiffly extended, plantar-flexed

Decorticate rigidity .... arms adducted and flexed, wrists and fingers flexed; legs extended, internally rotated, plantar-flexed

Dysarthria .... imperfect articulation of speech due to problems of muscular control resulting from central or peripheral nervous system damage

Dysphasia .... impairment in speech consisting of lack of coordination and inability to arrange words in their proper order

Extinction .... disappearance of conditioned response

Fasciculation .... rapid continuous twitching of resting muscle without movement of limb

Flaccidity .... loss of muscle tone, limp

Graphesthesia .... ability to "read" a number by having it traced on the skin

Hemiplegia .... loss of motor power (paralysis) on one side of the body, usually caused by a stroke; paralysis occurs on side opposite the lesion

Lower motor neuron .... motor neuron in the peripheral nervous system with its nerve fiber extending out to the muscle and only its cell body in the central nervous system

Myoclonus .... rapid sudden jerk of a muscle

Nuchal rigidity .... stiffness in cervical neck area

Nystagmus .... back-and-forth oscillation of the eyes

Opisthotonos .... prolonged arching of back, with head and heels bent backward, and meningeal irritation

Paralysis .... decreased or loss of motor function due to problem with motor nerve or muscle fibers

Paraplegia .... impairment or loss of motor and/or sensory function in the lower half of the body

Paresthesia .... abnormal sensation (e.g., burning, numbness, tingling, prickling, crawling skin sensation)

Point localization .... ability of the person to discriminate exactly where on the body the skin has been touched

Proprioception .... sensory information concerning body movements and position of the body in space

Spasticity .... continuous resistance to stretching by a muscle due to abnormally increased tension with increased deep tendon reflexes

Stereognosis .... ability to recognize objects by feeling their form, size, and weight while the eyes are closed

Tic .... repetitive twitching of a muscle group at inappropriate times (e.g., wink, grimace)

Tremor .... involuntary contraction of opposing muscle groups resulting in rhythmic movement of one or more joints

Two-point discrimination .... ability to distinguish the separation of two simultaneous pinpricks on the skin

Upper motor neuron .... nerve located entirely within the central nervous system

STUDY GUIDE

After completing the reading assignment and the media assignment, write or draw the answers in the spaces provided.

1. List the major function(s) of the following components of the central nervous system:

   Cerebral cortex—frontal lobe _____

   Cerebral cortex—parietal lobe _____

   Cerebral cortex—temporal lobe _____

   Cerebral cortex—Wernicke area _____

   Cerebral cortex—Broca area _____

   Basal ganglia _____

   _____

   Thalamus _____

   Hypothalamus _____

   _____

   Cerebellum _____

   Midbrain _____

   Pons _____

   Medulla _____

   Spinal cord _____

2. List the primary sensations mediated by the 2 major sensory pathways of the CNS.

3. Describe 3 major motor pathways in the CNS, including the type of movements mediated by each.

4. Differentiate an upper motor neuron from a lower motor neuron.

5. List the 5 components of a deep tendon reflex arc.

6. List the major symptom areas to assess when collecting a health history for the neurologic system.

7. List and describe 3 tests of cerebellar function.

8. Describe the method of testing the sensory system for pain, temperature, touch, vibration, and position.

9. Define the 4-point grading scale for deep tendon reflexes.

10. Which vertebral level is assessed when eliciting each of these reflexes?

   Biceps reflex _____   Quadriceps reflex _____

   Triceps reflex _____   Achilles reflex _____

   Brachioradialis reflex _____

11. List the components of the neurologic recheck examination that are performed routinely on hospital-ized persons being monitored for neurologic deficit.

12. List the 3 areas of assessment on the Glasgow Coma Scale.

Fill in the labels indicated on the following illustrations.

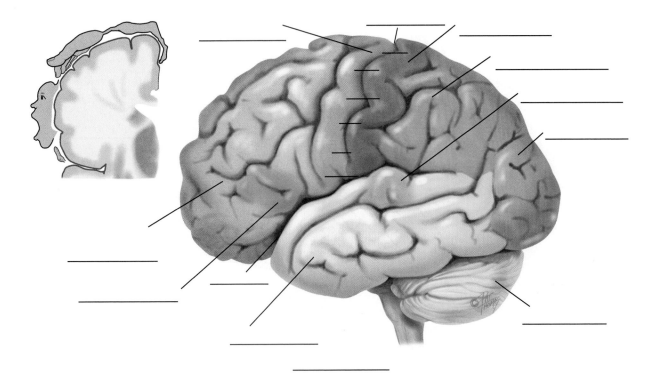

(© Pat Thomas, 2006.)

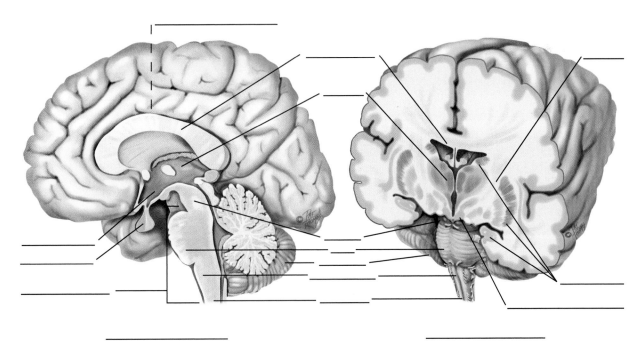

(© Pat Thomas, 2006.)

Fill in the Roman numeral and name of each cranial nerve, and then write S (sensory), M (motor), or MX (mixed).

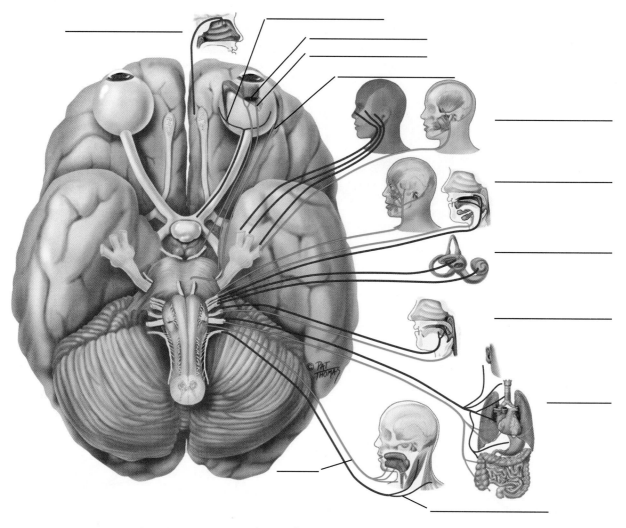

(© Pat Thomas, 2006.)

CLINICAL JUDGMENT QUESTIONS

This test is for you to check your own mastery of the content. The answers are provided in Appendix A.

1. During the assessment of a 4-week-old infant, you note the response in this photo as you move your finger up lateral side of foot. What is your next action?

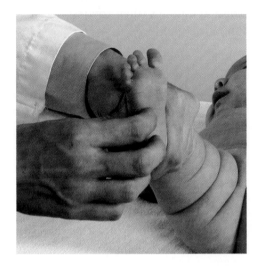

   a. This response should have disappeared by this age; alert another examiner.
   b. Move on with the examination; this is an expected response.
   c. Ask the parent if they were informed of any concerns at the birth of the baby.
   d. Test for nuchal rigidity to assess for suspected infection of meninges.
   e. Measure pulse oximetry to determine level of oxygen to tissues.

2. You are supervising a student caring for a 46-year-old man admitted to hospital with hypothermia following a boating accident. He was in the water 6 hours before rescue, wearing a floating device keeping his head out of water. You expect the student to know control of body temperature is located in:

   a. Wernicke's area
   b. The thalamus.
   c. The cerebellum.
   d. The hypothalamus.

3. During the neurologic exam, you place a key in the person's hand with their eyes closed and ask them to identify the object. This measures the ability of:

   a. Stereognosis.
   b. Graphesthesia
   c. Two-point discrimination
   d. Kinesthesia.

4. During an outpatient examination, you ask the person to stand with feet together, arms at sides, eyes closed, and hold position about 20 seconds. This text demonstrates intactness of:

   a. Cerebral cortex.
   b. Cerebral medulla
   c. Motor system
   d. Cerebellum.

5. Mr. G. is a 54-year-old man with parkinsonism. Which description of his speech would contribute to the expected findings?

   a. A garbled manner
   b. Loud, urgent
   c. Slow, monotonous
   d. Word confusion

6. Which of the following are correct examination techniques when testing the biceps reflex? **Select all that apply.**

   a. Locate and place your thumb on the person's biceps tendon.
   b. Strike the tendon just above the outside of the elbow.
   c. Expect the forearm to extend slightly in response to strike of reflex hammer.
   d. With the reflex hammer, strike over the target in person's antecubital fossa.
   e. Tell the person to let the arm "just go dead" as you suspend it by holding the upper arm.

7. During the examination of a 91-year-old woman, you note that the hands have a tremor as she reaches for her purse, and her head has a small yes-no nodding. There is no associated rigidity with movement. Which is your most accurate assessment?

   a. These are expected findings due to aging.
   b. These findings are associated with parkinsonism
   c. These findings are associated to Alzheimer disease.
   d. This woman should be referred to a neurologic specialist.

8. You are testing the DTRs of a 30-year-old woman. When striking the quadriceps reflex, you are unable to elicit a response. What is your next most appropriate action?

   a. Ask the woman to lock her fingers and "pull."
   b. Complete the exam, then test these reflexes again.
   c. Refer the woman to a specialist for further testing.
   d. Document these reflexes as "0" on a scale of 0 to 4+.

9. You test superficial reflexes on a 36-year-old woman. When you stroke up the lateral side of the sole and across the ball of the foot, you notice plantar flexion of the toes. How would you document this finding?

   a. Positive Babinski sign.
   b. Plantar reflex abnormal
   c. Plantar reflex present
   d. Plantar reflex absent

10. A 21-year-old woman has a head injury secondary to a blow on the head and is unconscious. During your assessment, what are the expected findings when you test her deep tendon reflexes?

    a. Reflexes will be normal.
    b. You will be unable to elicit any deep tendon reflexes.
    c. All deep tendon reflexes are diminished by present.
    d Some deep tendon reflexes are present depending on area of injury.

11. A fully alert normal person has a Glasgow Coma Scale of 15. Which assessments listed below contribute to the total score of the GCS? Check all that apply.

    a. Pupils equal and react to light and accommodation.
    b. Person's eyes open spontaneously during the assessment.
    c. Person wiggles the fingers when asked to do so.
    d. Person's blood pressure and pulse rate are within normal limits.
    e. Person is oriented to self, place, and time.

For questions 12–23, match Column B to Column A.

Column A: Cranial Nerve

12. _____ Olfactory
13. _____ Optic
14. _____ Oculomotor
15. _____ Trochlear
16. _____ Trigeminal
17. _____ Abducens
18. _____ Facial
19. _____ Acoustic
20. _____ Glossopharyngeal
21. _____ Vagus
22. _____ Spinal
23. _____ Hypoglossal

Column B: Function

a. Movement of the tongue
b. Vision
c. Lateral movement of the eyes
d. Hearing and equilibrium
e. Talking, swallowing, and sensory information from pharynx and carotid sinus
f. Smell
g. Extraocular movement, pupil constriction, down and inward movement of the eye
h. Mastication and sensation of face, scalp, cornea
i. Phonation, swallowing, tasting on the posterior third of tongue
j. Movement of trapezius and sternomastoid muscles
k. Down and inward movement of the eye
l. Tasting on the anterior two thirds of tongue, closing eyes

CRITICAL THINKING ACTIVITIES

Study the journal article on "Acute Ischemic Stroke" presented at the beginning of this chapter. Because strokes are so common in the United States, and because strokes are potentially so devastating, the improvement of lifestyle factors leading to stroke is crucial.

1. To understand the impact of lifestyle factors, take the following assessment tool for yourself:
   https://ninds.nih.gov/health-information/public-education/brain-basics/brain-basics-preventing-stroke?
   Discuss ways you can alter your lifestyle to decrease the risk of a future stroke when you are older.

2. Then, use the assessment tool again, considering an older person in your family or among your acquaintances. How do the summation scores differ from your personal assessment to this older person's assessment?

3. Finally, take on the role of the health care provider and formulate a teaching plan that addresses how the older person can reduce their risk of stroke.

SKILLS LABORATORY/CLINICAL SETTING

The purpose of the clinical component is to practice the neurologic regional examination on a peer in the skills laboratory or a patient in the clinical setting and to achieve the following.

Clinical Objectives

1. Demonstrate knowledge of the neurologic symptoms by obtaining a regional health history from a peer or patient.
2. Demonstrate examination of the neurologic system by assessing the cranial nerves, cerebellar function, sensory system, motor system, and deep tendon reflexes.
3. Record the history and physical examination findings accurately, reach an assessment of the health state, and develop a plan of care.

Instructions

Gather all equipment for a complete neurologic examination. Wash your hands. Practice the steps of the examination on a peer or on a patient in the clinical setting, giving appropriate instructions as you proceed. Record your findings using the regional write-up sheet that follows. The first section is intended as a worksheet; the last page is intended for your narrative summary recording using the SOAP format.

REGIONAL WRITE-UP—NEUROLOGIC SYSTEM

Date _____

Examiner _____

Patient _____ Age _____ Gender _____

Reason for visit _____

I. Health History

	No	Yes, explain
1. Any unusually frequent or unusually severe **headaches**?		
2. Ever had any **head injury**?		
3. Ever feel **dizziness**?		
4. Ever had any **seizures**?		
5. Any **tremors** in hands or face?		
6. Any **weakness** in any body part?		
7. Any problem with **coordination**?		
8. Any **numbness or tingling**?		
9. Any problem **swallowing**?		
10. Any problem **speaking**?		
11. **Past history** of stroke, spinal cord injury, meningitis, congenital defect, or alcoholism?		
12. Any environmental or occupational **hazards** (e.g., insecticides)?		

II. Physical Examination
A. Cranial nerves

II _____

III, IV, VI _____

V _____

VII _____

VIII _____

IX, X _____

XI _____

XII _____

B. **Motor system**
   1. Muscles
      Size, strength, tone _____
      Involuntary movements _____
   2. Cerebellar function
      Rapid alternative movements _____
      Finger-Nose-Finger test _____
      Heel to shin test _____
      Gait _____
      Romberg test _____

C. **Sensory system**
   1. Anterolateral tract
      Sharp or dull _____
      Light touch _____
   2. Posterior column tract
      Vibration _____
      Position (kinesthesia) _____
      Tactile discrimination
         Stereognosis _____
         Graphesthesia _____

D. **Reflexes**

	Bi	Tri	BR	P	A	PL (↑/↓)	Abd	Cre	Bab
R									
L									

0 = absent, 1+ = hypoactive, 2+ = normal, 3+ = hyperactive, 4+ = hyperactive with clonus, ↑ = dorsiflexion, ↓ = plantar flexion.

REGIONAL WRITE-UP—NEUROLOGIC SYSTEM

Summarize your findings using the SOAP format.

Subjective (reason for seeking care, health history)

Objective (physical examination findings)

Record reflexes on diagram below.

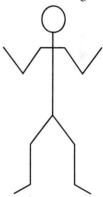

Assessment (assessment of health state or problem, diagnosis)

Plan (diagnostic evaluation, follow-up care, patient teaching)

NOTES

CHAPTER
25
Male Genitourinary System

PURPOSE

This chapter presents the structure and function of the male genitalia: the rationale and methods of inspection and palpation of these structures; and how to record the assessment accurately.

READING ASSIGNMENT

Jarvis: *Physical Examination and Health Assessment,* 9th ed., Chapter 25, pp. 685–714.

Suggested reading:
Bach, S., & Heavey, E. (2021). Resurgence of syphilis in the US. *Nurse Pract,* 46(10), 28–36.

GLOSSARY

Study the following terms after completing the reading assignment. You should be able to cover the definition on the right and define the term out loud.

Chancre .... red, round, superficial ulcer with a yellowish serous discharge that is a sign of syphilis

Condylomata acuminata .... soft, pointed, fleshy papules that occur on the genitalia and are caused by the human papillomavirus (HPV)

Cryptorchidism .... undescended testes

Cystitis .... inflammation of the urinary bladder

Epididymis .... structures composed of coiled ducts located over the superior and posterior surface of the testes, which store sperm

Epispadias .... congenital defect in which the urethra opens on the dorsal (upper) side of penis instead of at the tip

Hernia .... weak spot in the abdominal muscle wall (usually in the area of inguinal canal or femoral canal) through which a loop of bowel may protrude

Herpes genitalis .... a sexually transmitted infection characterized by clusters of small painful vesicles, caused by a virus

Heterosexism .... an unscientific expectation that heterosexuality is the expected norm and that individuals who are lesbian, gay, bisexual, or transgender are somehow abnormal

Homophobia .... an irrational fear of members of sexual and gender minority groups, resulting in negative feelings toward them

Hydrocele .... cystic fluid in tunica vaginalis surrounding the testis

Hypospadias .... congenital defect in which urethra opens on the ventral (under) side of penis rather than at the tip

MSM .... men having sex with men

Orchitis .... acute inflammation of testis, usually associated with mumps

Paraphimosis .... foreskin retracted and fixed behind the glans penis

Peyronie disease .... nontender hard plaques on the surface of penis, associated with painful bending of penis during erection

Phimosis .... foreskin is advanced and tightly fixed over the glans penis

Prepuce .... foreskin; the hood or flap of skin over the glans penis that often is surgically removed after birth by circumcision

Priapism .... prolonged, painful erection of penis without sexual desire

Spermatic cord .... collection of vas deferens, blood vessels, lymphatics, and nerves that ascends along the testis and through the inguinal canal into the abdomen

Spermatocele .... retention cyst in epididymis filled with milky fluid that contains sperm

Torsion .... sudden twisting of spermatic cord; a surgical emergency

Varicocele .... dilated tortuous varicose veins in the spermatic cord

Vas deferens .... duct carrying sperm from the epididymis through the abdomen and then into the urethra

STUDY GUIDE

After completing the reading assignment and the media assignment, you should be able to answer the following questions in the spaces provided.

1. Identify the structures that provide transport of sperm.

2. Describe the significance of the inguinal canal and the femoral canal.

3. List the pros and cons of circumcision of the male newborn.

4. Discuss ways of creating an environment that will provide psychological comfort for the patient and the examiner during examination of the male genitalia.

5. List teaching points to include with the teaching of testicular self-examination.

6. List laboratory tests to assess urinary function.

7. Discuss the rationale for making certain that the testes have descended in the male infant.

8. Contrast phimosis with paraphimosis and hypospadias with epispadias.

9. Describe the following lesions of the penis and genital area:

Tinea cruris

Herpes simplex type 2

Syphilitic chancre

Penile warts (HPV, condylomata acuminata)

10. Contrast the physical appearance and clinical significance of these scrotal lumps:

Epididymitis

Varicocele

Spermatocele

Testicular tumor

Hydrocele

11. Contrast the anatomic course and clinical significance of these hernias:

Indirect inguinal

Direct inguinal

Femoral

Fill in the labels indicated on the following illustrations.

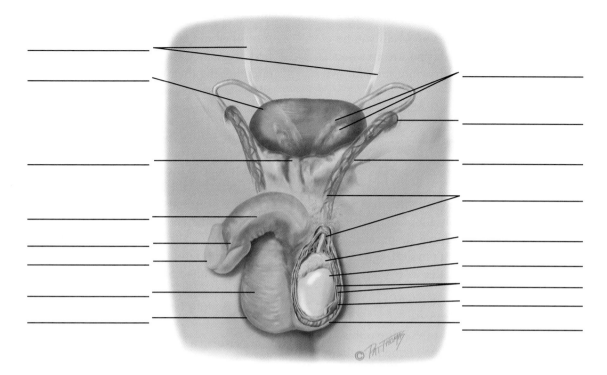

(© Pat Thomas, 2010.)

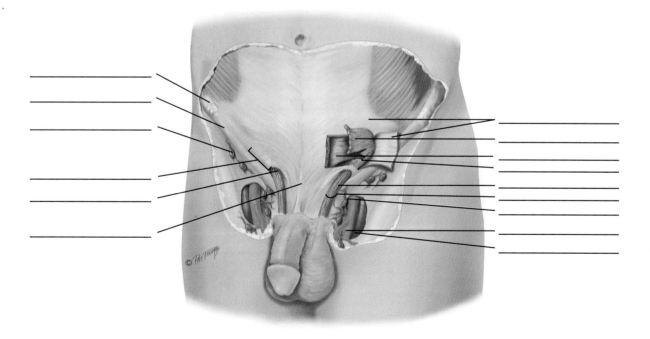

(© Pat Thomas, 2010.)

CLINICAL JUDGMENT QUESTIONS

This test is for you to check your own mastery of the content. Answers are provided in Appendix A.

1. During the health history, a man tells you he has trouble in starting his urine stream when he arrives at the toilet. This symptom is known as:

   a. Urgency.
   b. Dribbling.
   c. Frequency.
   d. Hesitancy.

2. A parent of three biologic daughters has a 10-year-old boy the family adopted at age 2 years. The parent is learning about raising boys and asks you the first physical sign of puberty in the male genitalia:

   a. Testes and scrotum begin to enlarge.
   b. Penis enlarges and lengthens.
   c. Dark coarse hair grows over entire pubis.
   d. Scrotal skin assumes same pigment as the abdomen and thighs.

3. During the health history, a 64-year-old man tells you he "never has sex anymore." Check the following appropriate follow-up questions you could use that are associated with withdrawal from sex. **Select all that apply.**

   a. "Have you been told about any side effects of your medications?"
   b. "Let's ask your provider for a blood test to detect decreased sperm production."
   c. "Would you say you have had feelings of depression in the last few months?"
   d. "How many alcohol drinks do you have each day?"
   e. "This is an expected outcome in aging men."
   f. "Have you experienced the loss of your spouse or your partner?"

4. A mother and father in the 7th month of their first pregnancy ask you about the benefits of circumcising their expected baby boy. Check all the facts you can share to help them with their decision.

   a. In the United States, circumcising baby boys is a proven way to prevent HIV transmission later in life.
   b. Removal of the foreskin decreases the incidence of urinary tract infections in very young infants.
   c. Most surgical risks of infant circumcision are minor and treatable.
   d. In the United States, circumcision protects against acquiring human papillomavirus and syphilis later in life.

5. You perform a genital examination on a 48-year-old man and note deeply pigmented wrinkled scrotal skin, with multiple, yellowish, 1-cm, firm, nontender nodules. What would be your next most appropriate action?

   a. Ask about any family history of testicular cancer in the father or brothers.
   b. Consider these sebaceous follicles an expected finding and proceed with the examination.
   c. Assess the scrotum using transillumination.
   d. Obtain a detailed history focusing on any scrotal abnormalities the man has noticed.

6. You perform a genital examination on a 25-year-old man and palpate testes that feel ovoid and movable yet somewhat sensitive to compression. What is your next most appropriate action?

   a. Ask another examiner to repeat the examination.
   b. Search for subcutaneous plaques that may be painful.

c. Ask the man if he has noticed anything unusual in his own exams.

d. Consider this an expected finding and proceed with the examination.

7. You are an advanced provider about to inspect and palpate a 55-year-old man for a suspected inguinal hernia. What is your best instruction to prepare this man?

   a. "Hold your breath and cough when I ask you to."

   b. "I will ask you to bear down when my gloved finger is in the inguinal canal."

   c. "I will ask you to turn you head and cough when my gloved finger is in the inguinal canal."

   d. "Please assume a lying-down position on the exam table for the hernia check."

8. You are about to examine the genitalia of a 93-year-old man who has an adhesion of the prepuce of the head of the penis, making the foreskin impossible to retract. You recognize this as:

   a. Paraphimosis.

   b. Phimosis.

   c. Smegma.

   d. Dyschezia.

9. During assessment of a newborn baby boy, you note the urethral meatus is positioned ventrally, on the underside of the penis. Your next best action is to: **Select all that apply.**

   a. Notice if the penis is straight or curved.

   b. Note that this is consistent with uncircumcised baby boys and proceed with the exam.

   c. Assure the parents that they can proceed with the planned circumcision at this time.

   d. Ask a physician or AP provider to repeat the examination.

10. A 1-month-old, uncircumcised boy comes to your clinic for a well-baby check-up. How would you proceed with the genital exam?

   a. Elicit the cremasteric reflex.

   b. Assess the glans for redness or lesions.

   c. Avoid retracting the foreskin.

   d. Note any dirt or smegma that has collected under the foreskin.

11. You are teaching a 19-year-old how to perform a testicular self-examination. Which of the following statements is your most appropriate?

   a. "A good time to examine your testicles is just before you take a shower."

   b. "If you notice an enlarged testicle or a firm lump, call your health care provider."

   c. "The testicle is egg shaped, feels soft, and has a spongy consistency."

   d. "Perform testicular self-exam at least once a week."

12. A 62-year-old man states his doctor told him he has an "inguinal hernia." He asks you to explain what a hernia is. Your best response is:

   a. Tell him not to worry and that most men his age develop hernias.

   b. Explain that a hernia is often the result of growth abnormalities that developed before he was born.

   c. Refer him to his physician for additional information because they made the initial diagnosis.

   d. Explain that a hernia is a loop of bowel protruding through a weak spot in the belly muscles.

13. You are caring for a person with jaundice from hepatitis. You expect the person's urine to be:

   a. Orange in color.

   b. Red from blood in urine.

   c. Normal, clear yellow.

   d. Dark gray in color.

CRITICAL THINKING ACTIVITIES

It may surprise you to learn that there is an alarming and continued increase in the incidence of syphilis in the United States. Read the article about the syphilis epidemic listed in the Suggested Readings. Consider the risk factors listed in the article concerning groups at higher risk of acquiring syphilis, as well as the assessment factors. Place yourself in the provider role to assess and teach a person with syphilis. Prepare a script for this teaching. Use the content in this article. Make your script nonjudgmental and free of medical jargon. Practice your delivery on a peer in your lab setting. The role of "patient" should be: (1) young sexually active woman having oral or vaginal sex; (2) man having oral, anal, or insertive sex; (3) person using illicit drugs, particularly methamphetamine; (4) pregnant woman.

SKILLS LABORATORY AND CLINICAL SETTING

Because of the need to maintain personal privacy, it is likely that you will not practice the male genitalia examination on a classmate. Your practice will likely be with a teaching mannequin in the skills laboratory or with a male patient in the clinical setting. Before you proceed, discuss the feelings that may be experienced by the man and the examiner and methods to increase the comfort of both. Make sure you have discussed the steps of the examination with your instructor before examining a patient.

Clinical Objectives

1. Demonstrate knowledge of the signs and symptoms related to the male genitalia by obtaining a pertinent health history.
2. Inspect and palpate the penis and scrotum.
3. Palpate the inguinal region for hernia.
4. Teach testicular self-examination.
5. Record the history and physical examination findings accurately, reach an assessment of the health state, and develop a plan of care.

Instructions

Prepare the examination setting, and gather your equipment. Wash your hands; wear gloves during the examination. Practice the steps of the examination on a male patient in the clinical setting, giving appropriate instructions as you proceed. Record your findings using the regional write-up sheet that follows. The front of the page is intended as a worksheet; the back of the page is intended for your narrative summary recording using the SOAP format.

REGIONAL WRITE-UP—MALE GENITOURINARY SYSTEM

Date _____

Examiner _____

Patient _____ Age _____ Gender _____

Reason for visit _____

I. Health History

	No	Yes, explain
1. Any urinary **frequency, urgency,** or awakening during night to urinate?	_____	
2. Any **pain** or **burning** associated with urination?	_____	
3. Any **trouble starting urine stream**?	_____	
4. Urine **color cloudy** or **foul-smelling**? **Red-tinged** or **bloody**?	_____	
5. Any **problem controlling your urine**?	_____	
6. Any **pain** or **sores** on penis?	_____	
7. Any **lump** in testicles or scrotum?	_____	
Do you perform testicular self-examination?	_____	
8. Are you in a relationship now involving intercourse?	_____	
Use a contraceptive? Which one?	_____	
9. Any contact with a partner who has any sexually transmitted infection? Was this treated with antibiotics?	_____	

II. Physical Examination

A. **Inspect and palpate penis.**
Skin condition _____
Glans _____
Urethral meatus _____
Shaft _____

B. **Inspect and palpate scrotum.**
Skin condition _____
Testes _____
Spermatic cord _____
Transillumination (if indicated) _____

C. **Inspect and palpate for hernia.**
Inguinal canal _____
Femoral area _____

D. **Palpate inguinal lymph nodes.** _____

E. **Teach testicular self-examination.** _____

REGIONAL WRITE-UP—MALE GENITOURINARY SYSTEM

Summarize your findings using the SOAP format.

Subjective (reason for seeking care, health history)

Objective (physical examination findings)

Assessment (assessment of health state or problem, diagnosis)

Plan (diagnostic evaluation, follow-up care, patient teaching)

Anus, Rectum, and Prostate

PURPOSE

This chapter presents the structure and function of the anus and rectum and the male prostate gland, the methods of inspection and palpation of these structures, and how to record the assessment accurately.

READING ASSIGNMENT

Jarvis: *Physical Examination and Health Assessment*, 9th ed., Chapter 26, pp. 715–730.

Suggested reading:
Dunlap, J. J., & Dunlap, B. S. (2021). Constipation. *Gastroenterology Nursing*, 44(5), 361–364.

GLOSSARY

Study the following terms after completing the reading assignment. You should be able to cover the definition on the right and define the term out loud.

Constipation .... decrease in stool frequency with difficult passing of very hard, dry stools

Fissure .... painful longitudinal tear in tissue (e.g., in the superficial mucosa at the anal margin)

Hemorrhoid .... flabby papules of skin or mucous membranes in the anal region caused by a varicose vein of the hemorrhoidal plexus

Human papillomavirus
(HPV) .... a double-stranded DNA virus that enters the nuclei of the squamous and basal cells in oral, nasal, genital, and anal regions; transmitted through vaginal, anal, and oral intercourse

Melena .... blood in the stool

Pruritus .... itching or burning sensation in the skin

Steatorrhea .... excessive fat in the stool, as in gastrointestinal malabsorption of fat

Valves of Houston .... set of 3 semilunar transverse folds that cross half the circumference of the rectal lumen

STUDY GUIDE

After completing the reading assignment and the media assignment, answer the following questions in the spaces provided.

1. State the length of the anal canal and the rectum in the adult and describe the location of these structures in the lower abdomen.

2. Describe the size, shape, and location of the male prostate gland.

3. List a few examples of high-fiber foods of the soluble type and insoluble type. What advantages do these foods have for the body?

4. List screening measures that are recommended for early detection of colon–rectal cancer and prostate cancer.

5. State the method of promoting anal sphincter relaxation to aid palpation of the anus and rectum.

6. Describe the normal physical characteristics of the prostate gland that would be assessed by palpation:

   Size

   Shape

   Surface

   Consistency

   Mobility

   Sensitivity

7. Define the condition *benign prostatic hypertrophy*, list the usual symptoms that a man experiences with this condition, and describe the physical characteristics.

Fill in the labels indicated on the following illustrations.

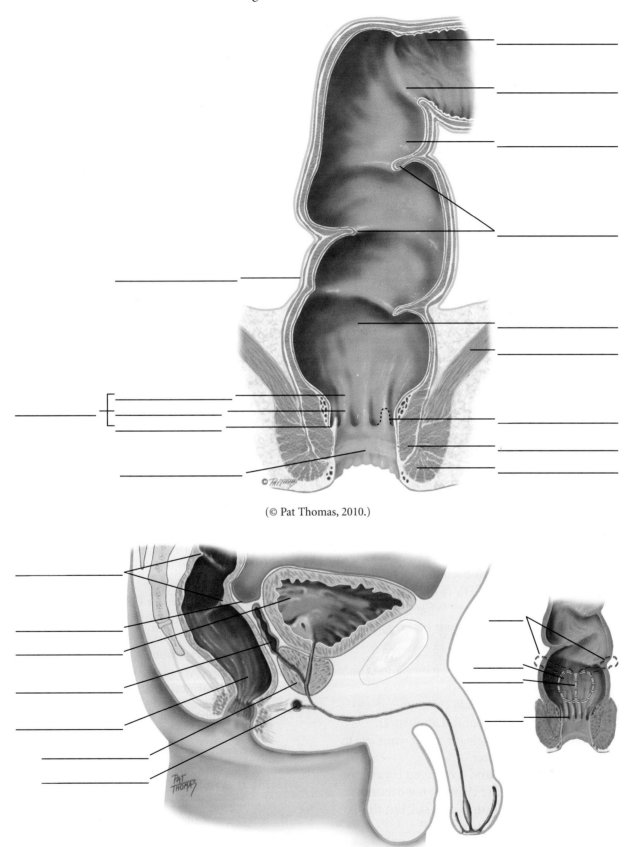

(© Pat Thomas, 2010.)

CLINICAL JUDGMENT QUESTIONS

This test is for you to check your own mastery of the content. Answers are provided in Appendix A.

1. During history collection, a 66-year-old man tells you he has trouble urinating, and his provider says his prostate gland is enlarged. He says, "Why do I even have a prostate gland?" Which is your best response?

   a. "It makes a thin, milky fluid to help the sperm stay alive during intercourse."
   b. "The prostate gland often shrinks as you grow older, so your urine troubles can get better."
   c. "The prostate gland secretes mucus into the rectum to help you pass stool."
   d. "The prostate gland passes a substance into the urine to make it more acidic and less likely to get infected."

2. During telephone triage, a new mother calls you to report her newborn has just passed a dark green "poop, the first one." The newborn is 30 hours of age. Your best response would be:

   a. "The dark green color may show blood in the stool."
   b. "The dark green color may show distress in the baby."
   c. "The baby should have passed the first stool within 12 hours after birth."
   d. "The dark green stool shows the rectum and anus are open and working."

3. A 60-year-old man has been told he has benign prostatic hypertrophy. His close friend just died from prostate cancer. "What if this happens to me!" What is your best response? **Select all that apply.**

   a. "The swelling in your prostate gland is only temporary and will go away."
   b. "Your provider will add chemotherapy to your treatment to control any cancer."
   c. "It would be unlikely for a man your age to have prostate cancer."
   d. "Your prostate gland is enlarged because of expected hormone changes, not cancer."
   e. "Your friend's death is very sad, but this is not a risk for you personally."

4. You inspect the perianal area of a 38-year-old woman and note: anal pigment darker than surrounding skin, anal opening closed, a shiny, blue skin sac. The woman reports pain with bowel movements and an occasional spot of red blood. These findings most likely indicate:

   a. A type of skin cancer in the anal area.
   b. A pilonidal cyst.
   c. Thrombosed hemorrhoids.
   d. Early stage of rectal prolapse.

5. While teaching a 63-year-old man with a family history of colorectal cancer (his father), you cover lifestyle factors to reduce future CRC risk. Which foods are helpful to reduce CRC risk?

   a. High in protein
   b. High in fiber
   c. High in fat
   d. High in carbohydrates

6. Lifestyle factors account for one-half of cases of CRC. To help a person reduce future CRC risk, **Select all that apply.**

   a. Stop smoking
   b. Annual colonoscopy
   c. Stop heavy alcohol drinking
   d. Meditation or yoga
   e. Daily fruit and vegetable intake
   f. Keeping a healthy weight
   g. Daily exercise
   h. Annual blood test for CRC marker
   i. Biennial ultrasound of lower abdomen

7. An advanced practitioner prepares to palpate the anus and lower rectum. Which approach to palpation is correct?

   a. Instruct the person that this will be a painful procedure.
   b. Place pad of examiner's index finger gently on anal opening.
   c. Insert examiner's extended index finger at a right angle to the anus.
   d. Insert examining finger back toward sacrum of patient's back.

8. During rectal examination, the practitioner palpates a firm, irregularly shaped mass along the mucosal wall. What is the practitioner's most appropriate response?

   a. Refer the patient to a specialist for further assessment.
   b. Ask the person to return in 1 month for a repeat assessment.
   c. Proceed with the exam; this is most likely a clump of stool.
   d. Pursue an ultrasound examination of lower abdomen.

CRITICAL THINKING ACTIVITIES 1

Communication is a crucial component of every patient encounter. Read the suggested article on p. 243 by Dunlap and Dunlap (2021). In a small discussion group during your laboratory, address these topics in the article:
- Compare the causes of primary (functional) constipation and secondary constipation.
- What further assessment tests are needed when constipation is present?
- List nonpharmacologic interventions to employ with constipation.
- Many older people experience constipation. Some discuss it freely; others do not discuss it unless pressed. Think about the older adults with whom you have had experience—how did you react to their discussions of constipation?

CRITICAL THINKING ACTIVITIES 2

Colon cancer is the third-highest cause of cancer death in the United States, but many cases are preventable with screening measures. Search the website at https://www.cdc.gov/cancer/colorectal/basic_info/what-is-colorectal-cancer.htm
- Choose materials that are most helpful to you in patient teaching, considering health literacy.
- Choose a family member or family friend older than 45 years, and practice patient teaching with this person. Concentrate on risk factors, symptoms, and screening measures.
- Bring your results back to laboratory for group discussion.

SKILLS LABORATORY AND CLINICAL SETTING

Perianal inspection is performed routinely in the hospital and outpatient setting. Digital rectal examination is less commonly performed and accomplished by an advanced practice provider.

Clinical Objectives

1. Demonstrate knowledge of the signs and symptoms related to the ano/rectal area by obtaining a pertinent health history.
2. Inspect the perianal region. When appropriate, palpate the anus and rectum.
3. Test any stool specimen for occult blood.
4. Record the history and physical examination findings accurately.

Instructions

Prepare the examination setting and gather your equipment. Wash your hands, wear gloves during the examination, and wash hands again after removing gloves. Practice the steps of the examination on a patient in the clinical setting, giving appropriate instructions as you proceed. Record your findings using the regional write-up sheet that follows. Note that only the worksheet is included in this chapter. Your narrative summary recording using the SOAP format can be included with the narrative summary of the genitalia.

REGIONAL WRITE-UP—ANUS, RECTUM, AND PROSTATE GLAND

Date _____

Examiner _____

Patient _____ Age _____ Gender _____

Reason for visit _____

I. Health History

	No	Yes, explain
1. Bowels move **regularly**? How often?	____	_____
Usual color? Hard or soft?	____	_____
2. Any **change** in usual bowel habits?	____	_____
Constipation, diarrhea	____	_____
3. Ever had **black or bloody stools**?	____	_____
4. Take any medications?	____	_____
5. Any **rectal itching, pain, or hemorrhoids**?	____	_____
6. Any family history of **colon–rectal polyps or cancer**?	____	_____
7. Describe usual amount of high-fiber foods in diet.	____	_____

II. Physical Examination

A. Inspect the perianal area.

Skin condition _____

Sacrococcygeal area _____

Note skin integrity while patient bears down. _____

B. **Palpate anus and rectum.** (When Indicated.)

Anal sphincter _____

Anal canal _____

Rectal wall _____

Prostate gland (for males)

Size _____

Shape _____

Surface _____

Consistency _____

Mobility _____

Any tenderness _____

Cervix (for females) _____

C. **Examine the stool.**

Visual inspection _____

Test for occult blood _____

REGIONAL WRITE-UP—ANUS, RECTUM, PROSTATE

Summarize your findings using the SOAP format.

Subjective (reason for seeking care, health history)

Objective (physical examination findings)

Assessment (assessment of health state or problem, diagnosis)

Plan (diagnostic evaluation, follow-up care, teaching)

Female Genitourinary System

PURPOSE

This chapter presents the structure and function of the female genitalia, the methods of inspection and palpation of the internal and external structures, the procedures for collection of cytologic specimens, and the ways to record the assessment accurately.

READING ASSIGNMENT

Jarvis: *Physical Examination and Health Assessment*, 9th ed., Chapter 27, pp. 731–768.

Suggested reading:

Davis, N. J., Wyman, J. F., Gubitosa, S., et al. (2020). Urinary incontinence in older adults. *Am J Nursing*, *120*(1), 57–62.

Gogineni, V., Waselewski, M. E., Jamison, C. D., et al. (2021). The future of STI screening and treatment for youth. *BMC Public Health*, *21*, 1–9. https://doi.org/10.1186/s12889-021-12091-y.

GLOSSARY

Study the following terms after completing the reading assignment. You should be able to cover the definition on the right and define the term out loud.

Adnexa .... accessory organs of the uterus (i.e., ovaries and fallopian tubes)

Amenorrhea .... absence of menstruation; termed secondary amenorrhea when menstruation has begun and then ceases; most common cause is pregnancy

Bartholin glands .... vestibular glands located on either side of the vaginal orifice that secrete a clear lubricating mucus during intercourse

Bloody show .... dislodging of thick cervical mucus plug at end of pregnancy that is a sign of beginning of labor

Caruncle .... small, deep red mass protruding from urethral meatus, usually due to urethritis

Chadwick sign .... bluish discoloration of cervix that occurs normally in pregnancy at 6 to 8 weeks' gestation

Chancre .... red, round, superficial ulcer with a yellowish serous discharge that is a sign of syphilis

Clitoris .... small, elongated erectile tissue in the female, located at anterior juncture of labia minora

Cystocele .... prolapse of urinary bladder and its vaginal mucosa into the vagina with straining or standing

Dysmenorrhea .... abdominal cramping and pain associated with menstruation

Dyspareunia .... painful intercourse

Dysuria .... painful urination

Endometriosis .... aberrant growths of endometrial tissue scattered throughout pelvis

Fibroid .... (myoma) hard, painless nodule in uterine wall that causes uterine enlargement

Gonorrhea .... sexually transmitted infection (STI) characterized by purulent vaginal discharge (or may have no symptoms)

Hegar sign .... softening of cervix that is a sign of pregnancy, occurring at 10 to 12 weeks' gestation

Hematuria .... red-tinged or bloody urine

Hymen .... membranous fold of tissue partly closing vaginal orifice

Leukorrhea .... whitish or yellowish discharge from vaginal orifice

Menarche .... onset of first menstruation, usually between 11 and 13 years of age

Menopause .... cessation of menses, usually occurring around 48 to 51 years of age

Menorrhagia .... excessively heavy menstrual flow

Multipara .... condition of having 2 or more pregnancies

Nullipara .... condition of first pregnancy

Papanicolaou test .... (Pap test) painless test used to detect cervical cancer

Polyp .... cervical polyp is bright red, soft, pedunculated growth emerging from os

Rectocele .... prolapse of rectum and its vaginal mucosa into vagina with straining or standing

Rectouterine pouch .... (cul-de-sac of Douglas) deep recess formed by the peritoneum between the rectum and cervix

Salpingitis .... inflammation of fallopian tubes

Skene glands .... paraurethral glands

Vaginitis .... inflammation of vagina

Vulva .... external genitalia of female

STUDY GUIDE

After completing the reading assignment and the media assignment, answer the following questions in the spaces provided.

1. Discuss ways of creating an environment that will provide psychological comfort for both the patient and practitioner during the female genitalia examination.

2. Discuss selection, preparation, and insertion of the vaginal speculum.

3. Describe the appearance or sketch these normal variations of the cervix and os:

   Nulliparous

   Parous

   Stellate lacerations

   Cervical eversion

   Nabothian cysts

4. List the steps in the procedure of obtaining these specimens:

   Ecto- and Endocervical specimen using "broom"

   Endocervical specimen using cytobrush

   Cervical scrape using spatula

5. Discuss the procedure and rationale for bimanual examination and list normal findings for the cervix, uterus, and adnexa.

6. Describe the appearance or sketch the appearance of the following abnormalities of the cervix:

Chadwick sign

Erosion

Polyp

Carcinoma

7. List the characteristics of vaginal discharge associated with the following conditions of vaginitis:

Candidiasis (yeast infection)

Trichomoniasis

Bacterial vaginosis

Chlamydia

Gonorrhea

8. List the changes observed during the perimenopausal period.

9. Differentiate the signs and symptoms of these conditions of adnexal enlargement:

Ectopic pregnancy

Ovarian cyst

Fill in the labels indicated on the following illustrations.

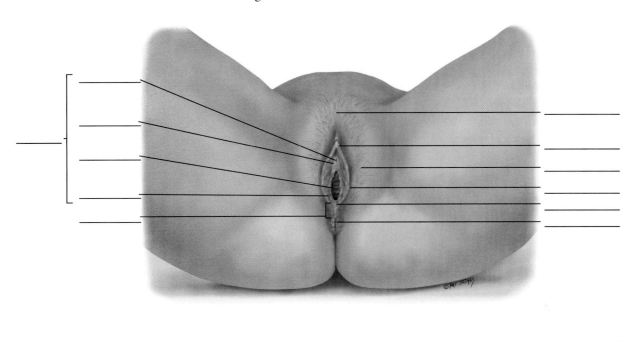

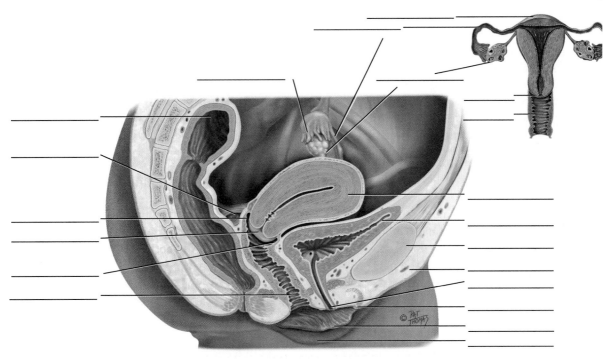

CLINICAL JUDGMENT QUESTIONS

This test is for you to check your own mastery of the content. Answers are provided in Appendix A.

1. You are beginning a health history for a 25-year-old female who comes to the clinic for her first pelvic examination. Her knees are jumpy, and her voice is a bit breathless. You choose to begin the history with questions about her menstrual period. What directs your question choice?

    a. If she is having her period now, she will have to go home and schedule another appointment.
    b. This is a good screening question to tell if she is pregnant.
    c. This question is a good test of memory to screen if she will be a reliable historian.
    d. Young women are used to discussing their menstrual periods, so this is a comfortable line of questioning to start.

2. A 48-year-old woman seeks care because of a depressed feeling, episodes of unusual heat, not sleeping well, and feeling exhausted and irritable. Her last menstrual period (LMP) was 14 days prior to this appointment. She describes these symptoms in detail, then states, "This can't be menopause, because I still have my periods." What is your next best response?

    a. "It sounds more like stress. Let's schedule an appointment with our psychotherapist here in the office."
    b. "Actually, 'perimenopause' can start well before your periods stop, and you may now be having symptoms of low estrogen."
    c. "How are things at work? Any new problems there that could cause stress?"
    d. "Have you noticed any vaginal dryness when having sex?"

3. An 11-year-old girl comes to your clinic for a sports physical and shows breast bud development. How can you help her understand usual growth and development? What is your best approach?

    a. Avoid commenting on her breasts because girls this age are very self-conscious.
    b. Ask her if her breasts are growing about the same way as other girls in her class.

    c. Tell her not to worry; by age 18 all girls will have their full breast development.
    d. Use Tanner's sexual development charts to show her where she is now in the stages and what to expect.
    e. Check her height and weight on the growth charts and tell her that after she gains more weight, her breasts will develop.

4. A 65-year-old woman tells you she "wets" herself a little when she sneezes or coughs. Your next best response is:

    a. "This sounds like 'stress incontinence' and usually is due to some weakness in the pelvic muscles."
    b. "This may be a sign of infection, so let's test a urine sample for bacteria."
    c. "This is called 'urge incontinence' and is usually due to an overactive bladder muscle."
    d. "This is a sign of blood in the urine, and we will need to refer you to a specialist."

5. A 25-year-old woman has some vaginal discharge and is worried she has a sexually transmitted infection (STI). What is your next best response?

    a. "Tell me more about the discharge: Color? Smell? Amount?"
    b. "Have you been having sex with a new partner?"
    c. "How about condoms? Do you use one every time you have sex?"
    d. "This is normal for some time within the menstrual cycle. Don't worry."

6. When discussing sexuality or sexual feelings with teenagers, a permission statement helps to communicate that it is normal and healthy to think or to feel a certain way. Which of the following would you choose to be a permission statement?

    a. "It's OK that girls your age are having sex."
    b. "Often girls your age have questions about sex and sexual activity. What questions do you have?"

c. "Now I want to ask you some questions about sexual activity. I ask all girls these questions."

d. "Do you use condoms every time you have sex?"

7. You are preparing a patient for a pelvic examination in the lithotomy position. What measures can you employ to ease comfort? **Select all that apply.**

a. Elevate patient's head and shoulders to keep eye contact during the exam.

b. Place patient's arms up and behind the head.

c. Position a chaperone standing by the patient's head.

d. Make sure bladder is empty before the exam.

e. Position the buttocks 6 inches up from the edge of the table so patient will not feel as if falling off.

f. State, "Now I'm going to . . ." before each step in the exam.

g. Touch the inner thigh before you directly touch the vulva.

8. Which of the following describes a normal and expected finding when inspecting the adult female's external genitalia?

a. Occasional yellowish, 1-cm nodules that are firm and nontender.

b. Swelling in the perineum just before the onset of menses.

c. Redness of the labia majora.

d. A yellow-green discharge at midcycle.

9. You are examining a 1-day-old baby girl following an uncomplicated vaginal delivery. The mother is present, and both are to be discharged to return home. During the exam, you note the baby's labia majora are swollen, the clitoris appears large, there is a small amount of mucoid discharge, and the vaginal opening is difficult to see. What is your next best action?

a. Ask to have the pediatrician check the baby in 2 days to make sure the genitalia decrease in size.

b. Refer the baby to a specialist to evaluate ambiguous genitalia.

c. Request an order for estrogen levels on the baby.

d. Proceed with the exam; this is a normal finding.

10. The provider palpates the adnexa on a 23-year-old woman who presents to the clinic following two missed menstrual periods. The findings regarding the adnexa are: nonpalpable ovaries; a firm, smooth uterine wall; a fallopian tube that feels firm and pulsating. What is your next best action?

a. Refer the woman promptly to the ED.

b. A pulsating fallopian tube occasionally is present due to the nearby iliac artery. Proceed with the exam.

c. Schedule a return appointment in 2 weeks to recheck the findings.

d. Request an ultrasound image to confirm presence of ovaries and both fallopian tubes.

11. Underline the findings that are normal and expected.

The provider examines the internal cervix and its os on a 36-year-old woman who has had 3 full-term pregnancies—all vaginal deliveries. The findings are: slit-like appearance of the os; occasional small, smooth yellow nodules on the cervix; thick, opaque, stringy cervical secretions; foul smelling secretions.

12. Underline the findings that are normal and expected.

The provider performs a bimanual examination on a 54-year-old woman. The findings are: cervix feels smooth; cervix feels hard; cervix is equally rounded; cervix does not move with examiner's finger movement; cervical movement produces some pain.

13. You are caring for a 32-year-old woman who presents to the clinic with a vaginal discharge. She has not had vaginal intercourse for 5 years before arrival. She reports ___A___. Your physical examination reveals ___B___. You suspect she has ___C___.

(A) Subjective Findings	(B) Objective Findings	(C) Condition
1—No further significant symptoms	1—Red and swollen vulva and vagina. Thick, white, curdy, non-smelling discharge	1—Trichomoniasis
2—Urinary frequency and painful urination	2—Reddened vaginal walls with tiny red spots	2—Chlamydia
3—Urinary frequency and intense itching	3—Tenderness on moving cervix	3—Candidiasis (Moniliasis)
4—Intense itching, recent treatment for bronchitis	4—Purulent vaginal discharge, no further abnormal exam findings	4—Gonorrhea

CRITICAL THINKING ACTIVITIES

1. Read the Davis article covering the common condition of urinary incontinence occurring in older adults. One type, stress incontinence, occurs in women of all ages, especially athletes!
1. Differentiate between Urge incontinence and Stress incontinence.
2. How would you frame an assessment by health history for an older adult with incontinence?
3. Discuss the ways incontinence can lead to social isolation, strain on caregivers, falls, pressure injuries, and depression.

2. Read and study the Gogineni, Waselewski article on screening youth for common STIs—chlamydia and gonorrhea. Study the representative quotes listed in Table 2 in the article.
1. Answer the research questions for yourself: Would it be hard for you to get TESTED? Would it be hard for you to get TREATED, if positive? Where would you go for treatment? If you got chlamydia or gonorrhea, would you tell your sexual partner?
2. Now discuss these questions as if you were an underresourced person. What are the barriers to care?
3. What is the incidence of these common STIs in youth aged 15 to 24 years? What are the risks of untreated infections?
4. In many sites, a woman can collect her own vaginal swab specimen and bring it in for testing for STIs. What advantages do you see with this technique?

SKILLS LABORATORY AND CLINICAL SETTING

Because of the need to maintain personal privacy, it is not likely you will practice the female genitalia examination on a peer. Your practice likely will be with a teaching mannequin in the skills laboratory or with a woman in the clinical setting under the guidance of a preceptor. Before you proceed, discuss the feelings that may be experienced by the woman and examiner and methods to increase the comfort of both. With your instructor, discuss methods of positioning the woman, steps in using the vaginal speculum, steps in procuring specimens, and methods of infection control precautions.

Clinical Objectives

1. Demonstrate knowledge of the signs and symptoms related to the female genitalia by obtaining a pertinent health history.
2. Demonstrate measures to increase the woman's comfort before and during the examination.
3. Demonstrate knowledge of infection control precautions before, during, and after the examination.
4. Inspect and palpate the external genitalia.
5. Using the vaginal speculum, gather materials for cytologic study.
6. Inspect and palpate the internal genitalia.
7. Record the history and physical examination findings accurately, reach an assessment of the health state, and develop a plan of care.

Instructions

Prepare the examination setting and gather your equipment. Collect the health history before the patient disrobes for the examination. Wash your hands, wear gloves during the examination, and wash hands again after removing gloves. Practice the steps of the examination on a patient in the clinical setting, giving appropriate instructions as you proceed. Record your findings using the regional write-up sheet that follows. The first section is intended as a worksheet; the last page is intended for your narrative summary recording using the SOAP format. Collection of data for the rectal examination is sometimes indicated with the examination of female genitalia; see Chapter 25 for the regional write-up sheet for the rectal examination.

NOTES

REGIONAL WRITE-UP—FEMALE GENITOURINARY SYSTEM

Date _____

Examiner _____

Patient _____ Age _____ Gender _____

Reason for visit _____

I. Health History

	No	Yes, explain
1. Date of last menstrual period?		
Age at first period? Usual cycle?		
Duration? Usual amount of flow?		
Any pain or cramps with period?		
2. Ever been **pregnant**? How many times?		
Describe pregnancy(ies).		
Any complications?		
3. Periods slowed down or **stopped**?		
4. How often are **gynecologic checkups**?		
Date of last Pap test? Results?		
5. Any problems with **urinating**?		
6. Any unusual **vaginal discharge**?		
7. **Sores or lesions** in genitals?		
8. In a relationship now involving intercourse?		
9. Use a contraceptive? Which one?		
10. Any contact with partner who has a sexually transmitted infection?		
11. Any precautions to reduce risk for STIs?		
12. Taking any medications?		
Any hormone therapy?		

II. Physical Examination
A. **Inspect external genitalia.**
Skin color and mucous membranes _____

Hair distribution _____ Structures symmetric? _____

Clitoris _____ Labia _____

Urethral opening _____ Vaginal opening _____

Perineum _____

Any lesions? _____

B. **Palpate external genitalia.**
Bartholin glands _____

Perineum _____

Assess for vaginal wall bulging or urinary incontinence. _____

Discharge, color, odor, consistency _____

C. **Speculum examination**

Inspect cervix and os

Color _____ Position _____

Size _____ _____Surface _____

Discharge, color, odor, consistency _____

Nabothian cysts? _____ IUD string, if present _____

Obtain cervical smears and cultures.

Vaginal pool _____ Cervical scrape _____ Endocervical specimen _____

Other (if indicated) _____

Complete acetic acid wash _____

Inspect vaginal wall as speculum is removed. _____

D. **Bimanual examination**

Cervix

Consistency _____ Mobility _____

Tenderness with motion _____

Uterus

Size and shape _____ Consistency _____

Position _____ Mobility _____

Tenderness _____

Adnexa

Able to palpate? (Be honest.) _____

Size and shape of ovaries _____

Tenderness _____ Masses _____

Rectovaginal examination _____

REGIONAL WRITE-UP—FEMALE GENITOURINARY SYSTEM

Summarize your findings using the SOAP format.

Subjective (reason for seeking care, health history)

Objective (physical examination findings)   Record findings on diagram below.

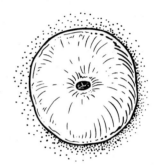

Assessment (assessment of health state or problem, diagnosis)

Plan (diagnostic evaluation, follow-up care, patient teaching)

NOTES

CHAPTER
28

The Complete Health Assessment: Adult

PURPOSE

This chapter presents the methods of integrating the regional examinations so that you will be able to conduct a complete physical examination on a well young adult.

READING ASSIGNMENT

Jarvis: *Physical Examination and Health Assessment,* 9th ed., Chapter 28, pp. 769–784.

CLINICAL OBJECTIVES

1. Demonstrate skills of inspection, percussion, palpation, and auscultation.

2. Demonstrate correct use of instruments, including assembly, manipulation of component parts, and positioning of the patient.

3. Use appropriate terminology and correctly pronounce medical terminology with the clinical instructor and adapt terms for the patient.

4. Choreograph the complete examination in a systematic manner, including integration of certain regional assessments throughout the examination (e.g., skin, musculoskeletal system).

5. Coordinate procedures to limit position changes for the examiner and patient.

6. Describe accurately the findings of the examination, including normal and abnormal findings.

7. Demonstrate appropriate infection control measures.

8. Recognize and maintain the privacy and dignity of the patient.
   a. Adequately explain what is being done while limiting small talk.
   b. Consider patient's anxiety and fears.
   c. Consider your own facial expressions and comments.
   d. Demonstrate confidence, empathy, and a gentle manner.
   e. Acknowledge and apologize for any discomfort caused.
   f. Provide for privacy and warmth at all times.
   g. Determine comfort level, pausing if patient becomes tired.
   h. Wash hands and don gloves appropriately.
   i. Allow adequate time for each step.
   j. Briefly summarize findings to the patient and thank the patient.

INSTRUCTIONS

The key to success in this venture is **practice**; you should conduct at least **three** complete physical examination practices in your preparation for this final examination proficiency. You will be assigned a peer "patient" for the examination. You should prepare your own notecard "outline" for the examination. You may refer to this minimally during the examination, but overdependence on your notes will constitute failure. You will have 45 minutes in which to conduct the examination (not including setup). Genitalia examination is omitted. With adequate practice, you will have no difficulty completing the examination in the allotted time.

Prepare the examination setting. Arrange for proper lighting. If you are using a hospital bed instead of an examination table, make sure to adjust the bed height during the examination to allow for proper body mechanics and for the patient's ease in getting into and out of the bed. Arrange for patient gown, bath blankets, and drapes.

Gather your equipment. The following items are needed for a complete physical examination. Check with your clinical instructor for any items that you may omit for your own examination proficiency.

Scale with height attachment	Nasal speculum
Sphygmomanometer with appropriately sized cuff	Tongue depressor
	Pocket vision screener
Stethoscope with bell and diaphragm endpieces (or tunable diaphragm)	Flexible tape measure
	Ruler marked in centimeters
Alcohol wipes for cleaning equipment	Reflex hammer
Thermometer	Sharp object (split tongue blade)
Flashlight or penlight	Cotton balls
Otoscope	Disposable gloves
Ophthalmoscope	Hand sanitizer

Record your findings using the write-up sheets that follow. Your clinical instructor may ask you to write your findings in narrative format. Remember to use appropriate medical terminology and concise phrases.

Following the examination worksheet, a sample form used in an ambulatory care setting has been included. You may use it for your write-up.

COMPLETE PHYSICAL EXAMINATION

Date _____

Examiner _____

Patient _____ Gender _____ Age _____

Occupation _____ Reason for visit _____

General Survey of Patient

1. Appears stated age _____
2. Level of consciousness _____
3. Skin color _____
4. Nutritional status _____
5. Posture and position _____
6. Obvious physical deformities _____
7. Mobility: gait, use of assistive devices, ROM of joints, involuntary movement _____
8. Facial expression _____
9. Mood and affect _____
10. Speech: articulation, pattern, content appropriate, native language _____
11. Hearing _____
12. Personal hygiene _____

Measurement and Vital Signs

1. Weight _____
2. Height _____
3. Waist circumference _____
4. Body mass index _____
5. Vision using Snellen eye chart
   Right eye _____ Left eye _____ Correction? _____
6. Radial pulse, rate, and rhythm _____
7. Respirations, rate, depth _____
8. Blood pressure
   Right arm _____ (sitting or lying?)
   Left arm _____ (sitting or lying?)
9. Temperature _____
10. Pain assessment _____

Stand in Front of Patient, Patient Sitting

Skin

1. Hands and nails _____
2. (For remainder of examination, examine skin with corresponding region.)
   Color and pigmentation _____
   Temperature _____
   Moisture _____
   Texture _____
   Turgor _____
   Any lesions _____

Head and Face

1. Scalp, hair, cranium _____
2. Face (cranial nerve VII) _____
3. Temporal artery, temporomandibular joint _____
4. Maxillary sinuses, frontal sinuses _____

Eyes

1. Visual fields (cranial nerve II) _____
2. Extraocular muscles, corneal light reflex _____
   Cardinal positions of gaze (cranial nerves III, IV, VI) _____
3. External structures _____
4. Conjunctivae _____
   Sclerae _____
   Corneas _____
   Irides _____
5. Pupils _____
6. Ophthalmoscope, red reflex _____
   Disc _____
   Vessels _____
   Retinal background _____

Ears

1. External ear _____
2. Otoscope, ear canal _____
   Tympanic membrane _____
3. Hearing (cranial nerve VIII), whispered voice test _____

Nose

1. External nose _____
2. Patency of nostrils _____
3. Speculum, nasal mucosa _____
   Septum _____
   Turbinates _____

Mouth and Throat

1. Lips and buccal mucosa _____
   Teeth and gums _____
   Tongue _____
   Hard and soft palate _____
2. Tonsils _____
3. Uvula (cranial nerves IX, X) _____
4. Tongue (cranial nerve XII) _____

Neck

1. Symmetry, lumps, pulsations _____
2. Cervical lymph nodes _____
3. Carotid pulse (bruits if indicated) _____
4. Trachea _____
5. ROM and muscle strength (cranial nerve XI) _____

Move to Back of Patient, Patient Sitting

    6. Palpate thyroid gland_____

Chest and Lungs, Posterior and Lateral

    1. Thoracic cage configuration _____
       Skin characteristics _____
       Symmetry _____
    2. Symmetric expansion _____
       Tactile fremitus _____
       Lumps or tenderness _____
    3. Spinous processes _____
    4. Percussion over lung fields _____
    5. CVA tenderness _____
    6. Breath sounds _____
    7. Adventitious sounds _____

Move to Front of Patient

Chest and Lungs, Anterior

    1. Respirations and skin characteristics _____
    2. Symmetric expansion, tactile fremitus, lumps, tenderness _____
    3. Percuss lung fields _____
    4. Breath sounds _____
    5. Inspect and palpate breasts (male only) _____

Upper Extremities

    1. ROM and muscle strength, shoulder _____
       Elbow _____
       Wrist and hand _____
    2. Epitrochlear nodes _____

Breasts (female)

    1. Symmetry, mobility, dimpling _____
    2. Supraclavicular and infraclavicular areas _____

Patient Supine, Stand at Patient's Right

Breasts (female)

    1. Breast palpation _____
    2. Nipple _____
    3. Axillae and regional nodes _____
    4. Teach breast self-examination _____

Neck Vessels

    1. Jugular venous pulse _____
    2. Jugular venous pressure, if indicated _____

Heart

    1. Precordium: pulsations and heave _____
    2. Apical impulse _____
    3. Precordium, thrills _____

    4. Apical rate and rhythm _____

    5. Heart sounds _____

Abdomen

    1. Contour, symmetry _____

       Skin characteristics _____

       Umbilicus and pulsations _____

    2. Bowel sounds _____

    3. Vascular sounds _____

    4. Percussion _____

    5. Light and deep palpation _____

    6. Palpation of liver, spleen, kidneys, aorta _____

    7. Abdominal reflexes, if indicated _____

Inguinal Area

    1. Femoral pulse _____

    2. Inguinal nodes _____

Lower Extremities

    1. Symmetry _____

       Skin characteristics, hair distribution _____

    2. Pulses, popliteal _____

       Posterior tibial _____

       Dorsalis pedis _____

    3. Temperature, pretibial edema _____

    4. Toes _____

    5. ROM and muscle strength, hips _____

Patient Sitting Up

Lower Extremities

    1. ROM and muscle strength, knees _____

       Ankles and feet _____

Neurologic

    1. Sensation, face _____

       Arms and hands _____

       Legs and feet _____

    2. Position sense _____

    3. Stereognosis or graphesthesia _____

    4. Cerebellar function, finger to nose _____

    5. Cerebellar function, heel to shin _____

    6. Deep tendon reflexes

       Biceps _____   Triceps _____

       Brachioradialis _____   Patellar _____

       Achilles _____

    7. Babinski reflex _____

Patient Standing Up

Musculoskeletal

1. Walk across room _____
   Walk, heel to toe _____
2. Walk on tiptoes, and then walk on heels _____
3. Romberg sign _____
4. Shallow knee bend _____
5. Touch toes _____
6. ROM of spine _____

Male Genitalia

1. Penis and scrotum _____
2. Testes and spermatic cord _____
3. Inguinal hernia _____
4. Teach testicular self-examination _____

Male Rectum

1. Perianal area _____
2. Rectal walls and prostate gland (if indicated) _____
3. Stool for occult blood (if indicated) _____

Female Patient in Lithotomy Position

Female Genitalia and Rectum

1. Perineal and perianal areas _____
2. Vaginal speculum: cervix and vaginal walls _____
3. Procure specimens _____
4. Bimanual: cervix, uterus, and adnexa _____
5. Rectovaginal (if indicated) _____
6. Stool for occult blood (if indicated) _____

Closure

1. Help patient sit up.
2. Thank patient and depart.

Comprehensive Adult History and Physical*

Date of Visit: _____ *Medical Record #:* _____

Patient name _____

Preferred Name _____ *Pronouns:* _____

Address: _____

Telephone: (home) _____ *(mobile)* _____

Date of Birth: _____ *Age:* ____ *Gender:* _____

Provider: _____

Sex assigned at birth: male   female

Language _____ *Interpreter present:* ☐ Yes ☐ No

Reliability: ☐ Adequate ☐ Inadequate

History of Present Illness

Past Medical History

☐ HTN	☐ Asthma/COPD	☐ Seizure Disorder	☐ Breast Disease
☐ DM	☐ GERD	☐ Renal Disease	☐ Anemia
☐ CVD/CAD	☐ Hepatitis	☐ Thyroid Disorder	☐ Transfusions
☐ CVA	☐ Osteoporosis	☐ Bleeding Disorder	☐ Psychiatric
☐ CA	☐ Arthritis	☐ Infectious Disease	☐ Childhood Illnesses

Other/Details of Above:

Past Surgical History/Trauma/Hospitalization

☐ T & A: *Other/Details:*

☐ Appendectomy:

☐ Cholecystectomy:

☐ Hernia repair:

☐ Hysterectomy:

☐ Laparotomy:

☐ Cesarean section:

☐ Biopsy: _____ ☐ ORIF: _____

Medications

☐ OTC

☐ Vitamins

☐ Supplements/Herbals

Allergies

☐ Drugs

☐ Environment

☐ Foods ☐ Latex

☐ IV Contrast

Reproductive History

Menstrual: Age at menarche _____ LMP _____

Interval _____ Duration _____ Flow _____

☐ Reg ☐ Irreg ☐ Cramping ☐ Intermenstrual Bleeding ☐ PMS

Obstetrical: G _____ T _____ P _____ A _____ L _____

Complications: _____

Menopause: Age _____ Abnl Bleeding: _____

Symptoms: _____

Hormones: ☐ ERT ☐ HRT ☐ topical _____

Contraceptives: _____

Sexual Activity:

☐ same sex   ☐ opposite sex   ☐ abstinent

☐ single partner   ☐ multiple partners   ☐ >4 lifetime partners

STD hx:_____

Concerns:

Adapted from Loretz, L. (2005). *Primary care tools for clinicians.* St. Louis: Elsevier.

Comprehensive Adult History and Physical - 2*

Medical record #: _____

Date of Birth: _____   Date of Exam: _____

Social History

Marital Status: ☐ Single   ☐ Married   ☐ Partnered
☐ Divorced   ☐ Widowed   ☐ Other _____

Cohabitants:_____

Children: _____

Education: _____

Occupation: _____

Interests/Activities: _____

Exercise: ☐ Aerobic ☐ Weights_____

Diet: ☐ Balanced ☐ Calcium _____

Sleep/Rest: _____ ***Caffeine:*** ☐ No ☐ Yes cups/day _____

Tobacco: ☐ No ☐ Yes PPD _____ # Years _____ Quit Year _____

Smoking in home: ☐ Yes ☐ No _____

ETOH: ☐ Yes ☐ No ☐ Daily ☐ Weekly ☐ Monthly # drinks_____

Recreational Drugs: _____

Support Systems/Coping Skills: ☐ Adequate   ☐ Inadequate

Family History

☐ ***Family History Unknown***

Father:_____

Mother: _____

Siblings: _____

MGF: _____

MGM:_____

PGF: _____

PGM: _____

Other:_____

_____

_____

Cultural/Religious Influences: _____

_____

Health Maintenance History

Exam	Last Date	Results	N/A	Refused	Exam	Last Date	Results	N/A	Refused
Pap test					Dental				
Mammogram					Vision				
SBE/TSE					Hearing				
Stool guaiac					Lipid Profile				
Flex sig/Colonoscopy					FBS				
CXR					PSA				
ECG					PPD				

Immunizations (dates):

Td	MMR/titers		Hep B		Polio
Varicella vaccine/chickenpox		Influenza		Pneumovax	

Safety:

☐ Seatbelt Use   ☐ Cycling Helmet   ☐ Sunscreen   ☐ Occupational

☐ Smoke Detectors   ☐ Housing   ☐ Dom. Violence   ☐ Firearms

Review of Systems (Check box at left if all systems negative.)

Comments/Details:

☐ ***General:*** ☐ fever   ☐ chills   ☐ night sweats   ☐ fatigue   ☐ unexplained weight loss   ☐ weight gain

☐ ***Skin:*** ☐ pruritus   ☐ rash   ☐ hair loss   ☐ worrisome lesion   ☐ pigment change   ☐ moles   ☐ sweating   ☐ dry skin   ☐ nail change

☐ ***HEENT:*** ☐ headache   ☐ dizziness   ☐ earache   ☐ hearing loss   ☐ tinnitus   ☐ vision change   ☐ eye pain/sensitivity
☐ excessive tearing   ☐ eyeglasses/contact use   ☐ glaucoma   ☐ rhinorrhea   ☐ nasal congestion   ☐ postnasal drip   ☐ sinus pain
☐ nosebleeds   ☐ hay fever   ☐ sore throat   ☐ mouth sores   ☐ hoarseness   ☐ toothache   ☐ bleeding gums   ☐ dentures

☐ ***Breast:*** ☐ pain   ☐ lumps   ☐ discharge   ☐ history of breast disease   ☐ implants

☐ ***Pulmonary:*** ☐ cough   ☐ sputum   ☐ hemoptysis   ☐ SOB   ☐ pain with respiration   ☐ wheezing   ☐ cyanosis

☐ ***CV:*** ☐ chest pain   ☐ palpitations   ☐ DOE   ☐ orthopnea   ☐ PND   ☐ diaphoresis   ☐ syncope   ☐ heart murmur   ☐ leg edema

☐ ***PVD:*** ☐ claudication   ☐ varicose veins   ☐ phlebitis   ☐ coldness of hands/feet   ☐ leg ulcers

☐ ***GI:*** ☐ dysphagia   ☐ heartburn   ☐ change in appetite   ☐ food intol   ☐ nausea   ☐ vomiting   ☐ hematemesis   ☐ abdominal pain   ☐ bloating
☐ flatulence   ☐ diarrhea   ☐ constipation   ☐ melena   ☐ jaundice   ☐ dark urine   ☐ BRBPR   ☐ change in BM   ☐ hemorrhoids   ☐ hernia

☐ ***GU:*** ☐ dysuria   ☐ urgency   ☐ frequency   ☐ hematuria   ☐ nocturia   ☐ polyuria   ☐ suprapubic pain   ☐ flank pain   ☐ incontinence   ☐ lesions
♂ ☐ hesitancy   ☐ dribbling   ☐ decreased force stream   ☐ testicular pain   ☐ testicular mass/swelling   ☐ penile discharge   ☐ erectile dysfunction
♀ ☐ vaginal itch   ☐ abnl vaginal discharge   ☐ vaginal dryness   ☐ dyspareunia   ☐ sexual dysfunction   ☐ abnl vaginal bleeding

☐ ***Endocrine:*** ☐ polyuria   ☐ polydipsia   ☐ polyphagia   ☐ heat/cold intol   ☐ tremor   ☐ lump in throat   ☐ unexplained wt change   ☐ hair changes

☐ ***Heme:*** ☐ anemia   ☐ easy bruising   ☐ swollen glands   ☐ bleeding of skin/mucous membranes   ☐ freq infections   ☐ allergies   ☐ delayed healing

☐ ***MSK:*** ☐ joint pain (location _____)   ☐ stiffness   ☐ restriction of motion   ☐ swelling   ☐ erythema
☐ bony deformity   ☐ myalgia   ☐ muscle cramps   ☐ weakness   ☐ antalgic gait   ☐ back pain

☐ ***Neuro:*** ☐ focal weakness   ☐ paralysis   ☐ numbness   ☐ tremor   ☐ seizure   ☐ syncope   ☐ gait disturbance   ☐ memory loss   ☐ aphasia

☐ ***Psych:*** ☐ anxiety   ☐ panic attacks   ☐ depression   ☐ mood changes   ☐ irritability   ☐ nervousness   ☐ decreased libido
☐ eating disorder   ☐ sleep disturbance   ☐ suicidal thoughts   ☐ impaired judgment   ☐ hallucinations   ☐ confusion

*Adapted from Loretz, L. (2005). *Primary care tools for clinicians*. St. Louis: Elsevier.

Comprehensive Adult History and Physical - 3*

Medical record #: _____

Date of Birth: _____ *Date of Exam:* _____

Physical Exam

N = Normal A = Abnormal (Check appropriate box)	N	A
1. General Appearance: age • LOC • nutrition • development • mobility • affect • speech • hygiene		
2. Skin: hydration • color • texture • hair • nails • lesions		
3. Head: shape • size • symmetry • scalp • TMJ • lesions		
4. Eyes: lids • conjunctiva • sclera		
Extraocular Muscles		
Visual fields		
Pupils: size, reaction to light and accommodation		
Fundi		
5. Ears: pinna • canals • TMs • hearing		
6. Nose: patency • nares • sinuses • nasal mucosa • septum • turbinates		
7. Mouth: lips • gums • teeth • mucosa • palate • tongue		
8. Throat: pharynx • tonsils • uvula		
9. Neck: ROM • symmetry • palpation • thyroid • trachea • carotids • jugular veins • lymph nodes		
10. Breasts: size • symmetry • skin • nipples • palpation • nodes		
11. Chest/Lungs: excursion • palpation • percussion • auscultation		
12. Cardiac: PMI • palpation • rate • rhythm • S1 • S2 • murmurs • gallops • bruits • extra sounds		
13. Abdomen: appearance • bowel sounds • bruits • percussion • palpation • liver • spleen • flank • suprapubic • hernia		
14. Anorectal: perianal		
digital rectal (if indicated)		
stool guiac (if indicated)		
prostate exam (if indicated)		
15. Female Genitalia: perineum • labia • urethral meatus • introitus		
Internal: vaginal mucosal • cervix		
Bimanual: vagina • cervix • uterus • adnexa		
16. Male Genitalia: penis • scrotum • testes • hernia		
17. Lymph Nodes: cervical • subclavian • axillary • inguinal • other		
18. Musculoskeletal: *Back/Spine:* ROM • palpation		
Upper Extremity: ROM • strength • palpation		
Lower Extremity: ROM • strength • palpation		
19. Peripheral Vascular: Upper extremity: pulses • appearance • temp		
Lower extremity: pulses • appearance • temp		
20. Neurologic: cranial nerves • motor • sensory • cerebellar • reflexes • gait • mental status		

Vitals

Ht _____ Wt _____ Temp _____ Resp _____ Pulse _____

BP (R arm) sitting _____ supine _____
BP (L arm) sitting _____ supine _____

Visual Acuity

Right   /   Left   /

Corrective lenses ☐ Yes   ☐ No

Document Abnormals (by number)/Comments

Lab/Studies

Assessment and Plan

*Adapted from Loretz, L. (2005). *Primary care tools for clinicians.* St. Louis: Elsevier.

Comprehensive Adult History and Physical - 4*

Medical record #: _____

Date of Birth: _____ *Date of Exam:* _____

Assessment and Plan (continued)

Periodic Health Screening Plan

Exam	Performed	Scheduled	N/A	Refused
Breast Exam				
Mammogram				
Pap Test				
Prostate exam				
Testicular exam				
Digital rectal with stool guaiac				
Flexible Sigmoidoscopy/Colonoscopy				
Bone Density				

Immunizations

Immunizations current: ☐ Yes ☐ No

Vaccine	Given	Planned	Refused
Td			
Hepatitis B			
Influenza			
Pneumonia			
Other:			

Lab/Studies Ordered

☐ CXR   ☐ Lipids   ☐ Creat/BUN   ☐ HbA$_1$C
☐ ECG   ☐ CBC/diff   ☐ LFTs   ☐ TSH
           ☐ Electrolytes ☐ FBS   ☐ UA/UC

☐ Other:

Health Counseling (check if discussed, describe any intervention)

☐ Smoking cessation _____

☐ Alcohol/Drug Use _____

☐ Diet/Weight _____

☐ Vitamins/Calcium _____

☐ Periodic Dental/Vision care _____

☐ Exercise/Sleep _____

☐ Sun exposure _____

☐ Seatbelts/Helmets _____

☐ Stress/Family issues _____

☐ Safety: Weapons/ Domestic Violence _____

☐ BSE/TSE _____

☐ Sexual issues/risks _____

☐ Contraception _____

☐ Living Will/Power of atty/DNR_____

*Adapted from Loretz, L. (2005). *Primary care tools for clinicians.* St. Louis: Elsevier.

_____

Provider's Signature   Date

☐ Note dictated/written

NOTES

CHAPTER
29

The Complete Physical Assessment: Infant, Young Child, and Adolescent

PURPOSE

This chapter presents the methods of integrating the health history and physical examination of those of varying ages. You will note specific developmental and behavioral items to address.

READING ASSIGNMENT

Jarvis: *Physical Examination and Health Assessment*, 9th ed., Chapter 29, pp. 785–794.

CLINICAL OBJECTIVES

1. Demonstrate skills of inspection, percussion, palpation, and auscultation.

2. Demonstrate correct use of instruments, including assembly, manipulation of component parts, and positioning of the patient.

3. Use appropriate terminology and correctly pronounce medical terminology with the clinical instructor and adapt it for the patient and caregiver.

4. Choreograph the complete examination in a systematic manner, including integration of certain regional assessments throughout the examination (e.g., skin, musculoskeletal).

5. Coordinate procedures to limit position changes for the examiner and patient.

6. Describe accurately the findings of the examination, including normal and abnormal findings.

7. Demonstrate appropriate infection control measures.

8. Recognize and maintain the privacy and dignity of the patient.
   a. Adequately explain what is being done in an age-appropriate manner.
   b. Consider the patient's and caregiver's anxiety and fears.
   c. Consider your own verbal and nonverbal communication.
   d. Demonstrate confidence, empathy, and a gentle manner.
   e. Acknowledge and apologize for any discomfort caused.
   f. Provide for privacy and warmth at all times.
   g. Determine comfort level, pausing if patient becomes tired.
   h. Wash hands and don gloves appropriately.
   i. Allow adequate time for each step.
   j. Briefly summarize findings to patient and caregiver, and thank patient and caregiver for their time.

INSTRUCTIONS

If your clinical instructor has arranged for you to perform a complete health assessment on an infant or young child, please review the instructions on p. 262 of the preceding chapter. Please review the age-appropriate considerations found throughout Jarvis: *Physical Examination and Health Assessment*, 9th ed.

Following this, you will find age-appropriate forms for assessment findings: Pediatric Initial Health Questionnaire to be completed with the caregiver; 0- to 1-month Well-Child Visit; 5-Year Well-Child Visit; and 15- to 17-Year Well Visit. For each form, note the age-specific points for Daily Activities, Health History, Development, and Anticipatory Guidance, in addition to the examination findings. If you do not perform these examinations, find a partner in your laboratory group and discuss these points thoroughly. State the rationale for including each point.

Pediatric Initial Health Questionnaire*

Date of Visit: _____

Your Name: _____   Relationship to Child: _____

Child's Name: _____   Preferred name/Nickname: _____

THIS FORM IS FOR MEDICAL RECORD USE ONLY AND WILL REMAIN CONFIDENTIAL. PLEASE ANSWER EACH QUESTION TO THE BEST OF YOUR ABILITY.

Vital Information

Child's Birth date _____

Birthplace: City/State _____

Hospital _____   Other _____

Primary Caregiver 1: _____   Birth date: _____

Relationship to child: _____

Occupation: _____

Primary Caregiver 2 (if applicable): _____   Birth date: _____

Relationship to child: _____

Occupation: _____

Names of brothers and sisters   Birth dates

_____

_____

_____

_____

Was child adopted? ☐ Yes ☐ No   At what age? _____

If adopted, country of origin _____

Religious Preference _____

Pregnancy

Number of pregnancies before this one: _____

How long was this pregnancy? _____ weeks

How many months pregnant when prenatal care was begun? _____

Were there any of the following illnesses or problems?

☐ Rubella (measles)   ☐ Accident/injury   ☐ Bleeding

☐ High blood pressure   ☐ Swelling   ☐ Gestational diabetes

☐ Excessive weight gain ☐ Other infections

Explain: _____

Medicines or drugs used during pregnancy: _____

_____

_____

Smoking while pregnant: ☐ Yes ☐ No

If yes, how many packs per day _____

Alcohol while pregnant: ☐ None ☐ <1 per week ☐ >1 per week

Birth

How long was labor? _____   Was labor induced? _____

At delivery (check all that apply):

☐ Breech (feet or bottom first)   ☐ Cesarean section ☐ VBAC

☐ Breathed and cried immediately ☐ Resuscitated   ☐ Oxygen

Did baby require:

☐ special nursery ☐ blood transfusion ☐ antibiotics ☐ lights

Did baby have:

☐ breathing problems ☐ Jaundice ☐ other _____

At birth:

Weight: _____   Length: _____   Apgar score _____

Discharge weight: _____   Length of hospital stay: _____

Describe any problems: _____

_____

_____

Living Situation

Who does the child live with: _____

Other members of household: _____

Age of home or apartment: _____   Any pets? _____

Has any parent, brother, or sister died? _____   Who? _____

Cause of death _____   Age _____

Please check the box of your child's blood relatives who have ever had any of the following conditions; circle examples in parentheses or write in name of disease, if known:	Father	Mother	Father's side	Mother's side	Siblings
Headaches (migraine, cluster, tension)					
Eye Disease (blindness, tumor, glaucoma)					
Ear Disease (deafness, infections, defects)					
Allergies (eczema, hay fever)					
Lung Disease (asthma, cystic fibrosis, bronchitis) . .					
Tuberculosis					
High Blood Pressure					
High Cholesterol					
Heart Attack (age _____)					
Heart Disease					
Anemia (Sickle Cell, other)					
Bleeding Disorders (hemophilia)					
Stomach or Duodenal Ulcers					
Liver or Gallbladder Disease (hepatitis)					
Intestinal Disease (colitis, polyps)					
Kidney Disease (nephritis, cysts, stones)					
Diabetes (Type_____)					
Thyroid Problems (goiter, nodules, hyper-, hypo-) . .					
Bone or Joint Disease (arthritis, osteoporosis)					
Muscle Weakness or Dystrophy					
Seizure Disorder (epilepsy)					
Neurologic Disorder					
Learning Disability					
Mental Retardation (Down syndrome, other)					
Mental Illness (depression, anxiety, other)					
Alcoholism or Drug Abuse					
Birth Defects (cleft lip, other deformity)					
Obesity					
Cancer: Blood cancer . . . . . (age___)					
Colon cancer . . . . . (age___)					
Breast cancer . . . . . (age___)					
Ovarian or cervical cancer (age___)					
Other cancer					
(Specify type and age_____)					

*Adapted from Loretz, L. (2005). *Primary care tools for clinicians.* St. Louis: Elsevier.

Pediatric Initial Health Questionnaire - 2*

Nutrition in Infancy

Feeding: Breast ❑   Duration _____ months/weeks

         Formula ❑   Type _____

❑ Vitamins   ❑ Fluoride   ❑ Iron   ❑ Uses pacifier

Problems: ❑ Vomiting   ❑ Colic   ❑ Diarrhea   ❑ Allergies

Solid foods: Age when started _____   Intolerances _____

Growth and Development

At what age did your child:

Sit alone _____   Walk alone _____   Feed self_____

Talk (2-3-word sentences) _____   Dress self _____

Toilet trained: Day _____   Night _____

School-age child: Current grade _____   Days missed this year _____

School problems: ❑ reading, writing   ❑ behavior   ❑ special needs

Are there any behavior problems at home?   ❑ Yes   ❑ No

Please describe: _____

_____

_____

_____

Medical History

Please check the diseases that your child has had and give age:

❑ Measles, Rubella _____   ❑ Anemia _____

❑ Mumps _____   ❑ Heart Disease _____

❑ Chickenpox _____   ❑ Allergies/Hay fever _____

❑ Whooping cough _____   ❑ Eczema _____

❑ Scarlet fever _____   ❑ Asthma _____

❑ Rheumatic fever _____   ❑ Pneumonia _____

❑ Convulsions/Seizures _____   ❑ Hepatitis _____

❑ Strep throat _____   ❑ Ear Infection _____

❑ Other illnesses _____

Has your child ever been injured?   ❑ Yes   ❑ No   Age _____

Injury _____

Any fractures?   ❑ Yes   ❑ No   Which bone(s)? _____

Any loss of consciousness or concussion?   ❑ Yes   ❑ No

Any accidental poisoning?   ❑ Yes   ❑ No   Age ___   Substance _____

Has your child ever had surgery?   ❑ Yes   ❑ No   Age _____

Type of operation _____

Has your child ever been hospitalized other than for

the above?   ❑ Yes   ❑ No

Describe:_____

Has your child ever had a blood transfusion?   ❑ Yes   ❑ No   Age ____

Does your child take any medications regularly?   ❑ Yes   ❑ No

Please list:_____

_____

_____

_____

Does your child take any of the following:

❑ Vitamins   ❑ Food supplements _____

Has your child worn:

❑ Glasses   ❑ Contact lenses   ❑ Dental braces   ❑ Leg braces

❑ Corrective shoes   ❑ Orthotics in shoes   ❑ Other braces

Is your child allergic to any medications?   ❑ Yes   ❑ No

If yes, please list the medication and child's reaction. _____

_____

_____

Is your child allergic to any foods?   ❑ Yes   ❑ No

If yes, please list the food and child's reaction. _____

_____

_____

Does your child have any other allergies?   ❑ Yes   ❑ No

If yes, please list the allergy and child's reaction. _____

_____

_____

Please check if your child has had:

❑ Frequent headaches   ❑ Crossed eyes

❑ Trouble hearing   ❑ More than two earaches a year

❑ Stuffy nose most of time   ❑ Frequent nosebleeds

❑ Chronic cough   ❑ More than 6 colds a year

❑ Heart murmur   ❑ Shortness of breath with exercise

❑ Frequent stomachaches   ❑ Constant or frequent fatigue

❑ Poor appetite   ❑ Frequent diarrhea or constipation

❑ Bloody, red, or brown urine   ❑ Frequent urination or accidents

❑ Joint pains or swelling   ❑ Frequent bed-wetting after age 5

❑ Inability to get to sleep   ❑ Dizziness or fainting spells

❑ Excessive thirst   ❑ Frequent nightmares or sleepwalking

❑ Signs of sexual   ❑ Excessive weight gain
    development before age 9

Other concerns: _____

_____

_____

Immunizations & Screenings

Please give approximate dates for each immunization, if known:

Series	#1	#2	#3	#4	#5
DtaP/DT					
Tetanus booster		■	■	■	■
Polio IPV/OPV			■		■
MMR			■	■	
Hib				■	
Hepatitis B				■	
Pneumococcal				■	
Varicella			■		
Meningococcal		■			
Influenza					
Hepatitis A			■		
HPV			■		
Rotavirus			■	■	■
COVID-19					

Please give approximate dates for the following, if done:

Test	No	Yes	Date(s)	Result
Lead blood test				
TB skin test				
Vision exam				
Hearing test				
Hemoglobin blood test				
Urine test				

*Adapted from Loretz L. (2005). Primary care tools for clinicians. St. Louis: Elsevier.

0- to 1-Month Well-Child Visit*

Date of Visit: _____

Child's Name: _____   Nickname: _____

Address: _____

Telephone: _____

Date of Birth: _____   Age: _____   Sex: ☐ Male ☐ Female

Provider: _____

Informant: _____

Relationship to child:_____

Interpreter present: ☐ Yes   ☐ No

Language _____

Measurements

Ht _____ _____ % Wt _____ _____ % OFC _____ _____ %

Temp _____   Pulse _____   Resp _____

Birth Data

Ht _____   Wt _____   OFC _____   Gest Age _____   Wks

L&D record on baby's chart?   ☐ Yes   ☐ No

Significant prenatal history on baby's chart?   ☐ Yes   ☐ No

Hepatitis B vaccine given in nursery?   ☐ Yes   ☐ No

Newborn Metabolic Screening

☐ Normal   ☐ Abnormal (specify):

Vision/Hearing

Newborn Hearing Screening

☐ Normal   ☐ Not screened   ☐ Abnormal (specify):

Vision concerns   ☐ No   ☐ Yes (explain)_____

Hearing concerns   ☐ No   ☐ Yes (explain)_____

Child Health History

Family/social history (refer to chart)   ☐ Completed   ☐ Updated

Parental concerns:_____

_____

Recent injury/illness/surgery/hospitalizations:

Allergies and reaction: _____

Medications: _____

Review of Systems

	N	AB
HEENT (eye discharge, thrush)		
Skin (rashes)		
CV (color)		
Resp (wheezing)		
GI (projectile vomiting/stools)		
GU (pain/stream/frequency)		
Neuromuscular (moves all extremities equally)		

Remainder of review of systems (unlisted) negative ☐

Daily Activities

Nutrition/Elimination

☐ Breast milk   # feedings/day _____

☐ Formula   # feedings/amount _____

☐ Iron/vitamins

Medication name/dose _____

stools/day _____   # voids/day _____

Sleep (arrangements/patterns) _____

Hygiene (cord/circ care)_____

Who does the child live with? _____

Daycare (if applicable). _____

Other caregivers. _____

Stresses for Caregivers _____

Environmental Risks—*Check if present*

☐ Lead risk   ☐ Guns in house/bldg   ☐ TB exposure

☐ Alcohol use in house/bldg   ☐ Housing inadequate   ☐ Domestic violence

☐ Smokers in house/bldg   ☐ Drug use in house/bldg   ☐ Other

Identified risks _____

Family and community resources.

_____

Mental Health/Behavior Risks:

☐ No concerns

☐ Concerns (explain) _____

Observation of parent/child interaction:

☐ Appropriate

☐ Not appropriate (explain)_____

Other:

Development

Personal/Social/Cognitive	N	AB
• Regards face		
• Smiles responsively		
Fine motor/adaptive		
• Follows to midline		
Language		
• Vocalizes		
• Responds to sound		
• "Ooo/aah"		
Gross motor		
• Lifts head 45°		
Breastfeeding		
• Latch-on/positioning		
• Quality of suck		

☐ Development screening tool, if used:

Name of tool _____

_____

☐ By observation/exam/ parent report. No tool used.

*Adapted from Loretz, L. (2005). *Primary care tools for clinicians*. St. Louis: Elsevier.

0- to 1-Month Well-Child Visit - 2*

Child's Name: _____

Physical Exam

WDL= within defined limits Ab = abnormal (check appropriate box)	WDL	Ab
1. General appearance:		
2. Skin: color • character • birthmarks • jaundice		
3. Nodes: cervical • axillary • inguinal		
4. Head: shape • AF size • PF size • sutures • scalp		
5. Eyes: tear ducts • EOM • red reflex • corneal light reflex • PERL • lids		
6. Vision: follows light, movement		
7. Ears: pinna • canals • TMs		
8. Hearing: responds to loud sound		
9. Nose: patency • nares		
10. Mouth: gums • tongue • frenulum • palate • mucosa • throat		
11. Neck: position • ROM • thyroid		
12. Chest: shape • symmetry • lungs • respiration rate • retractions		
13. CV: rate • rhythm • S_1 • S_2 • murmur • femoral pulses		
14. ABD: contour • umbilicus • liver • spleen • masses • anus • bowel sounds		
15. GU: ♀ labia • vaginal mucosa • discharge ♂ circ • penis • testes • hydrocele • hernia		
16. MS: ROM • Ortolani • spine		
17. Neuro: jitteriness • head control • posture • tone • DTRs • clonus • Babinski • Moro • TNR • suck • root • grasp • stepping crossed • extension • positive supporting		

Document Abnormals (by number):

Assessment

❏ Child well

❏ Additional diagnoses (specify):

Plan
Immunizations

Are immunizations on schedule? ❏ Yes ❏ No

*If not, catch-up plan?*_____

Vaccine education provided? ❏ Yes ❏ No

Response. _____

Immunizations ordered/given: ❏ Hepatitis B ❏ PCV

❏ DTaP ❏ IPV ❏ Hib ❏ Other _____

If immunization(s) due but not given, explain:

Anticipatory Guidance

✔ *Topics discussed*

Nutrition		
No solids		Spitting up/vomiting
Always hold to feed Never prop bottle		Encourage continuation of breastfeeding (if appropriate) on demand
No honey before one year		

Safety		
Car seat		Supervise sibling and pet interaction
Never leave unattended		Safe crib/sleep on back
Support head and neck		Smoke detectors
Sun protection		No smoking around baby
Hot water temp < 125° F		

Parenting		
Show affection to baby		Diarrhea care
Interact by responding to cry		Thermometer use
Never punish, jerk, or shake		When to call office
Day care concerns		Bulb syringe for congestion
Fever care		Infection risk reduction
Skin care		

Other:

Laboratory Tests (none routinely required at this age)

Additional Plan

Referrals

❏ *Smoking cessation class*

❏ *Breastfeeding class/support group*

❏ *Other:*

❏ *Encouraged smoking cessation*

❏ *Need for financial assistance*

❏ *Social services*

❏ *Requires additional health education*

❏ *Schedule 2-month visit*

Provider signature

❏ Note dictated

*Adapted from Loretz, L. (2005). *Primary care tools for clinicians.* St. Louis: Elsevier.

5-Year Well-Child Visit*

Date of Visit: _____

Child's Name: _____   *Nickname:* _____

Address: _____

Telephone: _____

Date of Birth: _____   *Age:* _____   *Sex:* ☐ *Male* ☐ *Female*   *Gender* _____

Provider: _____

Informant: _____   *Interpreter present:* ☐ *Yes*   ☐ *No*

Relationship to Child: _____   *Language* _____

Measurements

Ht _____ _____ %   Wt _____ _____ %   BP _____

Temp _____   Pulse _____   Resp _____

Vision/Hearing

Hearing								Vision
Right Ear				**Left Ear**				Glasses ☐ Yes ☐ No
500	1000	2000	4000	500	1000	2000	4000	Right eye /
								Left eye /

Right eye   /
Left eye   /
☐ Normal ☐ Abnormal ☐ Question validity/retest
Comments:
☐ Normal
☐ Refer to eye clinic
☐ Question validity/ retest

Vision concerns   ☐ No   ☐ Yes (explain) _____

Hearing concerns   ☐ No   ☐ Yes (explain) _____

Child Health History

Family/social history (refer to chart)   ☐ Completed   ☐ Updated

Parental concerns: _____

_____

Recent injury/illness/surgery/hospitalizations:

_____

Allergies: _____

Medications: _____

Review of Systems

	N	AB
HEENT		
Skin (rashes)		
CV (activity level)		
Resp (wheezing)		
GI (vomiting/stools)		
GU (pain on voiding/stream/bedwetting)		
Neuromuscular (headaches, limb pain)		

Remainder of review of systems (unlisted) negative ☐

Daily Activities

Nutrition: (variety/misses meals/wt concern) _____

Milk: (whole, 2%, 1%, skim) _____

Sleep: bedtime _____   awakes _____

Child Health History (continued)

Dental: (brushing frequency) _____

Last dental visit: _____

Exercise: _____

Recreation/Hobbies/TV: _____

Environmental Risks—Check if assessed

☐ Lead risk   ☐ Guns in house/bldg   ☐ TB exposure

☐ Alcohol use in house/bldg   ☐ Housing inadequate   ☐ Domestic violence

☐ Smokers in house/bldg   ☐ Drug use in house/bldg   ☐ Other

Identified risks _____

Family and community resources.

_____

Mental Health/Behavior Risks:

☐ No concerns

☐ Concerns (explain) _____

Observation of parent/child interaction:

☐ Appropriate

☐ Not appropriate (explain) _____

Other:

Development

Personal/social/cognitive	N	AB
• Dresses without help		
• Plays make believe		
• Plays board games		
Language		
• Names 4 colors		
• Counts 5 blocks		
• Understands 4 prepositions		
• Able to define 5 words		
• Speech all understandable		
Gross motor		
• Balances each foot 5 sec		
• Heel-to-toe walk		
Fine motor/adaptive		
• Copies square demonstrated		
• Copies +		
• Recognizes some letters		
• Draws a person with 6 parts		

☐ Developmental screening tool, if used:
Name of tool _____
_____

☐ By observation/exam/ parent report. No tool used.

*Adapted from Loretz, L. (2005). *Primary care tools for clinicians.* St. Louis: Elsevier.

5-Year Well-Child Visit - 2*

Child's Name: _____   Medical Record Number: _____

Physical Exam

WDL = within defined limits Ab = abnormal (check appropriate box)	WDL	Ab
1. General appearance:		
2. Skin: color • character • birthmarks		
3. Nodes: cervical • axillary • inguinal		
4. Head: shape • hair		
5. Eyes: EOM • red reflex • corneal light reflex • PERL • cross cover accommodation • fundi • lids		
6. Ears: pinna • canals • TMs		
7. Nose: patency • nares • turbinates		
8. Mouth: mucosa • tonsils • teeth • throat		
9. Neck: ROM • thyroid		
10. Chest: shape • symmetry • lungs • respiration rate		
11. CV: rate • rhythm • S_1 • S_2 • murmur • femoral pulses		
12. Abd: contour • liver • spleen • masses • anus • bowel sounds		
13. GU: ♀ labia • vaginal mucosa • urethra ♂ penis • testes • hernia		
14. MS: ROM • gait • spine		
15. Neuro: DTRs • clonus • motor strength • sensory		

Document Abnormals (by number):

Assessment

☐ Child well

☐ Additional diagnoses (specify):

Plan
Immunizations

Are immunizations on schedule? ☐ Yes ☐ No

If not, catch-up plan? _____

Vaccine education provided? ☐ Yes ☐ No

Response. _____

Immunizations ordered/given: ☐ Hepatitis B ☐ DTaP ☐ IPV
☐ Hib   ☐ MMR   ☐ Varicella   ☐ Influenza ☐ RV

If immunization(s) due but not given, explain:

Anticipatory Guidance

✔ Topics discussed	
Healthy Habits	

Limit TV	Food choices (friuts, vegetables, grains)
Safety: matches/poisons/guns	Safe after school environment
Safety: water/playground/stranger	Adequate sleep/physical activity
Safety: car seat/seat belt/ bike helmet	Curiosity about sex
	Infection risk reduction
Dental sealants	Eliminate lead risk

Social Competence	
School readiness	Family rules, respect, right from wrong
Praise, encourage	
Knows address and phone number	Anger control/conflict resolution

Family Relationships	
Affection	Know child's friends/families
Sibling relationships	Ethical role model

Other:

Laboratory Tests

☐ **Blood lead** (if never tested)   ☐ **UA** (optional)

☐ **Other**

Dental

☐ **Verbal referral for preventive dental visit**

Additional Plan

Referrals
☐ **Smoking cessation class**
☐ **Other:**

☐ **Encouraged smoking cessation**
☐ **Need for financial assistance/social services**
☐ **Requires additional health education**
☐ **Dental resource information given**
☐ **Schedule 6-year preventive visit**

_____
Provider Signature
☐ Note dictated

*Adapted from Loretz, L. (2005). *Primary care tools for clinicians.* St. Louis: Elsevier.

15- to 17-Year Well Visit*

Date of Visit: _____

Name: _____ Nickname/preferred name: _____

Address: _____

Telephone: _____

Date of Birth: _____ Age: _____ Gender: _____

Preferred pronoun: _____

Provider: _____

Informant (if applicable): _____ Interpreter present: ☐ Yes   ☐ No

Relationship: _____ Language _____

Measurements

Ht _____ _____ % Wt _____ _____ % BP _____

Temp _____ Pulse _____ Resp _____

Vision/Hearing

Vision concerns   ☐ No   ☐ Yes (explain) _____

Last vision screen: _____

☐ Contacts ☐ Glasses

Referral to eye clinic   ☐ Yes ☐ No

Hearing concerns   ☐ No   ☐ Yes (explain) _____

Last hearing screen: _____

Referral for hearing screen   ☐ Yes ☐ No

Health History

Family/social history (refer to chart)   ☐ Completed   ☐ Updated

Adolescent/parental concerns: _____

_____

Recent injury/illness/surgery/hospitalizations:

_____

Allergies: _____

Medications: _____

Review of Systems

	N	AB
HEENT		
Skin (rashes/acne)		
CV (dizziness, chest pain)		
Resp (wheezing)		
GI (vomiting/stools)		
GU (pain/stream)		
Neuromuscular (headaches)		

Remainder of review of systems (unlisted) negative ☐

Daily Activities

Nutrition: (variety/misses meals/wt concern) _____

Milk: (whole, 2%, 1%, skim) _____

Sleep: bedtime _____ awakes _____

Health History (continued)

Dental: _____

Exercise: _____

Recreation/Hobbies/TV: _____

Tobacco/Alcohol/Marijuana/Drugs/Driving: _____

Menstrual Hx (female):

Menarche _____ LMP _____ Regularity _____

Sexual History (activity, partners, birth control, STDs, pregnancy):

_____

Practices self-breast/testicular exam?:   ☐ Yes   ☐ No

Environmental Risks—

☐ Guns in house/bldg   ☐ TB exposure   ☐ Alcohol use in house/bldg

☐ Housing inadequate   ☐ Violence/rape   ☐ Smokers in house/bldg

☐ Drug use in house/bldg   ☐ Other:

Identified risks _____

Social support system:

_____

Mental Health/Behavior Risks:

☐ No concerns

☐ Concerns (explain) _____

Observation of parent/child interaction (if applicable):

☐ Appropriate

☐ Not appropriate (explain) _____

Other: _____

☐ Adolescent risk assessment tool (if used)

Development

	WDL	Ab	Comments:
School (employment) performance/attendance:			
Future plans, college, career			
Family relationships			
Ability to form/maintain peer relationships			
Dating/sexual activity			
Activities or sports involvement			
Emotional stability			

*Adapted from Loretz, L. (2005). *Primary care tools for clinicians.* St. Louis: Elsevier.

15- to 17-Year Well Visit - 2*

Child's Name: _____   Medical Record Number: _____

Physical Exam

WDL= within defined limits Ab = abnormal (check appropriate box)	WDL	Ab
1. General appearance:		
2. Skin: rash • acne		
3. Nodes: cervical • axillary • inguinal		
4. Head: scalp • hair		
5. Eyes: EOM • red reflex • corneal light reflex • PERL • lids		
6. Ears: pinna • canals • TMs		
7. Nose: patency • nares		
8. Mouth: gums • teeth/caries • occlusion • throat		
9. Neck: ROM • thyroid		
10. Chest: lungs • respiration rate		
♀ **Female:** Breasts • Tanner Stage: _____		
♂ **Male:** Gynecomastia		
11. CV: rate • rhythm • S1 • S2 • murmur • femoral pulses		
12. Abd: liver • spleen • masses • bowel sounds		
13. GU: ♀ labia • vaginal mucosa		
♂ penis • testes • hernia		
Tanner Stage: _____		
14. MS: ROM • spine • gait		
15. Neuro: DTRs • coordination • sensory • motor		

Document Abnormals (by number):

Assessment

☐ Adolescent well

☐ Additional Diagnoses (specify):

Plan

Immunizations

Are immunizations on schedule?   ☐ Yes ☐ No

If not, catch-up plan?_____

Immunizations ordered/given: ☐ Hepatitis B   ☐ Td   ☐ IPV
☐ MMR   ☐ Varicella   ☐ Meningococcal   ☐ HPV ☐ Influenza

If immunization(s) due but not given, explain:

Anticipatory Guidance

✔ *Topics discussed*

Healthy Habits

Self-protection	Alcohol
Weight management/food choices	Infection risk reduction
Sexual feelings	Adequate sleep/exercise
How to say no, abstinence	Athletic conditioning, weight training
Birth control, STDs, safe sex	Handle anger/conflict resolution
Tobacco	Weapons
Illicit drugs	Seat belts, bike helmets
Marijuana	Stress, nervousness, sadness

Social Competence

Family time	Social activities/groups/sports
Peer pressure/peer refusal	Respect parents' limits/consequences

Responsibility

Respect others	Rules, chores, responsibility
Ethical role model	Religious, cultural, volunteer activities

School Achievement

Attendance, homework	Frustrations, dropping out
Future plans, college, career	

Other:

Laboratory Tests

☐ **Hgb/Hct** (once in adolescence for menstruating females) _____

☐ **Urinalysis** (once in adolescence) _____

☐ **Other** (STD, Pap, TB, cholesterol if at risk) _____

Dental

☐ **Verbal referral for preventive dental visit**

Additional Plan

Referrals
☐ **Smoking cessation class**
☐ **Other:**

☐ **Encouraged smoking cessation**

☐ **Need for financial assistance/social services**

☐ **Requires additional health education**

☐ **Dental resource information given**

☐ **Schedule visit in 1 to 2 years**

Provider Signature

☐ Note dictated

*Adapted from Loretz, L. (2005). *Primary care tools for clinicians.* St. Louis: Elsevier.

CHAPTER 30

Bedside Assessment and Electronic Documentation

PURPOSE

This chapter presents the methods of integrating the regional examinations into the hospital setting. Selection and sequencing of the techniques provide an assessment that is efficient, thorough, and consistent with the assessments performed by nurses in the course of 24-hour care.

READING ASSIGNMENT

Jarvis: *Physical Examination and Health Assessment,* 9th ed., Chapter 30, pp. 795–802.

Suggested reading:
Oren, G. T., Lazzara, E. H., Keebler, J. R., et al. (2021). Dissecting communication barriers in healthcare: A path to enhancing communication resiliency, reliability, and patient safety. *J Patient Saf, 17*(8), e1465–e1471.

CLINICAL OBJECTIVES

1. Demonstrate skills of inspection, palpation, and auscultation.

2. Demonstrate correct use of instruments, including assembly, manipulation of component parts, and positioning of the patient.

3. Use appropriate terminology and correctly pronounce medical terminology with clinical instructor and adapt for patient.

4. Choreograph the examination in a systematic manner, including the integration of certain regional assessments throughout the examination (e.g., skin, musculoskeletal).

5. Coordinate procedures to limit position changes for examiner and patient.

6. Describe accurately the findings of the examination, including normal and abnormal findings.

7. Demonstrate appropriate infection control measures.

8. Recognize and maintain the privacy and dignity of the patient.
   a. Adequately explain what is being done while limiting small talk.
   b. Consider the patient's anxiety and fears.
   c. Consider your own facial expressions and comments.
   d. Demonstrate confidence, empathy, and a gentle manner.

e. Acknowledge and apologize for any discomfort caused.
f. Provide for privacy and warmth at all times.
g. Determine comfort level, pausing if the patient becomes tired.
h. Wash hands and don gloves appropriately.
i. Allow adequate time for each step.
j. Briefly summarize findings and thank patient.
9. Complete all procedures with attention to specifics of the technique, which allows clear and consistent replication of the procedures by others assessing the same patient.

INSTRUCTIONS

As with other assessments, this version of the head-to-toe examination requires a great deal of practice before you will feel truly confident. The good news about this sequence is that it is directly applicable to any inpatient clinical sites that you attend. If you are already attending clinicals, use any available time to practice this sequence on real patients.

You are responsible for recruiting a friend or classmate to act as your patient for this examination. You will have 20 minutes for this examination, not including setup. If you have practiced the individual regional assessments thoroughly and can complete this sequence three times, you will be able to complete it satisfactorily within the time allotted.

Prepare the examination setting. Arrange the lighting, furniture, and bed to allow for the most efficient and comfortable activity for yourself and your patient. Think carefully about the functions of the patient's hospital bed. It can be useful to raise the bed closer to your eyes and stethoscope, but you cannot expect the patient to get out of bed safely from that height. Position sheets, drapes, and blankets strategically to achieve the proper balance of modesty, efficiency, and comfort.

Gather and arrange your equipment before you begin. The following items are needed for this sequence, but your instructor may modify the equipment list slightly for your individual class or exercise:

Water (in a cup)	Ruler with millimeters
Watch with a second hand	Oxygen equipment (as indicated by your instructor)
Stethoscope	Doppler (as indicated by your instructor)
Blood pressure cuff	Bladder scanner (as indicated by your instructor)
Pulse oximeter	Standardized scales to calculate patient's fall risk and risk for skin breakdown
Penlight	Documentation forms (as included here, or provided by your instructor)

Verify with your instructor whether you should submit documentation of this assessment after your demonstration or documentation that you have prepared to reflect one of your earlier practice sessions.

Good luck!

COMPLETE INPATIENT REASSESSMENT

Date _____

Examiner _____

Patient _____ Age _____ Gender _____

Occupation _____ Reason for admission _____

Introduction
1. Check for flags or markers at doorway.
2. Introduce yourself.
3. Perform hand hygiene.
4. Make eye contact.
5. Offer water (if appropriate).
6. Check name band.
7. Ask appropriate interview questions, including current pain.
8. Elevate the bed to appropriate height.

General Appearance
1. Facial expression _____
2. Body position _____
3. Level of consciousness _____
4. Skin color _____
5. Nutritional status _____
6. Speech: articulation, pattern, content appropriate _____
7. Hearing _____
8. Personal hygiene _____

Measurement
1. Temperature _____
2. Pulse _____
3. Respiration _____
4. Blood pressure _____
5. Pulse oximetry _____
6. Weight on admission or daily weight, if indicated _____
7. Rate pain level on a scale of 0 to 10; note the ability to tolerate pain _____
8. Pain reassessment, if appropriate _____

Neurologic System
1. Glasgow Coma Scale:
   Eye opening _____
   Motor response _____
   Verbal response _____
2. Pupil size in millimeters and reaction
   a. R _____ b. L _____
3. Upper muscle strength
   a. R _____ b. L _____

4. Lower muscle strength

   a. R _____   b. L _____

5. Any ptosis, facial droop _____

6. Sensation (if indicated) _____

7. Communication _____

8. Ability to swallow _____

Respiratory

1. Oxygen by mask, nasal cannula; check fitting _____

2. Fio_2 _____

3. Respiratory effort _____

4. Auscultate breath sounds:

Anterior lobes:

   Right upper _____

   Left upper _____

   Right middle _____

   Right lower _____

   Left lower _____

Posterior lobes:

   Left upper _____

   Right upper _____

   Left lower _____

   Right lower _____

Cough and deep breathe; any mucus? Check the color and amount. _____

Educate on the use of incentive spirometry, if ordered.

Cardiovascular System

1. Auscultate rhythm at apex: regular or irregular? _____

2. Check apical versus radial pulse

3. Assess heart sounds in all auscultatory areas: first with diaphragm, repeat with bell.

4. Check capillary refill _____

5. Check pretibial edema

   a. R _____   **b.** L _____

6. Palpate posterior tibial pulse

   a. R _____   **b.** L _____

7. Palpate dorsalis pedis pulse

   a. R _____   **b.** L _____

8. Pulses by Doppler, if appropriate _____

9. IV fluid and rate, if present _____

Skin (may be integrated with rest of assessment)

1. Color _____

2. Temperature _____

3. Skin turgor _____

4. Note any lesions; check for any dressings _____

5. Note skin around IV site _____

6. Standardized scale regarding skin breakdown _____

7. Settings and application of specialized surface, if present _____

Abdomen

1. Contour of abdomen: flat, rounded, protuberant _____
2. Bowel sounds _____
3. Check any drains, if present; note amount and color of drainage _____
4. Inquire if passing flatus or stool _____
5. Can patient tolerate current diet? Should diet be advanced or changed? _____

Genitourinary

1. Inquire if voiding regularly _____
2. Urine for color, clarity, quantity _____
3. Bladder scan, if indicated _____

Activity

1. If on bed rest, check head of bed, risk for skin breakdown _____
2. Any SCDs or TED hose? SCDs must be hooked up/on _____
3. Transfer to chair or ambulate (if appropriate) _____
4. Note any assistance needed, how movement is tolerated, distance walked to chair, ability to turn __
   _____
5. Need for ambulatory aid or equipment _____
6. Standardized fall scale _____

Closure

1. Return bed to lowest position.
2. Verify that brakes are locked.
3. Make sure appropriate side rails are up.
4. Ensure call light is within reach.
5. Verify bed alarm, if indicated.
6. Thank the patient and let them know the plan for the day (e.g., any upcoming tests; when you will return).
7. Initiate or continue appropriate plan of care.
8. Document assessment.

The SBAR framework (Situation, Background, Assessment, Recommendation) is used in many hospital units to improve verbal communication and reduce medical errors. Practice with the SBAR form on the next page. It will keep your message concise and focused on the patient, yet give your colleague enough information to grasp the current situation and make a decision.

TELEMETRY UNIT SBAR

S	Patient name	Age	Allergies	Physician
	Room number	Admit date		Attending
	1 Dx	2 Dx	Code status	Consultants
	C/O		Advanced directive on chart?	

B	History			Isolation	Core Measures
	Surgery	Surgeon		Restraints	CHF MI PNA
	Anesthesia	Anesthesiologist	EBL	Fall risk	Vaccine - PNA Flu

A	Cardiac: BP/HR/Peripheral pulses/Edema/Heart sounds		Pain/sedation
	Current rhythm		Pain scale
	Daily wt?		Location
	DVT prophylaxis		Meds type and last dose

Pulmonary: Breath sounds/Secretions/SpO$_2$/UPAs/PIP/ Spontaneous VT & VE	Vent/bipap etc settings	Accu checks A1C
		Frequency
		Last results

GI NG/OGT	Diet GI Prophylaxis	Skin Wounds/drainage
BS Last BM		Staples
		Drains

GU Foley/void	Location
Output	Ducub photo on admission

IV Date inserted	Psych social
Fluids Gtts	

Meds	Pending orders

Na	Cl	BUN	gluc	mg	BNP	Coags INR	Hct	UA	CT CXR
K	Co	Cr	Ca	Phos	D dimer	PTT Next Lab	W Pl	Cultures	MRI Echo
Cardiac enz		1	2	3			Hgb		

R	DC Plan. Is pt informed of plan___24 hour orders reviewed___	Shift goals

Courtesy of Scrubs Magazine, The Nurses Guide to Good Living, at scrubsmag.com.

CHAPTER 31
Pregnancy

PURPOSE

This chapter presents the changes and function of the female genitalia during pregnancy; the methods of inspection and palpation of the internal and external structures, along with the pregnant abdomen; and how to record the assessment accurately.

READING ASSIGNMENT

Jarvis: *Physical Examination and Health Assessment,* 9th ed., Chapter 31, pp. 803-828.

Suggested reading:
MacLean, L. R. -D. (2021). Preconception, pregnancy, birthing, and lactation needs of transgender men. *Nurs Women's Health, 25*(2), 129–138.

GLOSSARY

Study the following terms after completing the reading assignment. You should be able to cover the definition on the right and define the term out loud.

Amniocentesis .... the transabdominal perforation of the amniotic sac for the purpose of obtaining a sample of amniotic fluid; helps identify genetic disorders, such as Down syndrome or sickle cell anemia

Amniotic fluid .... fluid in the sac surrounding the fetus in the person's uterus

Anemia .... condition in which the number of red blood cells/mm³ is less than normal

Antenatal testing .... consists of monitoring fetal growth, amniotic fluid volume, umbilical cord Doppler blood flow, and fetal monitoring via non-stress or contraction stress testing using a fetal monitor

Antepartum .... the period occurring before childbirth

Blastocyst .... the fertilized ovum; a specialized layer of cells around the blastocyst that becomes the placenta

Chadwick sign .... bluish purple discoloration of the cervix during pregnancy due to venous congestion

Chestfeeding .... feeding an infant from the chest

Chloasma .... the "mask of pregnancy"; butterfly-shaped pigmentation of the face

Chorionic villi sampling .... transabdominal or transvaginal sampling of trophoblastic tissue surrounding the gestational sac

Colostrum .... the precursor to milk that contains minerals, proteins, and antibodies

Corpus luteum .... "yellow body"; a structure on the surface of the ovary that is formed by the remaining cells in the follicle; acts as a short-lived endocrine organ that produces progesterone to help maintain the pregnancy in its early stages

Diastasis recti .... separation of the abdominal muscles during pregnancy, returning to normalcy following pregnancy

Engagement .... refers to when the widest diameter of the presenting part has descended into the pelvic inlet

Fetal lie .... orientation of the fetal spine to the pregnant person's spine

Goodell sign .... the softening of the cervix due to increased vascularity, congestion, and edema

Hegar sign .... occurs when the uterus becomes globular in shape, softens, and flexes easily over the cervix

Leopold maneuver .... external palpation of the pregnant abdomen to determine fetal lie, presentation, attitude, and position

Linea nigra .... a median line of the abdomen that becomes pigmented (darkens) during pregnancy

Morning sickness .... nausea and vomiting of pregnancy that usually begins between weeks 4 and 6, peaks between weeks 8 and 12, and resolves between weeks 14 and 16

Mucus plug .... mucus that forms a thick barrier in the cervix that is expelled at various times before or during labor

Multigravida .... a pregnant person who has previously carried a fetus to the point of viability

Multipara .... a person who has had two or more viable pregnancies and deliveries

Nägele rule .... a rule for calculating the estimated date of delivery; add 7 days to first day of the last menstrual period and subtract 3 months

Nuchal translucency .... the amount of fluid behind the neck of the fetus; also known as the nuchal fold. Fetuses at risk for Down syndrome tend to have a higher amount of fluid.

Position .... the location of a fetal part to the right or left of the pregnant person's pelvis

Postpartum .... the period occurring after delivery

Presentation .... the part of the fetus that is entering the pelvis first

Primigravida .... a person pregnant for the first time

Primipara .... a person who has had one pregnancy and delivery

Striae gravidarum .... "stretch marks" that may be seen on the abdomen and breasts (in areas of weight gain) during pregnancy

Ultrasound (US) image .... the use of sound waves to examine the fetus, amniotic fluid, and placenta in the uterus

Umbilical cord .... a ropelike structure containing blood vessels that connect the fetus to the placenta, carrying oxygen and nutrients from the pregnant person to the fetus and waste products away from the fetus

VBAC .... vaginal birth after cesarean delivery

STUDY GUIDE

After completing the reading assignment and the media assignment, write or draw the answers in the spaces provided.

1. Describe the function of the placenta.

2. Using Nägele rule, calculate the estimated date of delivery if the LMP is August 22.

3. Give examples of the following signs of pregnancy.

   Presumptive: _____

   Probable: _____

   Positive: _____

4. When can serum hCG be detected in blood? In urine?

5. Describe three physical and physiologic changes that are seen in the:

   First trimester: _____

   Second trimester: _____

   Third trimester: _____

6. Describe the "recommended" weight gain during pregnancy.

7. List the major concerns for teenage pregnancy.

8. List at least three risk factors concerning pregnant people over 35 years old.

9. Discuss how culture and genetics play a role in a person's pregnancy.

10. True or false: Please circle the best answer.

True	False	A person who has had a classic uterine incision is a good candidate for a VBAC.
True	False	A person who is pregnant for the first time is called a *primipara*.
True	False	The fetal period begins after the 9th gestational week.
True	False	Preeclampsia is seen only in the third trimester of pregnancy.
True	False	Vaginal bleeding in pregnancy always indicates a miscarriage.
True	False	Cervical incompetence is always accompanied by painful contractions.

11. What is the importance of fetal movement counting, and when should it be initiated?

12. Describe why it is important to ask pregnant people if they feel safe in their relationships and environment.

13. Label, list the order, and describe the purpose of the following maneuvers.

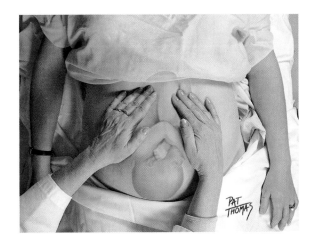

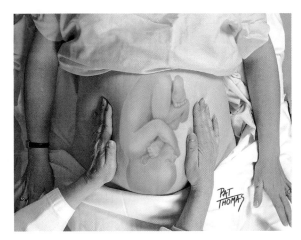

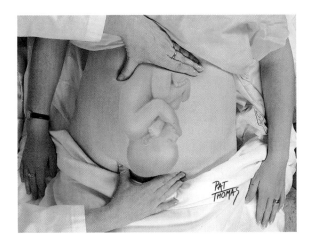

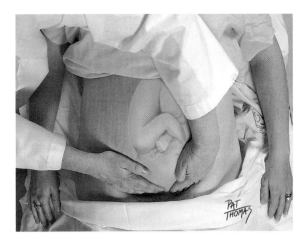

14. Describe the following for this figure.

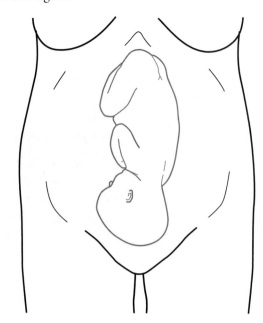

Fetal lie: _____

Fetal presentation: _____

Fetal position: _____

15. List the symptoms of preeclampsia.

16. List at least two reasons why fundal height may be small for gestational age.

17. List at least two reasons why fundal height may be large for gestational age.

18. Describe considerations and additional history questions for transgender men who are pregnant or who wish to become pregnant.

CLINICAL JUDGMENT QUESTIONS

This test is for you to check your own mastery of the content. Answers are provided in Appendix A.

1. During pregnancy, the body undergoes a number of normal physiologic changes to support the growing fetus. Identify normal skin changes that may occur during pregnancy. **Select all that apply.**

   a. Vascular spiders.
   b. Scars along easily accessed veins.
   c. Facial edema.
   d. Butterfly-shaped pigmentation of the face.
   e. Hyperpigmented line down the abdomen.
   f. Nevi that darken during pregnancy.

2. Transgender men:

   a. Should be counseled against becoming pregnant due to the increased risks associated with pregnancy after the gender confirming therapy is initiated.
   b. Should be counseled that initiation of testosterone therapy is adequate birth control to prevent pregnancy.
   c. Should receive high-quality peripartum care that affirms their gender and supports their emotional, physical, and psychological health.
   d. Should be referred to a reproductive specialist early in a pregnancy to avoid complications related to gender.

3. You are caring for a 5-day-old infant who was admitted to the NICU in the immediate postpartum period for unstable temperature, feeding difficulty, and seizures. The infant's mother is a 21-year-old with a 3-year history of opioid prescription abuse and a 1-year history of heroin use. Given your knowledge of opioid use in pregnancy, you know that:

   a. the infant is likely suffering from neonatal abstinence syndrome due to withdrawal from opioid medications.
   b. the mother will need to be treated for her drug addiction before the infant can be discharged to go home.
   c. the infant will likely require quiet time in the infant warmer because holding an infant with neonatal abstinence syndrome is not recommended.
   d. the infant will require opioid pain medications to curb the withdrawal symptoms but should be discharged soon.

4. Identify the following as presumptive, probable, or positive signs of pregnancy.

	Presumptive	Probable	Positive
Amenorrhea			
Enlarged uterus			
Fatigue			
FHTs			
Nausea			
Breast tenderness			
Cardiac activity on US			

5. Choose from the words below. Words may be used more than once or not at all.

The nurse should recognize that _____ and _____ are classic symptoms of preeclampsia, but _____ is not required for diagnosis. Onset and worsening of symptoms may be _____ and rapid intervention is necessary. _____ is a serious variant of preeclampsia.

Select from these words:

hypertension	elevated liver enzymes	sudden	eclampsia
hypotension	proteinuria	insipidus	HELLP

6–8. Use the following scenario to answer questions 6–8.

The nurse is caring for a 38-year-old female who is gravida 8, para 8. All spontaneous vaginal deliveries after 38 weeks gestation. She reports a history of preeclampsia with her last two pregnancies, with no long-term sequelae. She states the preeclampsia occurred "right at the end" of each pregnancy, though she does not remember specific information. She is 5'4" and weighs 225 pounds. Her prepregnancy weight was 180 pounds. She is 36 weeks gestation and is in active labor. Her due date was confirmed by US at 21 weeks gestation. FHTs 155 bpm with normal accelerations. Vital Signs: HR 110 bpm, RR 20 bpm, unlabored, BP 146/98, T 97.5°F. Currently rating pain at 2/10 at rest and 10/10 during contractions. Medical history of PPH with last pregnancy requiring blood transfusion. Routine medications include a prenatal vitamin.

6. Underline the information in the scenario that requires follow-up, may indicate potential risk for complications, or is abnormal.

7. PPH is the leading cause of death in pregnant people. What risk factors does the person described in the scenario have for PPH? **Select all that apply.**

   a. History of PPH.
   b. Cesarean delivery.
   c. Macrosomia.
   d. Multigravidity.
   e. Clotting issues.
   f. Hypertension.
   g. Pain.

8. The patient delivers a 7 lb, 8 oz baby 6 hours after labor began. Three hours after delivery, you notice significant bleeding soaking one pad every 15 minutes and estimate the total blood loss to be >1000 mL throughout the peripartum period. You: **Select all that apply.**

   a. Continue to monitor the patient, watching for any signs of hypovolemia or PPH. Standard postpartum care continues.
   b. Identify that the patient is having a PPH. Begin more frequent uterine massage and contact the provider immediately so that appropriate interventions can begin.
   c. Identify that the patient is at risk for PPH. Continue to monitor bleeding and notify the provider if >1500 mL of blood loss is estimated.
   d. Identify the patient as having a PPH. Avoid uterine massage so as not to disrupt normal uterine function and immediately contact the provider.
   e. Continue monitoring the patient and call the provider if signs of hypovolemia are seen. Continue supportive therapy.

9. Identify whether each of the following pregnancy-related changes are physiologic or pathologic.

	Physiologic	Pathologic
Mammary souffle		
Purulent nipple discharge		
Diastolic murmur 2/6		
Breast enlargement		
Decreased cardiac output		
Blood volume increase by 45%		
Slight hemodilution		
Increased pulse		

SKILLS LABORATORY AND CLINICAL SETTING

You are now ready for the clinical component of the pregnancy examination. Some clinical settings may arrange for a pregnant person to participate, or your practice setting may have available a pregnant teaching mannequin that you can use to practice your skills. If you have a pregnant person available, discuss the methods of examination that will be used. Maintain the patient's comfort and adequate positioning to prevent dizziness, nausea, and hypotension and to maintain adequate uterine blood flow.

Clinical Objectives

1. Demonstrate knowledge of the physical changes related to pregnancy in the first, second, and third trimesters.
2. Demonstrate obtaining a pertinent health history during the first prenatal visit.
3. Demonstrate cultural sensitivity during the examination.
4. Inspect and palpate the pregnant abdomen for uterine size and fetal position.
5. Demonstrate obtaining fetal heart tones.
6. Record the history and physical examination findings accurately; reach an assessment of the health state, estimated gestational age, and fetal position (when appropriate). Develop a plan of care.

Instructions

Prepare the examination setting and gather your equipment. Collect the health history before the person disrobes for the examination. Calculate the EDD. Wash your hands. Practice the steps of the examination on a person in the clinical setting, giving appropriate instructions and explanations as you proceed. Record your findings using the regional write-up sheet that follows. The first section is intended as a worksheet; the last page is intended for your narrative summary recording using the SOAP format. See Chapter 27 for the female genital examination.

NOTES

REGIONAL WRITE-UP—PREGNANT FEMALE

_____

Patient Name   Date

PRENATAL HISTORY QUESTIONNAIRE

Having a healthy baby is a special event. Once a baby is born, families take certain precautions to ensure the baby's health and safety. The unborn child deserves similar care.

QUESTIONNAIRE

The following questions will help in the care of your pregnancy. Please answer these questions as well as you can. All answers will remain private. If you need help answering the questions, please ask your health care provider. The first question relates to your family history. The next 7 questions will be about you, your baby's father, and both your families. When thinking about your families, please include your child (or unborn baby), mother, father, sisters, brothers, grandparents, aunts, uncles, nieces, nephews, and cousins.

Yes   No   1.   Will you be 35 years or older when the baby is due? Age when due: _____ .

Yes   No   2.   Are you and the baby's father related to each other (e.g., cousins)?

Yes   No   3.   Have you had three or more pregnancies that ended in miscarriage?

Yes   No   4.   Have you or the baby's father had a stillborn baby or a baby who died around the time of delivery?

Yes   No   5.   Do either you or the baby's father have a birth defect or genetic condition such as a baby born with an open spine (spina bifida), a heart defect, or Down syndrome?

Yes   No   6.   Does anyone in your family or anyone in the baby's father's family have a birth defect or condition that has been diagnosed as genetic or inherited, such as open spine (spina bifida), a heart defect, or Down syndrome?

Yes   No   7.   Where your ancestors came from may sometimes give us important information about the health of your baby. Are you or the baby's father from any of the following ethnic/racial groups: Jewish, African American, Asian, Mediterranean (Greek, Italian)?

Yes   No   8.   Have you or the baby's father ever been screened to see if you are carriers of the gene for any of the following: Tay-Sachs, sickle cell, thalassemia?

Sometimes, the unborn baby can be exposed to outside factors that can cause birth defects. The next 8 questions will give us important information about possible exposure to the baby.

Yes   No   9.   Have you had any x-rays during this pregnancy?

Yes   No   10.   Have you had any alcohol during this pregnancy?

              11.   Prior to your pregnancy, how often did you drink alcoholic beverages?
- ☐ Every day
- ☐ At least once a week, not daily
- ☐ At least once a month, not weekly
- ☐ Less than once a month
- ☐ I do not drink alcoholic beverages.

              12.   Prior to your pregnancy, about how many alcoholic beverages did you usually have per occasion? (1 = one can of beer, one wine cooler, one glass of wine, or one shot of liquor.)
- ☐ 3 or more
- ☐ 1 to 2
- ☐ I do not drink alcoholic beverages.

Yes   No   13.   Have you taken any over-the-counter, prescription, or "street" drugs during this pregnancy? If yes, list drugs.

_____

_____

Yes   No   14.   Have you ever sought and/or received treatment for alcohol or drug problems? If yes, how long ago?_____

Yes   No   15.   Do you think you are at increased risk for having a baby with a birth defect or genetic disorder?

Yes   No   16.   At any time during the first 2 months of your pregnancy, have you had a rash or a fever of 103° F or greater?

A test for HIV is strongly recommended for all pregnant people, regardless of your responses to the next questions. The test is voluntary. There are two reasons to be tested: [1] New medications are available to reduce the chance of an infected person passing HIV to her baby; and [2] most people do not know if they are infected with HIV until late in the disease. Sometimes other infections can put you and your baby at risk. The following questions will help your health care provider determine other areas for counseling and evaluation.

Yes   No   Unsure   17.   Have you or your sexual partners ever had a sexually transmitted infection (STI or VD) such as chlamydia, gonorrhea, syphilis, or herpes?

Yes   No   Unsure   18.   Have you ever had a serious pelvic infection or pelvic inflammatory disease (PID)?

Yes   No   Unsure   19.   Do you think any of your male sexual partners have ever had sex with other men?

Yes   No   Unsure   20.   Have you or your sexual partners ever used IV street drugs?

Yes   No   Unsure   21.   Have you had sex with two or more partners in the last 12 months?

Yes   No   Unsure   22.   Do you think any of your sexual partners may have HIV or AIDS?

Yes   No   Unsure   23.   Have you or your sexual partners ever had a blood transfusion?

How safe you feel in your daily living gives us important information about risks to you and your baby.
Please answer these questions as well as you can. All answers will remain private.

		24.	Do you feel safe....
Yes	No	-	in your personal relationship?
Yes	No	-	within your home?
Yes	No	-	in your own neighborhood?
Yes	No	-	other (specify)_____

Yes   No   25.   Have you ever had your feelings repeatedly hurt, been repeatedly put down, or experienced other kinds of hurting?

Yes   No   26.   Are you being or have you ever been hit, slapped, kicked, pushed, or otherwise physically hurt? If yes, by whom?
☐ Husband   ☐ Family member
☐ Ex-husband   ☐ Stranger
☐ Partner   ☐ Other (specify)_____
☐ Ex-partner

Yes   No   27.   Are you experiencing or have you ever experienced uncomfortable touching or forced sexual contact? If yes, by whom?
☐ Husband   ☐ Family member
☐ Ex-husband   ☐ Stranger
☐ Partner   ☐ Other (specify)_____
☐ Ex-partner

RM/603 REV 6/97

PRENATAL RECORD

DATE	NAME		PREFERRED PRONOUN	DOB		RACE	RELIGION	OCCUPATION	YEARS EDUCATION	RELATIONSHIP STATUS

PREFERRED PHONE		ADDRESS			REFERRAL SOURCE	PRIMARY CARE PROVIDER		PARTNER	PARTNER'S PHONE NUMBER

GYNECOLOGICAL HISTORY / MEDICAL HISTORY - CONTINUED

MENARCHE YRS	INTERVAL	☐ REGULAR ☐ IRREGULAR	DURATION DAYS		CARDIOVASCULAR

✔ IF NEGATIVE-DESCRIBE POSITIVE HISTORY

- PAP HISTORY
- INFERTILITY
- GYN DISORDER
- GYN SURGERY
- DES EXPOSURE
- PRIOR CONTRACEPTION
- BCP W/IN 90 DAYS CONCEP
- BREASTS
- OTHER GYN HX
- GONORRHEA
- SYPHILIS
- CHLAMYDIA
- HERPES-SELF/PARTNER
- OTHER STI/HIV

MEDICAL HISTORY - CONTINUED:
- CARDIOVASCULAR
- RESPIRATORY/TB
- GI
- GU
- METABOLIC
- NEURO
- PSYCH-EMOTIONAL
- HEPATITIS
- MUSCULOSKELETAL
- SKIN DISORDERS
- OTHER DISEASE/DX
- OPERATIONS
- TRANSFUSIONS
- ALLERGIES

FAMILY HISTORY - NOTE IF FATHER OF BABY
- DIABETES
- HYPERTENSION
- TWINS
- CONGENITAL ANOM
- OTHER FAMILY HX

MEDICAL HISTORY
✔ IF NEGATIVE-DESCRIBE POSITIVE HISTORY
- HEENT

PREVIOUS PREGNANCIES

NO.	DATE	LENGTH (WKS)	LABOR (HRS)	TYPE DELIVERY	ANES.	SEX	WEIGHT	WHERE DELIVERED	COMPLICATIONS-AP, IP, PP, NEONATAL	OUTCOME/NAME

PRESENT PREGNANCY HISTORY / PHYSICAL EXAMINATION DATE

LMP ☐ NORM ☐ ABNORM	LNMP	EDC	+ PG TEST TYPE DATE	✔ IF NEGATIVE-DESCRIBE POSITIVE FINDINGS

PLANNED PREGNANCY/OK?   PARTNER SUPPORTIVE?

✔ IF NEGATIVE-DESCRIBE POSITIVE HISTORY
- NAUSEA/VOMITING
- BLEEDING
- URINARY SX
- VAGINAL DISCHARGE
- INFECTION
- FEVER/RASH
- TOBACCO/SMOKING
- ETOH
- PHYSICAL/SEXUAL ABUSE

PHYSICAL EXAMINATION:
- HEIGHT
- WEIGHT
- B.P.
- HEENT
- NECK
- LUNGS
- BREASTS
- HEART
- ABDOMEN
- NEURO
- EXTREMITIES/SKIN

PELVIC EXAMINATION DATE
- EXT. GENITALIA
- VAGINA/CERVIX
- UTERUS-SIZE
- PELVIS
- ADNEXA
- BONY PELVIS/ADEQUATE?
- HEMORRHOIDS

PROVIDER SIGNATURE

FIRST TRIMESTER			DATE	PROBLEMS AND RISK FACTORS
	DATE	WEEKS	EDC/RANGE		
LMP					
LNMP					
OVU/CONCEP					
FIRST EXAM					
+ HCG URINE					
+ HCG SERUM					
FHT DOPPLER					
FHT FETOSCOPE					
FM					
ULTRASOUND					
ULTRASOUND					
ULTRASOUND					

ANTICIPATORY GUIDANCE

FIRST TRIMESTER	SECOND TRIMESTER	THIRD TRIMESTER

CLINIC PROCEDURES/OUTLINE PRENATAL CARE
HIV COUNSELING/TESTING
NUTRITION
VITAMINS/MINERALS
DENTAL/VISION CARE
WEIGHT GAIN
SEAT BELTS
EXERCISE
PRENATAL DIAGNOSIS
HAZARDS: SMOKING, ETOH, DRUGS, OVERHEATING, CATS,
    RAW MEAT, UNPASTEURIZED MILK
DISCOMFORTS/RELIEF MEASURES
WARNING SIGNS: BLEEDING, CRAMPS, ABDOMINAL
     PAINS, DYSURIA, ETC.
BROCHURES
	FETAL DEVELOPMENT/QUICKENING
	PARTNER/FAMILY/SIBLINGS
	HOSPITAL PRE-ADMISSION/TOUR?
	FEEDING PLANS (BREAST/BOTTLE)
	EXERCISES/BODY MECHANICS
	WARNING SIGNS: SROM, BLEEDING, PRE-TERM LABOR
	BABY'S CARE PROVIDER _____
	    NEWBORN CARE/ROOMING-IN
	    CIRCUMCISION
	BROCHURES
	PRENATAL CLASSES
	SUPPORT PERSON _____
	BIRTH PLANS/OPTIONS
	SEXUALITY
		DISCOMFORTS/RELIEF MEASURES
		WARNING SIGNS
		FETAL ACTIVITY MONITORING
		LABOR SIGNS: WHEN AND HOW TO CALL
		TRAVEL RESTRICTIONS
		LABOR & DELIVERY ROUTINE
		ELECTRONIC FETAL MONITORING
		ANESTHESIA/ANALGESIA
		EPISIOTOMY/PERINEAL INTEGRITY
		LABOR & DELIVERY COMPLICATIONS/OPERATIVE DELIVERY
		BREAST CARE
		CAR SEAT
		DISCUSS POST-TERM MANAGEMENT
		EARLY DISCHARGE/HELP AT HOME

DATE	MEDICATIONS	POSTPARTUM CONTRACEPTIVE PLANS	
	RHOGAM	☐ ORAL CONTRACEPTION	☐ LONG-ACTING CONTRACEPTION
		☐ STERILIZATION - DATE TUBAL FORM SIGNED _____	
		☐ BARRIER	☐ OTHER
DRUG ALLERGIES/REACTIONS ☐ NKA			
PATIENT NAME			

LABORATORY DATA

TYPE RH		RUBELLA	SEROLOGY	HBsAg	HIV	URINE			DIABETIC SCREEN ____ @ ____ WKS		SICKLE PREP	PPD/TINE
ANTIBODY SCREEN ____ @ ____ WKS ____ @ ____ WKS		HCT ____ @ ____ WKS ____ @ ____ WKS		HSV SEROLOGY I _____ II _____ MSAFP / MOM PAP DATE		CERVICAL CULTURES DATE CHLAMYDIA GC HSV STREP			GTT @ ____ WKS FBS 1 HR _____ 2 HR _____ 3 HR _____		OTHER COPY SENT _____ COPY SENT _____	

EDC	REVISED EDC	REVISED EDC	AGE	GRAVIDA	PARA		ABORTIONS			DEATHS		LIVING CHILDREN
					TERM	PRETERM	SPONT	ELEC	ECTOPIC	FETAL	NEONATAL	

WEIGHT AND FUNDAL HEIGHT GRAPH

DATE																								
WEEKS GESTATION	6	8	10	12	14	16	18	20	22	24	26	28	30	32	33	34	35	36	37	38	39	40	41	42	43

CM 40, FUNDAL HEIGHT 35, 30, 25, 20 — FUNDAL HEIGHT / WEIGHT curves; + 50 #, + 40 #, + 30 #, + 20 #, + 10 # (left and right axes 50 #, 40 #, 30 #, 20 #, 10 #)

PRENATAL VISITS

WEIGHT NON PG ____																									
BLOOD PRESSURE																									
BLOOD PRESSURE RE-CHECK																									
URINE PROTEIN/ GLUCOSE																									
FHR D-DOPPLER F-FETOSCOPE																									
PRESENTATION																									
ESTIMATE UTERINE SIZE																									
FETAL ACTIVITY																									
WEEKS GESTATION	6	8	10	12	14	16	18	20	22	24	26	28	30	32	33	34	35	36	37	38	39	40	41	42	43
FUTURE PARAMETERS TO CHECK						M S A F P OR TRIPLE SCREEN					HCT DIABETIC SCREEN RhNEG - ANTIBODY SCREEN ? RHOGAM											FETAL SURVEILLANCE			
SEE NOTE (✔)																									
RETURN WEEKS																									
INITIALS																									

PATIENT NO.   HOSPITAL

PATIENT NAME

D.O.B.

RISK FACTOR GUIDELINES	PROGRESS NOTES

PATIENT PROFILE
AGE > 34 OR PREGNANCY WITHIN 2 YEARS OF MENARCHE
OCCUPATION AND AVOCATION
DRUG ABUSE OR ADDICTION
   ALCOHOL
   SMOKING
   COCAINE
   MARIJUANA
   NARCOTICS
   SEDATIVES/HYPNOTICS
   SALICYLATES AND OTHER PGSI'S
   OTHER
LOW SOCIO-ECONOMIC STATUS
   WELFARE
   EDUCATION < 9TH GRADE
   CROWDED LIVING CONDITIONS
   OTHER
BODY HABITUS
   SMALL STATURE (< 5 FEET TALL)
   OBESE (BMI >30)
   UNDERWEIGHT (BMI <18.5)
   PREGNANT PERSON'S BIRTHWEIGHT (LOW BIRTH WEIGHT OR LARGE FOR DATES)
PARTNER
   MEDICAL OR SURGICAL DISORDERS
   DRUG, SMOKING OR ALCOHOL ABUSE
   OCCUPATION, AVOCATION, HOBBIES
   STI'S (HERPES, URETHRITIS)
   HIV RISK FACTORS

GYNECOLOGICAL HISTORY
UTERINE AND CERVICAL ABNORMALITIES
   PAST UTERINE SURGERY (NON-CESAREAN)
   UTERINE ANOMALIES (CONGENITAL ANOMALIES, DES STIGMATA, MYOMATA)
   CERVICAL LACERATIONS OR CONIZATIONS
MENSTRUAL HISTORY AND GESTATIONAL DATING
   IRREGULAR MENSES OR OLIGOMENORRHEA
   ORAL CONTRACEPTIVE USE PRIOR TO CONCEPTION

MEDICAL HISTORY
ANEMIA (HGB < 9.5 OR HCT < 30)
HEART DISEASE (SYMPTOMATIC OR ASYMPTOMATIC)
THROMBOEMBOLISM (DURING PREVIOUS PREGNANCY OR PRIOR TO
    CURRENT PREGNANCY)
ANTICOAGULANT USE
CHRONIC HYPERTENSION (BP > 140/90)
ASTHMA OR OTHER CHRONIC LUNG DISEASE
SEIZURE DISORDER (WITH OR WITHOUT ANTICONVULSANT USE)
DIABETES MELLITUS (GESTATIONAL OR PREGESTATIONAL)
HEPATITIS
HIV RISK FACTORS
CHRONIC RENAL DISEASE (BUN > 20, CREATININE > 1.2 AT FIRST PRENATAL
    VISIT)
PYELONEPHRITIS

OBSTETRICAL FACTORS
PARITY
   PRIMIGRAVIDA
   GRAND MULTIPARA (> 4)
PAST PREGNANCIES
   HABITUAL ABORTION (≥ 3)
   PREMATURE BIRTH (< 37 WEEKS)
   PREMATURE RUPTURE OF MEMBRANES
   LOW BIRTH WEIGHT INFANT (BIRTHWEIGHT < 10TH PERCENTILE FOR DATES)
   LARGE FOR DATES INFANT (BIRTHWEIGHT > 90TH PERCENTILE FOR DATES)
   FETAL OR NEONATAL DEATH
   CONGENITAL ANOMALIES
   SURVIVING NEUROLOGICALLY IMPAIRED INFANT
   CERVICAL INCOMPETENCY
   MIDFORCEP OR DIFFICULT DELIVERY (E.G., SHOULDER DYSTOCIA)
   ABNORMAL LABOR (ARREST OR PROTRACTION DISORDER OF FIRST OR
    SECOND STAGE)
   ANTEPARTUM HEMORRHAGE (PLACENTAL ABRUPTION, PLACENTA PREVIA)
   BLEEDING PRIOR TO 20 WEEKS
   RH ISOIMMUNIZATION
   PREGNANCY-INDUCED HYPERTENSION
   CESAREAN DELIVERY (LOW TRANSVERSE, LOW VERTICAL, CLASSIC,
    UNKNOWN)
   INTERVAL FROM LAST DELIVERY < 12 MONTHS
   ANESTHESIA INTOLERANCE OR REACTIONS

PRESENT PREGNANCY
EMOTIONAL STRESS
POOR COMPLIANCE
LATE REGISTRATION FOR CARE
UNCERTAIN DATES
FAILURE TO GAIN WEIGHT (< 1/2 # PER WEEK AFTER 12 WEEKS)
EXCESSIVE WEIGHT GAIN (> 2 # PER WEEK AFTER 12 WEEKS)
BLEEDING PRIOR TO 20 WEEKS
ANY NAUSEA AND VOMITING
PLACENTAL ABRUPTION
PLACENTA PREVIA
OTHER VAGINAL BLEEDING
PREMATURE RUPTURE OF MEMBRANES
POLYHYDRAMNIOS OR OLIGOHYDRAMNIOS
THREATENED PREMATURE LABOR

PATIENT NAME

RM 612 REV 5/97

CHAPTER
32

Functional Assessment of the Older Adult

PURPOSE

This chapter describes the functional assessment of the older adult using a systems perspective, including the normal changes of aging and ongoing chronic geriatric syndromes. Tools that may be used as part of the functional assessment of an older adult are described.

READING ASSIGNMENT

Jarvis: *Physical Examination and Health Assessment,* 9th ed., Chapter 32, pp. 829–839.

Suggested readings:
Gabauer, J. (2020). Mitigating the dangers of polypharmacy in community-dwelling older adults. *Am J Nurs, 120*(2), 36–42.
Zonsius, M. C., Cothran, F. A., & Miller, J. M. (2020). Acute care for patients with dementia. *Am J Nurs, 120*(4), 34–42.

GLOSSARY

Study the following terms after completing the reading assignment. You should be able to cover the definition on the right and define the term out loud.

Activities of daily living .... tasks that are necessary for self-care, such as eating/feeding, bathing, grooming, toileting, walking, and transferring

Advanced activities of daily living .... activities that a person performs as a family member or as a member of society or community, including occupational and recreational activities

Caregiver assessment .... assessment of the health and well-being of an individual's caregiver

Caregiver burden .... the perceived strain by the person who cares for an older, chronically ill, or disabled person

Domains of cognition .... domains included in mental status assessments, such as attention, memory, orientation, language, visuospatial skills, and higher cognitive functions

Environmental assessment ..... assessment of an individual's home environment and community system, including hazards in the home

Functional ability .... the ability of a person to perform activities necessary to live in the modern society; may include driving, using the telephone, or performing personal tasks such as bathing and toileting

Functional assessment .... a systematic assessment that includes assessment of an individual's activities of daily living, instrumental activities of daily living, and mobility

Geriatric assessment .... multidimensional assessment: physical examination and assessments of mental status, functional status, social and economic status, pain, and physical environment for safety

Home care .... supportive services provided in the home: skilled nursing care, primary care, therapy (physical, occupational, speech), social work, nutrition, case management, ADL assistance, durable medical equipment

Instrumental activities of daily living .... functional abilities necessary for independent community living, such as shopping, meal preparation, housekeeping, laundry, managing finances, taking medications, and using transportation

Katz Index of Independence in Activities of Daily Living .... an instrument used to measure physical function in older adults and the chronically ill

Lawton Instrumental Activities of Daily Living .... an instrument used to measure an individual's ability to perform instrumental activities of daily living; may assist in assessing one's ability to live independently

Physical performance measures .... tests that measure balance, gait, motor coordination, and endurance

Social domain .... the domain that focuses on an individual's relationships within family, social groups, and the community

Social networks .... informal supports accessed by older adults, such as family members and close friends, neighbors, church societies, neighborhood groups, and senior centers

Spiritual assessment .... assessment of an individual's spiritual health

STUDY GUIDE

After completing the reading, you should be able to answer the following questions in the spaces provided.

1. Differentiate the following, and provide two examples of each:

   Activities of daily living (ADLs)

   Instrumental activities of daily living (IADLs)

   Advanced activities of daily living (AADLs)

2. Discuss at least two disorders that may alter an older adult's cognition.

3. What are some indications of possible caregiver burnout?

4. Describe a method of assessing an older adult for depression.

5. Describe at least three contexts of care of an older adult.

6. How do falls affect older adults? Name some interventions.

7. List four ways in which driving cessation negatively affects the older adult.

8. Define an environmental assessment and list at least four common environmental hazards that may be found in an individual's home.

9. State the priority when assessing an older adult who is in pain.

10. Describe four nonpharmacologic interventions to improve sleep.

CRITICAL THINKING ACTIVITIES

Consider the importance of home safety, especially as it relates to fall risk in older adults. Go online and review home safety checklists from the AARP and the National Safety Council. Use the checklists to determine the safety of your home. As you walk around your home, make note of anything that may be a trip hazard or anything that could be considered unsafe. Use the same checklists to assess the safety of an older adult's home. Were there any differences between the assessments? Did you notice anything within the older adult's home that should be changed to assure safety and prevent falls? Did you assess the older adult's home differently than you did your own home?

CLINICAL JUDGMENT QUESTIONS

This test is for you to check your own mastery of the content. Answers are provided in Appendix A.

1. You are caring for an elderly woman with early dementia. Her family is concerned about her driving ability, reporting that she "sometimes gets lost on the way home," drives "really slow," and she "can't seem to see very well." Given your knowledge of warning signs for cessation of driving, you recommend:

   a. As long as she can still pass her driving test, she can continue to safely drive. There is no need to take her car away, as it will only upset her further.
   b. Driving requires executive function, good sensory perception, and good physical abilities. It is likely time to discuss the cessation of driving.
   c. Driving requires good sensory perception. I would recommend having her eyes tested. As long as she gets new glasses, she can keep driving.
   d. Cessation of driving is never easy. Perhaps recommend that she only drive during the day when it is light out so she can see better and only have her drive where she is familiar.

2. The nurse is caring for a 78-year-old female who reports difficulty sleeping. She says she wakes at least twice to urinate each night. She always goes to bed at a different time but wakes up promptly at 0700 without an alarm. Which of the following are recommended interventions to promote sleep? **Select all that apply.**

   a. Avoid all alcohol.
   b. Limit caffeine to two caffeinated drinks per day.
   c. Avoid caffeine after lunch.
   d. Take frequent naps up to 1 hour in length.
   e. Eat a large meal before bed.
   f. Adhere to a schedule.
   g. Open drapes/blinds during the day.
   h. Have a light snack before bed.
   i. Be active during the day.

Use the following scenario to answer questions 3–6.

The nurse is caring for an 86-year-old patient who was hospitalized with a urinary tract infection and acute confusion × 2 days. The patient was admitted for IV antibiotics. The nurse receives the following information during the shift report:

A.K. is an 86-year-old gentleman who lives at home with his wife. His brother died in Vietnam and his son died in the first Iraq war. He has a history of arthritis and had an MI 15 years ago. No history of dementia or cognitive impairment. He is alert and oriented to person and place only, but his cognition is improving. Upon admission, he was only oriented to person. His Timed Up and Go test was 14 seconds. His wife reports that he's fallen at home twice in the past 2 months. Upon physical exam, VS are as follows: HR 101 bpm, RR 26 bpm, shallow, BP 110/60. Lungs clear and equal bilaterally; normal S1S2 no extra sounds, no murmur. DTRs 1+ and equal. Difficulty with whispered voice test.

3. Underline any abnormal or concerning findings.

4. Highlight the changes expected with normal aging.

5. Early discharge planning is a crucial part of any hospitalization. Which of the following accurately describes the discharge for A.K.?

   a. A.K. can be discharged home with his spouse. Social work should be consulted to ensure they have adequate housing, meals, and social support, but it should not be an issue.
   b. A.K. will need a functional assessment to identify any areas of concern prior to discharge. Including his caregiver will be important to ensure adequate support at home.
   c. A.K. will likely need nursing home care upon discharge. He has declined significantly, and his spouse is also elderly, so she may not be able to care for him.
   d. A.K. should cease driving and consider moving to an adult living facility where he can have adequate transportation, meals, and social support. Returning home is not a good option.

6. Given the information in the scenario, which of the following is true regarding hospital at home care for A.K.

   a. A.K. would not be a candidate for a hospital at home. Any person over 85 years old with an elderly spouse is not appropriate given the lack of younger social support and care required during a home stay.
   b. A.K. would not benefit from a hospital at home. His acute confusion places him at risk to himself and others. A hospital environment with a sitter and restraints will ensure his safety throughout his hospitalization.
   c. A.K. is a candidate for hospital at home given his diagnoses and the lack of high acuity needs, but a full assessment would be required to ensure he meets qualifications and that it is an amenable choice for him and his caregiver.
   d. A.K. is a candidate for hospital at home and should not be admitted as an inpatient. Hospital at home can be used to avoid some in hospital complications such as nosocomial infection and should be considered for all elderly patients regardless of diagnosis.

7. Fill in the following blanks

   The nurse should recognize that a Timed Up and Go test greater than _____ seconds indicates a person is at high risk for _____. The person should be _____ to use their assistive devices (if applicable) and shoes _____ be worn.

8. Label the steps to the Timed Up and Go test in the correct order. (Not all items will be used.)

Sit down in chair
Turn around
Walk 15 feet
Rise from chair
Walk 10 feet
Walk back to chair
Walk to the other chair

9. Underline the areas of the environmental assessment below that are concerning for your 89-year-old patient who lives alone, has limited mobility, and uses a walker.

   M.K. lives in a single-story home in a safe neighborhood of town. Streetlights are present, though functionality was not assessed since it is daytime. The neighborhood has sidewalks, and the nearest fire station is four blocks away. M.K. no longer drives and the nearest bus stop is approximately 1 mile away. There is a grocery store within 2 miles. The house has no steps to enter. There are throw rugs in the entry way, the kitchen, and in each of the two bathrooms. The toilet is lower than standard, and there are no grab bars. Curtains are open and the home is well-lit. Old magazines and books are neatly stacked all over the floor.

10. Given the concerns identified in question 9, write 5 recommended changes to promote safety and independent living.

    1. _____
    2. _____
    3. _____
    4. _____
    5. _____

SKILLS LABORATORY AND CLINICAL SETTING

The purpose of this component is to practice a functional assessment of an older adult. If possible, complete at least two assessments in different settings (e.g., acute care, ambulatory clinic, assisted living, home setting), noting the differences between the settings and how you adapted the assessment based on the context of care.

Clinical Objectives

1. Correctly administer the Timed Up and Go Test to an older adult.
2. Demonstrate the ability to assess ADLs and IADLs in an older adult.
3. Analyze differences between functional assessment findings (either between two or more assessments you completed or with a partner who assessed a different person).
4. Identify potential causes of decreased functional ability in an older adult.
5. Measure caregiver strain in an adult caregiver of an older dependent adult.

Instructions

Functional Assessment of an Older Adult

Using the instructions and checklists below, complete a functional assessment of at least one older adult. If possible, assess at least two older adults in different settings (e.g., acute care hospital, ambulatory clinic, assisted living, home environment). Compare the results of each assessment. Did you identify areas of dependence? Were you able to observe each area, or was self-reporting used? What medical conditions, if any, lead to a decrease in independence for the older person? If only one assessment was completed, discuss your findings with a partner who assessed a different older adult. Note similarities and differences in your findings. Did context of care shape the results?

- **Timed Up and Go Test**
  - Equipment: arm chair, tape measure, tape, stopwatch.
  - Place a piece of tape 10 feet (3 m) away from the chair so that it is easily seen by the subject.
  - Instructions to the subject: "When I say go, you will stand up, walk to the line on the floor, turn around, walk back to the chair, and sit down. Please walk at your regular pace."
  - The subject should wear normal footwear and use any assistive device typically used during ambulation. You will begin timing when you say go and end when the subject has returned to a seated position. The subject should begin the test completely seated with their hips all the way to the back of the seat. Give the subject a practice run that is not timed so that the person understands the test.
  - Note gait, balance, and the amount of time it takes for the person to complete the test.
  - A result ≥12 seconds indicates an increased risk for falls.
- **Katz Index of Independence in Activities of Daily Living** and **Lawton Instrumental Activities of Daily Living Scale**
  - Review the questions on each scale. In the clinical setting, use the Katz ADL form and the Lawton IADL form to assess an older adult.

Katz Activities of Daily Living		
Activities Points (1 or 0)	**Independence** (1 point) NO supervision, direction, or personal assistance	**Dependence** (0 points) WITH supervision, direction, personal assistance, or total care
Bathing Points _____	(1 point) Bathes self completely or needs help in bathing only a single part of the body such as the back, genital area, or disabled extremity	(0 points) Needs help with bathing more than one part of the body or getting in or out of the tub or shower; requires total bathing
Dressing Points _____	(1 point) Gets clothes from closet and drawers and puts on clothes and outer garments complete with fasteners; may have help tying shoes	(0 points) Needs help with dressing self or needs to be completely dressed
Toileting Points _____	(1 point) Gets to toilet, gets on and off, arranges clothes, cleans genital area without help	(0 points) Needs help transferring to the toilet, cleaning self, or using bedpan or commode
Transferring Points _____	(1 point) Moves in and out of bed or chair unassisted. Mechanical transferring aids are acceptable	(0 points) Needs help in moving from bed to chair or requires a complete transfer
Continence Points _____	(1 point) Exercises complete self-control over urination and defecation	(0 points) Is partially or totally incontinent of bowel or bladder
Feeding Points _____	(1 point) Gets food from plate into mouth without help. Preparation of food may be done by another person	(0 points) Needs partial or total help with feeding or requires parenteral feeding
Total points = _____	6 = High (patient independent)	0 = Low (patient very dependent)

Adapted from Gerontological Society of America. Katz, S., Downs, T. D., Cash, H. R., et al. (1970). Progress in the development of the index of ADL. *Gerontologist, 10,* 20–30.

The Lawton Instrumental Activities of Daily Living Scale

A. Ability to Use Telephone
  1. Operates telephone on own initiative; looks up and dials numbers   1
  2. Dials a few well-known numbers   1
  3. Answers telephone, but does not dial   1
  4. Does not use telephone at all   0

B. Shopping
  1. Takes care of all shopping needs independently   1
  2. Shops independently for small purchases   0
  3. Needs to be accompanied on any shopping trip   0
  4. Completely unable to shop   0

C. Food Preparation
  1. Plans, prepares, and serves adequate meals independently   1
  2. Prepares adequate meals if supplied with ingredients   0
  3. Heats and serves prepared meals or prepares meals, but does not
  maintain adequate diet   0
  4. Needs to have meals prepared and served   0

D. Housekeeping
  1. Maintains house alone with occasional assistance (heavy work)   1
  2. Performs light daily tasks such as dishwashing, bed making   1
  3. Performs light daily tasks, but cannot maintain acceptable level of
  cleanliness   1
  4. Needs help with all home maintenance tasks   1
  5. Does not participate in any housekeeping tasks   0

E. Laundry
  1. Does personal laundry completely   1
  2. Launders small items, rinses socks, stockings, etc   1
  3. All laundry must be done by others   0

F. Mode of Transportation
  1. Travels independently on public transportation or drives own car   1
  2. Arranges own travel via taxi, but does not otherwise use public
  transportation   1
  3. Travels on public transportation when assisted or accompanied by
  another   1
  4. Travel limited to taxi or automobile with assistance of another   0
  5. Does not travel at all   0

G. Responsibility for Own Medications
  1. Is responsible for taking medication in correct dosages at correct time   1
  2. Takes responsibility if medication is prepared in advance in
  separate dosages   0
  3. Is not capable of dispensing own medication   0

H. Ability to Handle Finances
  1. Manages financial matters independently (budgets, writes checks,
  pays rent and bills, goes to bank); collects and keeps track of income 1
  2. Manages day-to-day purchases, but needs help with banking, major
  purchases, etc   1
  3. Incapable of handling money   0

Scoring: For each category, circle the item description that most closely resembles the client's highest functional level (either 0 or 1).

From Lawton, M. P., & Brody, E. M. (1969). Assessment of older people: self-maintaining and instrumental activities of daily living. *Gerontologist, 9,* 179–186. © The Gerontological Society of America.

Caregiver Assessment

Too often, health care workers fail to assess the caregivers of older dependent patients. Assessment of the caregiver is an integral part of identifying the needs of the older adult; it helps to assure that the caregiver is not suffering from burnout, depression, or increased stress. After completing your assessment and discussing it with the caregiver, discuss the results with a partner who assessed a different caregiver. Were there any significant differences? If so, what do you think contributed to the differences?

Modified Caregiver Strain Index

Identify an adult who is the primary caregiver for a dependent older adult. If you are unable to identify an adult caregiver of an older dependent adult, identify a caregiver to a disabled or dependent adult >18 years old. Administer the Modified Caregiver Strain Index. Discuss the results with the caregiver. While no specific cutoff for caregiver strain is identified, the higher the score, the more strain the caregiver is under and the more likely it is that the person will need assistance.

Modified Caregiver Strain Index

Directions: Here is a list of things that other caregivers have found to be difficult. Please put a checkmark in the columns that apply to you. We have included some examples that are common caregiver experiences to help you think about each item. Your situation may be slightly different, but the item could still apply.

	Yes, on a regular basis = 2	Yes, sometimes = 1	No = 0
My sleep is disturbed (For example, *the person I care for* is in and out of bed or wanders around at night)			
Caregiving is inconvenient (For example, helping takes so much time or it's a long drive over to help)			
Caregiving is a physical strain (For example, lifting in or out of a chair; effort or concentration is required)			
Caregiving is confining (For example, helping restricts free time or *I* cannot go visiting)			
There have been family adjustments (For example, helping has disrupted *my* routine; there has been no privacy)			
There have been changes in personal plans (For example, *I* had to turn down a job; *I* could not go on vacation)			
There have been other demands on my time (For example, other family members *need me*)			
There have been emotional adjustments (For example, severe arguments *about caregiving*)			
Some behavior is upsetting (For example, incontinence; *the person cared for* has trouble remembering things; or *the person I care for* accuses people of taking things)			
It is upsetting to find the person I care for has changed so much from his or her former self (For example, he or she is a different person than he or she used to be)			
There have been work adjustments (For example, *I* have to take time off *for caregiving duties*)			
Caregiving is a financial strain			
I feel completely overwhelmed (For example, *I* worry about *the person I care* for; *I* have concerns about how *I* will manage)			

Total Score =

Words appearing in *italics* represent modifications from Thornton, M., & Travis, S. S. (2003). Analysis of the reliability of the modified caregiver strain index. *The Journals of Gerontology, 58B*(2), S129. © The Gerontological Society of America. Reproduced by permission of the publisher.

NOTES

CHAPTER

33

Next-Generation NCLEX® (NGN) Examination– Style Unfolding Case Studies

Use the following case studies to apply the knowledge and skills learned in *Physical Examination and Health Assessment*, 9th edition. There will be 2 questions per section of the unfolding case study for a total of 6 questions per case study. Please note the questions are formatted in a style to represent those found on the Next-Generation NCLEX® (NGN) Examination. Answers are provided in Appendix B.

UNFOLDING CASE STUDY 1: PEDIATRIC HEALTH ASSESSMENT

Question 1: Highlight/Recognize Cues

Highlight any important cues in the Nurses' Notes and Vital Signs that require **immediate** follow up by the nurse.

Health History	Nurses' Notes	Vital Signs	Laboratory Results

1000: A 10-year-old male patient arrives at the Emergency Department (ED) via private car with his mother, who is his legal guardian. Mother reports that the patient was riding his bicycle without a helmet when the front tire entered a drain grid. Patient hit handlebars and then flew over top of bicycle to ground. Event was witnessed by mother who denies patient's loss of consciousness. Mother brought the patient directly from scene to ED. Patient is alert and acting appropriately for his age. Patient is crying, holding his stomach. Scrapes noted on bilateral forearms oozing blood, as well as an obvious deformity to his right lower leg. Immunizations are up to date per mother. NKDA. Denies significant PMH.

Health History	Nurses' Notes	Vital Signs	Laboratory Results

1000: Initial vital signs in triage

T: 98.2°F (36.8°C)/HR 140 bpm, regular/RR 22 bpm, crying/BP 142/72 mm Hg/Spo$_2$ 97% on RA

Pain: 6/10 using FACES scale

Weight: 27.2 kilograms

Question 2: Select All That Apply/Analyze Cues

The nurse is concerned about the patient's crying and reported pain level of 6/10. What factors may be the cause of the reported pain? **Select all that apply.**

1. Fear of the hospital environment
2. Right lower leg injury
3. Abdominal pain
4. Fracture to arm
5. Pain to face and head

Question 3: Drag and Drop Table/Recognize and Analyze Cues

Drag the cues in the Nurses' Notes and Glasgow Score Options to calculate the Glasgow Coma Scale below.

Health History	Nurses' Notes	Vital Signs	Laboratory Results

1015: Patient to room 18, placed in bed, supine, report given by triage nurse to RN who assumed care of patient. Primary trauma survey as follows:

A-airway intact/B-breathing Within Normal Limits (WNL)/C-capillary refill 2 s with pulses 2+ bilaterally/D-disability—alert and age appropriate; patient opens eyes spontaneously, answers most questions appropriately but at times is confused, obeys commands with purposeful movement/E-environment—clothes are damp from sweat and blood; patient's clothing is cut off with a gown placed and warm blankets applied/F-family presence—mother is worried and at patient's bedside/G-give comfort—right lower leg splinted; patient reassured with plan of care updated to both mother and patient.

Glasgow Score Options: 1, 2, 3, 4, 5, 6, 7, 8

Cues	Associated Score
1.	1.
2.	2.
3.	3.
Glasgow Score Calculation: _____	

Question 4: Multiple Response Select N/Analyze Cues

The nurse prepares to start the secondary survey of the patient. In addition to a head-to-toe examination, and using findings identified prior, the nurse will plan to perform focused assessments on which **four** of the following?

☐ Abdomen
☐ Heart
☐ Neurologic
☐ Thorax and lungs
☐ Peripheral vascular
☐ Musculoskeletal
☐ Skin
☐ Neck

Question 5: Highlight in Text/Recognize Cues

The nurse prepares to speak with the provider about the patient's assessment findings. From the 1045 note, **highlight the three symptoms from the nurses' note** and **highlight any abnormal vital signs in the flowsheet** to relay to the provider.

Health History	Nurses' Notes	Vital Signs	Laboratory Results

1045: Head-to-toe secondary survey complete. Patient log rolled with c-spine immobilization maintained. Back and spine WNL. IV established. IV fluid bolus initiated and labs sent. Patient with increased complaints of nausea and dry heaving. Abdominal distention is noted, and bowel sounds hypoactive with tenderness in the right upper quadrant upon palpation. X-ray of right leg at bedside.

Health History	Nurses' Notes	Vital Signs	Laboratory Results

1000: T 98.2°F (36.8°C)/HR 140 bpm, regular/RR 22 bpm, crying/BP 142/72 mm Hg/Spo$_2$ 97% on RA

1015: T 97.0°F (36.1°C)/HR 122 bpm/RR 20 bpm/BP 120/78 mm Hg/Spo$_2$ 96% on RA

1030: T 97.8°F (36.6°C)/HR 138 bpm/RR 20 pm/BP 118/72 mm Hg/Spo$_2$ 96% on RA

1045: T 97.8°F (36.6°C)/HR 138 bpm/RR 22 bpm/BP 99/70 mm Hg/Spo$_2$ 96% on RA

Question 6: Matrix Multiple Response/Analyze Cues/Prioritize Hypotheses

Select the **most likely** involved organ with the assessment finding in the table below. Each column must have at least one selection and each row may have more than one response option.

Symptoms	Liver	Spleen	Kidney(s)
Abdominal distention			
Nausea, dry heaving			
Tenderness RUQ abd with palpation			

Conclusion

Health History	Nurses' Notes	Vital Signs	Laboratory Results

Provider at bedside with FAST (focused assessment with sonography) performed. Findings suspicious of internal bleeding. Patient is taken to radiology for CT head/neck/chest/ abdomen/pelvis. CT abdomen is positive for liver laceration. CT head, neck, and chest are all normal. X-ray of right lower leg showing nondisplaced fibula fracture. IVF bolus finishing. Pt will remain NPO. Surgeon at bedside for consult.

Bonus Questions to Level Up With Critical Thinking

1. What could the vital sign trend be indicative of?
2. What lab values from a CBC, CMP, Type and Cross, coagulation profile, and lactate level are important for this patient and why?

UNFOLDING CASE STUDY 2: ADULT HEALTH ASSESSMENT

Question 1: Drag and Drop Cloze/Analyze Cues

Health History	Nurses' Notes	Vital Signs	Laboratory Results

0830: October 10th—A 41-year-old female arrives at the clinic today as a follow-up visit for wound check. The patient reports she was "getting ramen soup out of the microwave when it splashed on her arms." Accident occurred 10 days prior. Patient was seen in the ED with treatment for first- and second-degree splash burns.

Bandages to bilateral arms intact, dry, and clean. Patient has been applying over-the-counter antibiotic ointment to the areas and dressing twice per day. Complains of a "throbbing" pain, reports it as 5 out of 10. Describes pain as constant, nonradiating focused to round wound areas on bilateral arms, worse the past 2 days. Patient has not been changing the dressing the past 2 days as it seemed to make the pain worse.

T 100.0°F (37.8°C)/HR 86 bpm/RR 18 bpm/BP 138/78 mm Hg/Spo$_2$ 97% RA.

The nurse wants to ensure they have assessed the patient's pain completely. Drag and drop from the items below to finish what the nurse should document for the PQRST acronym related to pain: P_____, Q_____, R_____, S_____, T_____.

Answer Options

10 days
Changing the dressing
First- and second-degree burns
Nonradiating
5/10 on 0–10 numerical scale

100°F temperature
Throbbing
Constant
Bilateral arms

Question 2: Drag and Drop Rationale/Prioritize Hypotheses

Drag one potential risk and one assessment finding to complete the sentence for this patient.

The nurse knows the patient is at risk for _____ due to _____.

Potential Risk	Assessment Finding
Sleep deprivation	Wounds
Infection	Scarring from burn
Poor self-image	Pain
Poor pain control	Lack of proper dressing changes

Question 3: Highlight/Recognize Cues

Highlight the cues in the Health History note which puts the patient at an increased health risk.

Health History	Nurses' Notes	Vital Signs	Laboratory Results

Immunizations: Unknown Allergies: NKDA Height: 5'6 Weight: 180 lbs

Surgical hx: Tonsils and Adenoids, age 4; C-section ages 33 and 35

Health Conditions: Type 2 Diabetes, High cholesterol

Hospitalizations: Diabetic Ketoacidosis, age 16

Denies alcohol use presently or in past. Denies recreational drugs presently or in the past. Patient currently uses e-cigarettes on and off throughout the day; smoked cigarettes 1 ppd for 10 years prior.

Current medications: Metformin 1000 mg PO twice daily/Lispro insulin SQ before meals sliding scale/Triple antibiotic ointment to burns OTC twice daily/Atorvastatin 80 mg every evening.

Question 4: Select All That Apply/Analyze Cues

Health History	Nurses' Notes	Vital Signs	Laboratory Results

0900, October 10th: Patient was discharged with verbal and written instructions given. Patient verbalized understanding. Wound consult ordered and a home visit scheduled with the nurse in 2 days for wound check. Patient advised to continue with triple antibiotic ointment to wounds and dressing changes twice a day.

The nurse, in preparation for discharge, would add which items for patient education handouts? **Select all that apply.**

1. Smoking cessation
2. Medication compliance
3. Nonpharmacologic and pharmacologic pain options
4. Wound care
5. Daily nutrition charts

Question 5: Drag and Drop Table/Analyze Cues

Subjective and Objective data were obtained from the wound nurse's focused assessment.

Health History	Nurses' Notes	Vital Signs	Laboratory Results

1200, October 12th: S (situation): Wound nurse visit to patient's home for a wound follow-up assessment.

B (background): Patient at day 12 from occurrence of accidental burn. Had follow-up visit at day 10 with primary health care clinic. Patient has been treating bilat arm burn with triple antibiotic ointment and dressings twice per day. Reports taking OTC ibuprofen for pain.

A (assessment): Bilateral arms with full range of motion. 2+ radial pulses bilaterally, 2 s cap refill bilaterally. Varying degrees of healing to skin on both arms. Some blisters have popped and are oozing yellow drainage. Red streaks from the burns on right arm extending up to right elbow. Right arm is warm to touch.

Vital signs: T 101.5°F (38.6°C)/HR 100 bpm/RR 22 bpm/ BP 145/90 mm Hg/Spo_2 97% RA

Patient reports blood sugar at home running in the 300s and "running out of her insulin and is waiting for the refill to come via mail delivery".

R (recommendation): Patient sent to ED for evaluation of possible infection of wound.

Drag and drop from the list of subjective and objective findings below to place in the corresponding normal or abnormal finding column.

Normal Finding	Abnormal Finding

List of Subjective and Objective Findings

OTC ibuprofen for pain

Varying degrees of healing to skin on both arms

Bilat arms with full range of motion

2+ radial pulses

Two-second capillary refill

Blisters with yellow drainage

Red streaks from burn on right arm extending to right elbow

Right arm warm to touch

T 101.5°F (38.6°C)

HR 100 bpm

RR 22 bpm

BP 145/90 mm Hg

SpO_2 97% RA

Blood sugar running in 300s

Question 6: Multiple Response Select N/Analyze Cues/Recognize Hypotheses

Using the Subjective and Objective Findings list from Question 5, select **seven** assessments that correspond with the wound nurse's R (recommendation) to send the patient to the ED for possible infection of wound

☐ OTC ibuprofen for pain

☐ Varying degrees of healing to skin on both arms

☐ Bilat arms with full range of motion

☐ 2+ radial pulses

☐ Two-second capillary refill

☐ Blisters with yellow drainage

☐ Red streaks from burn on right arm extending to right elbow

☐ Right arm warm to touch

☐ T 101.5°F (38.6°C)

☐ HR 100 bpm

☐ RR 22 bpm

☐ BP 145/90 mm Hg

☐ SpO_2 97% RA

☐ Blood sugar running in 300s

Bonus Questions to Level Up With Critical Thinking

1. Describe why pathophysiologically a patient with diabetes is at an increased risk for proper wound healing?
2. What labs do you think would be ordered for the patient once they are sent to the ED as a recommendation from the wound nurse in relation to ruling out infection?

UNFOLDING CASE STUDY 3: OLDER ADULT HEALTH ASSESSMENT

Question 1: Drop Down Cloze/Recognize Cues/Analyze Cues

Health History	Nurses' Notes	Vital Signs	Laboratory Results

0800: Day 1 admission to cardiac floor, General Hospital, an 83-year-old is admitted for shortness of breath, chest pain, and positive for COVID.

Per family, patient is alert and oriented to person and place for baseline mental status. Lives with her daughter due to advanced dementia. Upon admission, patient is confused, only alert to person at this time. Tested positive for COVID 6 days prior to admission. Progression of illness and weakness brought patient via ambulance to the hospital for evaluation and care.

Vitals: T 99.0°F (37.2°C)/HR 105 bpm, irregular/RR 20 bpm/BP 122/68 mm Hg/SpO_2 95% on 2 L nasal cannula

The nurse wants to assess the patient's pain score to complete the vital signs. Utilizing the information from the nurses' notes, the nurse identifies two cues (options 1 and 2) that determine the pain assessment tool that should be used for this patient (option 3): ____1____, ____2_____, ____3_____.

Options for 1	Options for 2	Options for 3
Confused	Progression of illness	Numeric rating scale
Weakness	Positive COVID test	Faces Pain Scale
Shortness of breath	Advanced Dementia	Visual Analogue Scale
Chest Pain	HR 105 bpm, irregular	PAINAD Scale

Question 2: Drop Down Cloze/Recognize Cues/Analyze Cues

Complete the following sentences by choosing from the list of options.

When taking vital signs, the nurse noted the ____1____ pulse to be irregular. The nurse knows to follow up by auscultating the ____2_____ rate for ____3_____ minute(s).

Options for 1	Options for 2	Options for 3
Carotid	Carotid	One
Apical	Apical	Two
Radial	Radial	Three
Pedal	Aortic	Four

Question 3: Select All that Apply/Analyze Cues

Health History	Nurses' Notes	Vital Signs	Laboratory Results

0430: Day 2 of admission to cardiac floor, General Hospital, 83-year-old

Daughter remains at the bedside. Patient A&O x1 with increase work of breathing, clutching her chest. Focused assessment of the thorax, lungs, and heart performed. Patient is lifted upright in a high fowler position with oxygen increased to 5 L nasal cannula. Symmetrical lung expansion, lungs with bilateral inspiratory crackles auscultated. No crepitus. S_1-S_2 normal, not accentuated or diminished, S_3 gallop present. No carotid bruit.

VS: T- 101.0°F (38.3°C)/HR 122 bpm, irregular/RR 36 bpm/BP 101/70 mm Hg/Spo$_2$ 90% on 5 L nasal cannula

Provider notified of patient status. New orders received for STAT portable chest x-ray, EKG, troponin, BNP, and arterial blood gas. Call respiratory to place patient on heated high-flow oxygen. Transfer patient to Intensive Care Unit.

What **significant changes** in the patient's status from day 1 admission notes to day 2 admission notes will the nurse include in their report? (**Select all that apply.**)

1. Clutching her chest
2. A & O X1
3. Increased work of breathing, RR 36 bpm
4. Oxygen increased to 5 L nasal cannula, Spo$_2$ 90%
5. Bilateral inspiratory crackles auscultated
6. S3 gallop present
7. T 101.0°F (38.3°C)
8. HR 122 bpm, irregular, BP 101/70 mm Hg
9. Symmetrical lung expansion
10. COVID positive

Question 4: Multiple Response Grouping/Recognize Cues/Analyze Cues

Choose the finding(s) and abnormal finding(s) that correspond with each body system.

A. Body System	B. Normal Assessment Findings	C. Abnormal Assessment Finding
Thorax and lungs	☐ BP 105/70 ☐ Confusion ☐ Symmetrical lung expansion ☐ Clutching of chest ☐ No crepitus	☐ Bilateral inspiratory crackles ☐ Spo$_2$ 90% on 5 L nasal cannula ☐ HR in the 120s, irregular ☐ S$_3$ gallop ☐ T 101.0°F (38.3°C)
Heart	☐ BP 105/70 ☐ Bilateral inspiratory crackles ☐ Symmetrical lung expansion ☐ Clutching chest ☐ No carotid bruit	☐ Confusion ☐ RR 36 bpm ☐ HR 110 bpm, irregular ☐ S$_3$ gallop ☐ BP 105/70

Question 5: Highlight in Text/Recognize Cues

Highlight the cues the nurse should make note to follow up on in the Nurses' Notes

Health History	Nurses' Notes	Vital Signs	Laboratory Results

0930: Day 8 Follow-up visit post discharge from hospital, Primary Care Office

Patient follow-up visit after a 7-day hospitalization for COVID pneumonia and new onset atrial fibrillation. Daughter is with patient. Daughter reports she has hired someone to help with her mother until the patient regains some of her strength. Using walker with gait belt.

Patient is alert and oriented to person and place, which daughter reports is her baseline. Denies any complaints of pain. Skin tear noted to right lower extremity. Lungs with fine crackles bilaterally. Heart S$_1$-S$_2$, not accentuated or diminished, regular rhythm, 74 bpm. Grade 2/6 Murmur heard at apex. 1+ pitting edema to bilateral lower extremities. Appetite slowly improving. Daughter denies recent fever. Denies any falls. Denies any issues with current medications.

Question 6: Drop Down Cloze/Analyze Cues

Complete the following sentence by choosing from the list of options.
   The nurse knows a murmur heard at the apex suggests a problem with the _____.

Drop Down Options
Mitral valve
Aortic valve
Tricuspid valve
Pulmonary valve

Bonus Questions to Level Up With Critical Thinking

1. Describe what pneumonia versus congestive heart failure would look like in a patient, i.e., pathophysiology of condition, subjective findings, assessment findings.
2. The patient had baseline confusion from dementia history. What else can cause acute confusion or an increase in confusion from baseline?

APPENDIX A

Answers to Clinical Judgment Questions

CHAPTER 1: EVIDENCE-BASED ASSESSMENT

1. a, b, e, f, h	6. first	11. a, c, e
2. c, d, e	7. second	12. b
3. d	8. third	13. a
4. c	9. second	
5. a	10. third	

CHAPTER 2: CULTURAL ASSESSMENT

1. a	5. d	9. a
2. c	6. b	10. c
3. c	7. d	11. c
4. d	8. a, b	

CHAPTER 3: THE INTERVIEW

1. a	4. d	7. a, c, e
2. a, b, d	5. a, c, g	8. b
3. a	6. c	

9.

Statement	Therapeutic	Nontherapeutic
I'm sure everything will be fine.		X
You sound upset. Please tell me more about what happened today.	X	
Dr. Daniels knows what he is talking about. Just follow his recommendations.		X
What are the pros and cons of surgery?	X	
If I were you, I would get another opinion before having surgery.		X
Why did you wait so long to see the doctor after the symptoms began?		X
You must not eat or drink anything after midnight except for small sips of water to take your morning pills.	X	
No need to cry. Let's move on to a different topic.		X

10.

Behavior	Positive	Negative
Tapping a pen rhythmically on the table.		X
Warm smile while leaning slightly forward.	X	
Moderate tone of voice and rate of speech.	X	
Frequently crossing and uncrossing legs.		X
Arms crossed over chest.		X
Standing by the client's bed.		X

CHAPTER 4: THE COMPLETE HEALTH HISTORY

1. a, b, d, e, h
2. d
3. a, c, g
4. d
5. The client comes to the clinic for "shortness of breath after climbing stairs." He is a 49-year-old male construction worker who upon further questioning reports chest pain with exertion, fatigue, and a stomach ache. Upon talking to the patient, you note that he appears pale and clammy. His hands are cool to the touch and he is audibly wheezing.
6. The client comes to the clinic for "shortness of breath after climbing stairs." He is a 49-year-old male construction worker who upon further questioning reports chest pain with exertion, fatigue, and a stomach ache. Upon talking to the patient, you note that he appears pale and clammy. His hands are cool to the touch and he is audibly wheezing.
7. a, c, d, f
8. c

9. When completing the health history on a young child, additional information is collected. Identify whether the following information is collected regardless of age or only collected on children.

Information	Always Collected	Children only
Perinatal history		X
Reason for seeking care	X	
Immunization status	X	
Medications	X	
Developmental milestones		X
Family history	X	

CHAPTER 5: MENTAL STATUS ASSESSMENT

1. a
2. b
3. c
4. c
5. a, d, f
6. a, b, c
7. Answers will vary.
8. b
9. h
10. c
11. f
12. e
13. a
14. d
15. g

16. __2__ Check hearing and vision.
    __4__ Ask orientation questions.
    __5__ Supplemental mental status examination (e.g., Mini-Cog, MMSE, MoCA)
    __1__ Note general appearance
    __3__ Give patient four words to remember for the Four Unrelated Words Test

17.

Characteristic	Delirium	Dementia	Depression
Sudden onset	X		
Impaired memory	X	X	
Level of consciousness not altered		X	X
Characterized by rapid emotional swings	X		
Reversible with proper treatment	X		X

CHAPTER 6: SUBSTANCE USE ASSESSMENT

1. b
2. b
3. c
4. c
5. a, c, d
6. b
7. a, b, e

8.

Characteristic	Alcohol	Marijana	Opiates	Cocaine
Pinpoint pupils			X	
Reddened eyes		X		
Pupillary dilation				X
Loss of balance	X	X		
Slurred speech	X		X	
Talkativeness	X			X

9.

Characteristic	Alcohol	Marijuana	Opiates	Cocaine
Irritability	X	X	X	X
Dilated pupils			X	
Hallucinations	X			
Fatigue				X
Hand tremors	X			

CHAPTER 7: FAMILY VIOLENCE AND HUMAN TRAFFICKING

1. b
2. a
3. b
4. c
5. b, c, d, e
6. b
7. a, c, d, f
8. a, d, f, h
9. are not, likely, effective

CHAPTER 8: ASSESSMENT TECHNIQUES AND SAFETY IN THE CLINICAL SETTING

1. c
2. a
3. a, b, e, f
4. c
5. a
6. b
7. a, c, e, f
8. d

9. The best position for this patient is <u>High Fowler's</u>. To complete the assessment, you should <u>complete a focused assessment</u> and <u>pause as necessary and provide breaks</u>.

10.

Position	Inpatient	Outpatient	Both
Supine			X
Lithotomy		X	
Semi-fowler's	X		
Sims'	X		
Dorsal recumbent			X

CHAPTER 9: GENERAL SURVEY AND MEASUREMENT

1. c
2. E.K. is a 39-year-old female who appears stated age, is alert and oriented, and appears well-nourished. <u>Facial grimace with movement</u>. <u>Pronounced limp with walking</u>. Height and weight appear normal for age and gender. No body odor. Good personal hygiene.
3. L.M. is an 89-year-old male who appears stated age, is alert and oriented <u>to person and place only</u>, and able to answer questions. <u>Wide, shuffling gait</u> noted. Kyphosis. No body odor noted. Clothing appropriate for season and age.
4. D.F. is an 18-month-old female. Appears stated age. Pronounced lordosis. Wide, unsteady gait. <u>Arm span shorter than height</u>. <u>Frontal bossing noted</u>.
5. The nurse should recognize that <u>lordosis</u>/kyphosis is normal for toddlers, while lordosis/<u>kyphosis</u> is normal for older adults. Other changes with aging include <u>loss of</u>/gain in subcutaneous fat in the face and extremities. Older adults lose height due to changes in the long bones/<u>vertebrae</u>.
6. a

CHAPTER 10: VITAL SIGNS

1. c
2. a, c
3. d
4. declines, lower, less
5. c
6. b
7. b
8. b, c, d, f, h

9.

Finding	Normal	Abnormal
Rectal temperature 37.7°C	X	
Respiratory rate 20 bpm, even	X	
Respiratory rate 9 bpm		X
Pulse 80 bpm, 2+, irregular		X
Temperature 35°C		X

10.

1 Palpate the artery if possible and apply coupling gel. If artery is not palpable, apply gel to the correct anatomical position.
2 Turn on Doppler flowmeter.
3 Touch the probe to skin, holding it perpendicular to the artery.
4 Once you hear the pulsatile whooshing, inflate the cuff until the sound disappears.
5 Continue inflation 20–30 mm Hg beyond the point at which the sound disappears
6 Slowly deflate the cuff noting the point at which sound is first heard. This is the systolic pressure.
7 Rapidly deflate the cuff allowing the blood to dissipate.

CHAPTER 11: PAIN ASSESSMENT

1. c
2. a
3. d
4. b
5. a, c, d, f, h
6. a, b, d, e, h, i

7.

Physiological Change	Acute Pain	Chronic Pain
Depression		X
Nausea	X	
Fear	X	
Isolation		X
Limited functioning		X
Tachycardia	X	

8. Mu-opioid receptors found in the <u>brainstem</u> lead to respiratory depression while mu-receptors located in the dorsal horn are responsible for pain <u>modulation</u> and those located in the ventral tegmental area are responsible for <u>pleasure</u>.
9. You are caring for a 62-year-old male who is receiving morphine to treat pain related to metastatic bone cancer. The patient also has chemotherapy-induced peripheral neuropathy. Vital signs: HR 124, regular; RR 30 bpm, shallow; BP 148/88, R arm, lying down. Complains of burning pain in bilateral feet, rated at 8/10.

CHAPTER 12: NUTRITION ASSESSMENT

1. a   2. a, c, f, g, i, l, m   3. a, c, e

4. A.L. is 54 inches tall and weighs 93 pounds. Vital signs: HR 85, RR 20, BP 110/80. Her <u>BMI is 22.4 which puts her in the 96th percentile</u>. Her total cholesterol is 165 mg/dL, her LDL is 99 mg/dL, and her <u>HDL is 35 mg/dL</u>. Her fasting glucose was <u>101 mg/dL</u>.
5. b
6. <u>Marasmus</u> is caused by inadequate protein intake, while <u>kwashiorkor</u> is caused by diets high in calories, but deficient in protein. A patient with <u>maramus/kwashiorkor mix</u> often has an emaciated appearance due to prolonged inadequate intake of protein and calories due to starvation.
7.

	Vitamin A	Vitamin B6	Vitamin D	Thiamine	Calcium
Rickets			X		X
Peripheral neuropathy		X		X	
Pale conjunctiva		X			
Bitot spots	X				
Osteomalacia			X		X
Dry skin	X				

8. K.L. is a 52-year-old female who comes to the clinic today for her annual checkup. During the history, she reports no recent changes to diet and has no acute concerns. Her current medications include <u>simvastatin (for high cholesterol), metformin (oral hypoglycemic)</u>, calcium supplement, fish oil supplement, and a multivitamin. Weight 205 pounds. Height 5'4". BMI 35.2. <u>WC 41 inches</u>. Vital signs: HR 89, RR 20, <u>BP 138/90</u>. Lungs are clear to auscultation. Mild edema bilateral lower extremities. All lab values are within normal limits.
9. a
10. a, b, c, d, e, f

CHAPTER 13: SKIN, HAIR, AND NAILS

1. c	13. c	24. c
2. d	14. a	25. a
3. b	15. b, d	26. b
4. a	16. a, b, c	27. d
5. d	17. a	28. b
6. a	18. c	29. a
7. b	19. b	30. g
8. a	20. c	31. c
9. a	21. a	32. f
10. c	22. a	33. d
11. b	23. b	34. e
12. c		

CHAPTER 14: HEAD, FACE, NECK, AND REGIONAL LYMPHATICS

1. c	9. a	16. h
2. c	10. a, b	17. g
3. b	11. a	18. i
4. a	12. b	19. j
5. a, b, d	13. c	20. b
6. c	14. e	21. d
7. d	15. f	22. a
8. d		

CHAPTER 15: EYES

1. a, c	6. a	11. c, g
2. c	7. a	12. a, b, d
3. a	8. c	13. b
4. a, c	9. a, b, c	14. a, b, d, e
5. a, c, d	10. b, c	

CHAPTER 16: EARS

1. b, c	6. a	11. a
2. c	7. b	12. c
3. a	8. c	13. a
4. d	9. c	
5. b	10. d	

CHAPTER 17: NOSE, MOUTH, AND THROAT

1. c	6. b	11. b, c, d
2. a, b	7. d	12. c
3. d	8. b, d	13. a
4. c	9. c	14. c
5. b	10. a	

CHAPTER 18: BREASTS, AXILLAE, AND REGIONAL LYMPHATICS

1. b, c	6. c	11. b, d
2. a	7. c	12. b
3. c	8. b	13. a, b, c
4. c	9. a, d	
5. c	10. a, b, d	

CHAPTER 19: THORAX AND LUNGS

1. b	8. d	15. b
2. d	9. c	16. e
3. d	10. d	17. a
4. a	11. e	18. d
5. d	12. a	19. f
6. b	13. c	20. c
7. d	14. d	21. b

22.

Assessment finding	Left-sided pneumothorax	Left-sided pneumonia
Dullness to percussion on the left side		X
Decreased breath sounds on the left side	X	
Coarse crackles on the left side		X
Decreased tactile fremitus on the left side	X	
Lag in expansion on the left side	X	X

23. Condition C, Assessment Finding D.

CHAPTER 20: HEART AND NECK VESSELS

1. c	8. c	15. d
2. b	9. b	16. e
3. c	10. b, d	17. c
4. b	11. d	18. f
5. d	12. c	19. a
6. a, c, d	13. a, b, d	20. b
7. a	14. b	21. d

22. S_1 is best heard at the <u>apex</u> of the heart, whereas S_2 is loudest at the <u>base</u> of the heart. S_1 coincides with the pulse in the <u>carotid artery</u> and coincides with the <u>R</u> wave if the patient is on an ECG monitor.

23. B, A, A

CHAPTER 21: PERIPHERAL VASCULAR SYSTEM AND LYMPHATIC SYSTEM

1. c	4. d	7. b
2. c	5. a	8. d
3. c	6. d	9. b

10. a. iv; b. iii; c. i; d. ii

11. You are assessing a woman with a history of <u>breast cancer</u>. She underwent a <u>right mastectomy 2 months ago</u> and is getting <u>radiation therapy</u>. She is concerned because her <u>right arm is swollen</u>, and she thinks she may have a blood clot. Your examination reveals <u>firm, non-pitting edema</u>. Her arm <u>pulses are 2+ bilaterally</u>. Her <u>skin is warm</u> and there are <u>no areas of redness or tenderness</u>.

12.

1. You are caring for a patient who presented to the emergency department with right leg pain. She reports <u>acute, sudden onset of very severe pain</u>, and your physical exam reveals <u>pallor, coolness, and pulselessness</u> in the right leg. You suspect the patient has <u>acute arterial insufficiency,</u> and your next action is to <u>contact the provider immediately.</u>

13.

Finding	Peripheral Artery Disease	Chronic Venous Insufficiency	Acute Deep Vein Thrombosis
Thin, shiny, hairless skin	X		
Thick skin with brown discoloration		X	
Red, warm skin			X
Hair loss	X		
Bilateral diminished pulses	X		
Varicose veins		X	
Unilateral edema			X

14. A 62-year-old man presents with complaints of <u>pain in calf in multiple positions</u>. You examine his legs and note <u>unilateral swelling and warmth</u>. You are concerned he may be experiencing <u>Acute DVT</u>.

CHAPTER 22: ABDOMEN

1. c	6. a, b, c	11. d
2. a	7. a	12. b
3. c	8. d	13. d
4. b	9. b	14. a
5. c, e, f, g	10. c	15. d

16. You are examining a patient with a distended abdomen. The patient has a history of <u>cirrhosis</u> and type 2 diabetes. The shape of the abdomen is <u>protuberant</u> with a <u>single, uniform curve</u>. The patient's <u>flanks are bulging slightly,</u> and the <u>skin appears shiny and taut</u>. The patient has no <u>tenderness</u> to palpation.

CHAPTER 23: MUSCULOSKELETAL SYSTEM

1. a, c, f, h, j	8. i	14. n
2. 2, 5, 4	9. d	15. l
3. d	10. a	16. h
4. b, f, g	11. j	17. f
5. b	12. m	18. c
6. e	13. k	
7. g		

19.

Change in the Musculoskeletal System	Expected	Not expected
Boggy metacarpophalangeal joints		X
Kyphosis	X	
Lordosis		X
Flexion in hips	X	
Flexion in knees	X	
Osteoarthritis		X

20.

	Infant	Toddler	Preschool/school age	Pregnant woman
Lordosis		X		X
Varus position of feet/legs (flexible)	X	X	X	
Valgus position of feet/legs (flexible)	X	X	X	
Cervical flexion				X

21. The client comes to the clinic with reports of <u>bilateral swelling and pain of the DIP joints in her fingers</u>. She also complains of <u>fatigue and weight loss</u> for the past year. VS: HR 86 bpm, regular, RR 18 bpm, unlabored, <u>Temperature 100.5°F,</u> BP 110/78. Upon physical examination, the <u>DIP joints are tender and warm with limited range of motion bilaterally</u>. Full ROM in all other joints. Muscle strength—able to maintain flexion against resistance. <u>Atrophy noted in interosseous muscles of hands bilaterally</u>.

22. The client most likely has <u>rheumatoid arthritis</u> which is an <u>inflammatory condition</u> typically involving <u>symmetric</u> joints in the <u>feet</u> and <u>hands</u>.

23.

Potential Steps	Appropriate steps
1. Position self in front of client so entire torso is visible.	
2. Note level of shoulders, scapulae, and iliac crests.	2
3. Position self behind client so full spine is visible.	1
4. Note level of shoulders, ribs, and superior iliac spine.	
5. Ask client to bend at the waist and reach for toes.	3
6. Note level of superior iliac spine while bent forward.	
7. Note level of shoulders, ribs, and iliac crests while bent forward.	4

CHAPTER 24: NEUROLOGIC SYSTEM

1. b
2. d
3. a
4. d
5. c
6. a. d
7. a
8. a
9. c
10. a
11. b, c, e
12. f
13. b
14. g
15. k
16. h
17. c
18. l
19. d
20. i
21. e
22. j
23. a

CHAPTER 25: MALE GENITOURINARY SYSTEM

1. d
2. a
3. a, c, d, f
4. b, c
5. b
6. d
7. b
8. b
9. a, d
10. c
11. b
12. d
13. a

CHAPTER 26: ANUS, RECTUM, AND PROSTATE

1. a
2. d
3. d, e

4. c
5. b
6. a, c, e, f, g

7. b
8. a

CHAPTER 27: FEMALE GENITOURINARY SYSTEM

1. d
2. b
3. d
4. a

5. a
6. b
7. a, c, d, f, g
8. a

9. d
10. a

11. The findings are: <u>slit-like appearance of the os; occasional small smooth yellow nodules on</u> the cervix; <u>thick opaque stringy cervical secretions; foul smelling secretions.</u>

12. The findings are:<u> cervix feels smooth;</u> cervix feels hard; <u>cervix is equally rounded;</u> cervix does not move with examiner's finger movement; cervical movement produces some pain.

13. You are caring for a 32-year-old woman who presents to the clinic with a vaginal discharge. She has not had vaginal intercourse for 5 years before arrival. A. She reports (4) <u>intense itching</u>, <u>recent treatment for bronchitis.</u> B. Your physical examination reveals (1) <u>red and swollen vulva and vagina. Thick, white, curdy, nonsmelling discharge.</u> C. You suspect she has (3) So–A = 4, B = 1, C = 3 <u>Candidiasis (Moniliasis).</u>

CHAPTER 31: PREGNANCY

1. a, d, e

2. c

3. a

4.

	Presumptive	Probable	Positive
Amenorrhea	X		
Enlarged uterus		X	
Fatigue	X		
FHTs			X
Nausea	X		
Breast tenderness	X		
Cardiac activity on US			X

5. The nurse should recognize <u>proteinuria</u> and <u>hypertension</u> are classic symptoms of preeclampsia, but <u>proteinuria</u> is not required for diagnosis. Onset and worsening of symptoms may be <u>sudden</u> and rapid intervention is necessary. <u>HELLP</u> is a serious variant of preeclampsia.

6. The nurse is caring for a <u>38-year-old</u> female who is <u>gravida 8, para 8</u>. All spontaneous vaginal deliveries after 38 weeks gestation. She reports a <u>history of preeclampsia</u> with her last two pregnancies with no long-term sequelae. She states the preeclampsia occurred "right at the end" of each pregnancy, though she does not remember specific information. She is <u>5'4"</u> and weighs <u>225 pounds. Her pre pregnancy weight was 180</u> pounds. She is <u>36 weeks gestation</u> and is <u>in active labor.</u> Her due date was confirmed by US at 21 weeks gestation. FHTs 155 bpm with normal accelerations. Vital signs: <u>HR 110 bpm</u>, RR 20 bpm,

unlabored, <u>BP 146/98</u>, T 97.5°F. Currently rating pain at 2/10 at rest and 10/10 during contractions. <u>Medical history of PPH</u> with last pregnancy <u>requiring blood transfusion</u>. Routine medications include a prenatal vitamin.

7. a, d   8. b

9.

	Physiologic	Pathologic
Mammary souffle	X	
Purulent nipple discharge		X
Diastolic murmur 2/6		X
Breast enlargement	X	
Decreased cardiac output		X
Blood volume increase by 45%	X	
Slight hemodilution	X	
Increased pulse	X	

CHAPTER 32: FUNCTIONAL ASSESSMENT OF THE OLDER ADULT

1. b   2. b, c, f, g, h, i

3. and 4. The nurse is caring for an 86-year-old patient who was hospitalized with a urinary tract infection and acute confusion x 2 days. The patient was admitted for IV antibiotics. The nurse receives the following information during shift report: A.K. is an 86-year-old gentleman who lives at home with his wife. His brother died in Vietnam and his son died in the first Iraq war. He has a history of arthritis, and he had an MI 15 years ago. No history of dementia or cognitive impairment. He is <u>alert and oriented to person and place only,</u> but his cognition is improving. Upon admission he was only oriented to person. His <u>Timed Up and Go test was 14 seconds</u>. His wife reports that he's <u>fallen at home twice</u> in the past 2 months. Upon physical exam, VS are as follows <u>HR 101 bpm, RR 26 bpm, shallow</u>, BP 110/60. Lungs clear and equal bilaterally; normal S1S2 no extra sounds, no murmur. DTRs 1+ and equal. Difficulty with whispered voice test.

5. b   6. c

7. The nurse should recognize that a Timed Up and Go test greater than <u>12</u> seconds indicates a person is at high risk for <u>falls</u>. The person should be <u>allowed</u> to use normal assistive devices and shoes <u>should</u> be worn.

8.

Sit down in chair	5
Turn around	3
Walk 15 feet	
Rise from chair	1
Walk 10 feet	2
Walk back to chair	4
Walk to the other chair	

9. M.K. lives in a single-story home in a safe neighborhood of town. Streetlights are present though functionality was not assessed since it is daytime. The neighborhood has sidewalks, and the nearest fire station is 4 blocks away. M.K. no longer drives and the <u>nearest bus stop is approximately 1 mile away</u>. There is a grocery store within 2 miles. The house has no steps to enter. There are <u>throw rugs in the entry way, the kitchen, and in each of the two bathrooms</u>. The <u>toilet is lower than standard and there are no grab bars</u>. Curtains are open and the home is well-lit. <u>Old magazines and books are neatly stacked all over the floor.</u>

10.
1. Remove throw rugs since they are a tripping hazard.
2. Ask the person about social support and transportation. Provide referral to resources as appropriate.
3. Recommend reorganization of magazines to get them off the floor as they are trip hazards.
4. Consider a renovation to place a standard height toilet or use a raised toilet seat addition.
5. Put grab bars in the bathroom.

Answers to Next-Generation NCLEX® (NGN) Examination–Style Unfolding Case Studies

UNFOLDING CASE STUDY 1: PEDIATRIC HEALTH ASSESSMENT

Question 1: Highlight/Recognize Cues

Highlight any important cues in the Nurses' Notes and Vital Signs that require **immediate** follow-up by the nurse.

Health History	Nurses' Notes	Vital Signs	Laboratory Results

1000: A 10-year-old male patient arrives at the Emergency Department (ED) via private car with his mother, who is his legal guardian. Mother reports that the patient was riding his bicycle without a helmet when the front tire entered a drain grid. Patient hit the handlebars and then flew over top of the bicycle to the ground. Event was witnessed by the mother who denies patient's loss of consciousness. Mother brought the patient directly from the scene to the ED. Patient is alert and acting appropriately for his age. Patient is crying, holding his stomach. Scrapes noted on bilateral forearms oozing blood, as well as an obvious deformity to his right lower leg. Immunizations are up to date per mother. NKDA. Denies significant PMH.

Health History	Nurses' Notes	Vital Signs	Laboratory Results

1000: Initial vital signs in triage

T 98.2°F (36.8°C)/HR 140 bpm, regular/RR 22 bpm, crying/BP 142/72 mm Hg/Spo$_2$ 97% on RA

Pain 6/10 using FACES scale

Weight: 27.2 kilograms

Question 2: Select All That Apply/Analyze Cues

The nurse is concerned about the patient's crying and reported pain level of 6/10. What factors may be the cause of the reported pain? **Select all that apply.**

1. Fear of the hospital environment
2. Right lower leg injury
3. Abdominal pain
4. Fracture to arm
5. Pain to face and head

    Answers: 1, 2, 3

Question 3: Drag and Drop Table/Recognize and Analyze Cues

Drag the cues in the Nurses' Notes and Glasgow Score Options to calculate the Glasgow Coma Scale below.

Health History	Nurses' Notes	Vital Signs	Laboratory Results

1015: Patient to room 18, placed in bed, supine, report given by triage nurse to RN who assumed care of patient. Primary trauma survey as follows:

A-airway intact/B-breathing Within Normal Limits (WNL)/C-capillary refill 2 s with pulses 2+ bilaterally/D-disability—alert and age appropriate; patient opens eyes spontaneously, answers most questions appropriately but at times is confused, obeys commands with purposeful movement/E-environment—clothes are damp from sweat and blood; patient's clothing is cut off with a gown placed and warm blankets applied/F-family presence—mother is worried and at patient's bedside/G-give comfort—right lower leg splinted; patient reassured with plan of care updated to both mother and patient.

Glasgow Score Options: 1, 2, 3, 4, 5, 6, 7, 8

Cues	Associated Score
1. Patient opens eyes spontaneously	1. 4
2. Answers most questions, but at times is confused	2. 4
3. Obeys commands with purposeful movement	3. 6
Glasgow Score Calculation: ___14_____	

Question 4: Multiple Response Select N/Analyze Cues

The nurse prepares to start the secondary survey of the patient. In addition to a head-to-toe examination, and using findings identified prior, the nurse will plan to perform focused assessments on which **four** of the following?

☑ Abdomen
☐ Heart
☑ Neurologic
☐ Thorax and lungs
☑ Peripheral vascular
☑ Musculoskeletal
☐ Skin
☐ Neck

Question 5: Highlight in Text/Recognize Cues

The nurse prepares to speak with the provider about the patient's assessment findings. From the 1045 note, **highlight the three symptoms from the nurses' note** and **highlight any abnormal vital signs in the flow-sheet** to relay to the provider.

Health History	Nurses' Notes	Vital Signs	Laboratory Results

1045: Head-to-toe secondary survey complete. Patient log rolled with c-spine immobilization maintained. Back and spine WNL. IV established. IV fluid bolus initiated and labs sent. Patient with increased complaints of nausea and dry heaving. Abdominal distention is noted, and bowel sounds hypoactive with tenderness in the right upper quadrant upon palpation. X-ray of right leg at bedside.

Health History	Nurses' Notes	Vital Signs	Laboratory Results

1000: T 98.2°F (36.8°C)/HR 140 bpm, regular/RR 22 bpm, crying/BP 142/72 mm Hg/Spo$_2$ 97% on RA

1015: T 97.0°F (36.1°C)/HR 122 bpm/RR 20 bpm/BP 120/78 mm Hg/Spo$_2$ 96% on RA

1030: T 97.8°F (36.6°C)/HR 138 bpm/RR 20 pm/BP 118/72 mm Hg/Spo$_2$ 96% on RA

1045: T 97.8°F (36.6°C)/HR 138 bpm/RR 22 bpm/BP 99/70 mm Hg/Spo$_2$ 96% on RA

Question 6: Matrix Multiple Response/Analyze Cues/Prioritize Hypotheses

Select the **most likely** involved organ with the assessment finding in the table below. Each column must have at least one selection and each row may have more than one response option.

Symptoms	Liver	Spleen	Kidney(s)
Abdominal distention	X	X	
Nausea, dry heaving	X	X	X
Tenderness RUQ abd with palpation	X		

Bonus Questions to Level Up With Critical Thinking

1. What could the vital sign trend be indicative of?
   a. **Answer:** Hypovolemic shock
2. What lab values from a CBC, CMP, Type and Cross, coagulation profile, and lactate level are important for this patient and why?
   a. **Answer:** CBC: Hematocrit and Hemoglobin; CMP: all components for a patient baseline of the kidney and liver functions and electrolytes; Type and Cross: blood type to determine for the patient if a blood transfusion is needed; Coagulation Profile: PT, PTT, and INR all important (if the liver is injured) as it can effect bleeding times putting the patient at an increased risk of uncontrolled bleeding; Lactate: to assess level as a marker for tissue perfusion or hypoperfusion.

UNFOLDING CASE STUDY 2: ADULT HEALTH ASSESSMENT

Question 1: Drag and Drop Cloze/Analyze Cues

Health History	Nurses' Notes	Vital Signs	Laboratory Results

0830: October 10th—A 41-year-old female arrives at the clinic today as a follow-up visit for wound check. The patient reports that she was "getting ramen soup out of the microwave when it splashed on her arms." Accident occurred 10 days prior. Patient was seen in the ED with treatment for first- and second-degree splash burns.

Bandages to bilateral arms intact, dry, and clean. Patient has been applying over-the-counter antibiotic ointment to the areas and dressing twice per day. Complains of a "throbbing" pain, reports it as 5 out of 10. Describes pain as constant, nonradiating focused to round wound areas on bilateral arms, worse the past 2 days. Patient has not been changing the dressing the past 2 days as it seemed to make the pain worse.

T 100.0°F (37.8°C)/HR 86 bpm/RR 18 bpm/BP 138/78 mm Hg/Spo$_2$ 97% RA.

The nurse wants to ensure they have assessed the patient's pain completely. Drag and drop from the items below to finish what the nurse should document for the PQRST acronym related to pain:
P: Changing the dressing, **Q:** Throbbing, **R:** Nonradiating, **S:** 5/10 on 0–10 numerical scale, **T:** Constant.

Question 2: Drag and Drop Rationale/Prioritize Hypotheses

Drag one potential risk and one assessment finding to complete the sentence for this patient.
   Answer: The nurse knows the patient is at risk for <u>Infection</u> due to <u>Wounds</u>.

Potential Risk	Assessment Finding
Sleep deprivation	Wounds
Infection	Scarring from burn
Poor self-image	Pain
Poor pain control	Lack of proper dressing changes

Question 3: Highlight/Recognize Cues

Highlight the cues in the Health History note which puts the patient at an increased health risk.

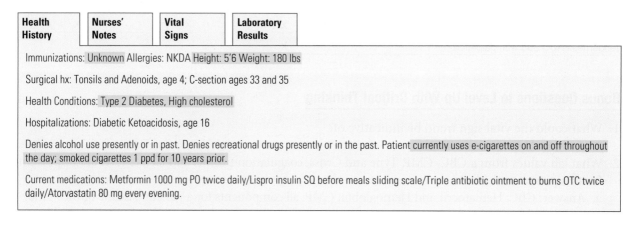

Health History	Nurses' Notes	Vital Signs	Laboratory Results

Immunizations: Unknown Allergies: NKDA Height: 5'6 Weight: 180 lbs

Surgical hx: Tonsils and Adenoids, age 4; C-section ages 33 and 35

Health Conditions: Type 2 Diabetes, High cholesterol

Hospitalizations: Diabetic Ketoacidosis, age 16

Denies alcohol use presently or in past. Denies recreational drugs presently or in the past. Patient currently uses e-cigarettes on and off throughout the day; smoked cigarettes 1 ppd for 10 years prior.

Current medications: Metformin 1000 mg PO twice daily/Lispro insulin SQ before meals sliding scale/Triple antibiotic ointment to burns OTC twice daily/Atorvastatin 80 mg every evening.

Question 4: Select All That Apply/Analyze Cues

Health History	Nurses' Notes	Vital Signs	Laboratory Results

0900, October 10th: Patient was discharged with verbal and written instructions given. Patient verbalized understanding. Wound consult ordered and a home visit scheduled with the nurse in 2 days for wound check. Patient advised to continue with triple antibiotic ointment to wounds and dressing changes twice a day.

The nurse, in preparation for discharge, would add which items for patient education handouts? **Select all that apply.**

1. Smoking cessation
2. Medication compliance
3. Nonpharmacologic and pharmacologic pain options
4. Wound care
5. Daily nutrition charts

   Answers: 1, 3, 4

Question 5: Drag and Drop Table/Analyze Cues

Subjective and Objective data were obtained from the wound nurse's focused assessment.

Health History	Nurses' Notes	Vital Signs	Laboratory Results

1200, October 12th: S (situation): Wound nurse visit to patient's home for a wound follow-up assessment.

B (background): Patient at day 12 from occurrence of accidental burn. Had follow-up visit at day 10 with primary health care clinic. Patient has been treating bilat arm burn with triple antibiotic ointment and dressings twice per day. Reports taking OTC ibuprofen for pain.

A (assessment): Bilateral arms with full range of motion. 2+ radial pulses bilaterally, 2-second cap refill bilaterally. Varying degrees of healing to skin on both arms. Some blisters have popped and are oozing yellow drainage. Red streaks from the burns on right arm extending up to right elbow. Right arm is warm to touch.

Vital signs: T 101.5°F (38.6°C)/HR 100 bpm/RR 22 bpm/BP 145/90 mm Hg/Spo$_2$ 97% RA

Patient reports blood sugar at home running in the 300s and "running out of her insulin and is waiting for the refill to come via mail delivery."

R (recommendation): Patient sent to ED for evaluation of possible infection of wound.

Drag and drop from the list of subjective and objective findings below to place in the corresponding normal or abnormal finding column.

Normal Finding	Abnormal Finding
OTC ibuprofen for pain	Varying degrees of healing to skin on both arms
Bilat arms with full range of motion	Blisters with yellow drainage
2+ radial pulses	Red streaks from burn on right arm extending to right elbow
Two-second capillary refill	Right arm warm to touch
Spo$_2$ 97% RA	T 101.5°F (38.6°C)
	HR 100 bpm
R 22 bpm	BP 145/90 mm Hg
	Blood sugar running in the 300s

Question 6: Multiple Response Select N/Analyze Cues/Recognize Hypotheses

Using the Subjective and Objective Findings list from Question 5, select **seven** assessments that correspond with the wound nurse's R (recommendation) to send the patient to the ED for possible infection of wound

☐ OTC ibuprofen for pain
☑ Varying degrees of healing to skin on both arms
☐ Bilat arms with full range of motion
☐ +2 radial pulses
☐ Two-second capillary refill
☑ Blisters with yellow drainage
☑ Red streaks from burn on right arm extending to right elbow
☑ Right arm warm to touch
☑ T 101.5°F (38.6°C)
☑ HR 100 bpm
☐ RR 22 bpm
☑ BP 145/90 mm Hg
☐ Spo$_2$ 97% RA
☑ Blood sugar running in 300s

Bonus Questions to Level Up With Critical Thinking

1. Describe why pathophysiologically a patient with diabetes is at an increased risk for proper wound healing.
    a. **Answer:** Elevated blood sugar impairs the immune system's ability to repair and replace cells.
2. What labs do you think would be ordered for the patient once they are sent to the ED as a recommendation from the wound nurse in relation to ruling out infection?
    a. **Answer:** CBC: for white blood cell count; blood culture: to make sure there are no bacteria growing in the blood; wound culture: to assess what bacteria are growing in the wound and to help determine proper antibiotic; lactic acid: as a measurement to ensure the patient is not septic from the infection.

UNFOLDING CASE STUDY 3: OLDER ADULT HEALTH ASSESSMENT

Question 1: Drop Down Cloze/Recognize Cues/Analyze Cues

Health History	Nurses' Notes	Vital Signs	Laboratory Results

0800: Day 1 admission to cardiac floor, General Hospital, an 83-year-old is admitted for shortness of breath, chest pain, and positive for COVID.

Per family, patient is alert and oriented to person and place for baseline mental status. Lives with her daughter due to advanced dementia. Upon admission, patient is confused, only alert to person at this time. Tested positive for COVID 6 days prior to admission. Progression of illness and weakness brought patient via ambulance to the hospital for evaluation and care.

Vitals: T-99.0°F (37.2°C)/HR-105 bpm, irregular/RR-20 bpm/BP-122/68 mm Hg/Spo_2 95% on 2 L nasal cannula.

The nurse wants to assess the patient's pain score to complete the vital signs. Utilizing the information from the nurses' notes, the nurse identifies two cues (options 1 and 2) that determine the pain assessment tool that should be used for this patient (option 3): _____1_____, _____2_____, _____3_____.
    Answers:

Options for 1	Options for 2	Options for 3
Confused	Advanced Dementia	PAINAD Scale

Question 2: Drop Down Cloze/Recognize Cues/Analyze Cues

Complete the following sentences by choosing from the list of options.
    When taking vital signs, the nurse noted the _____1_____ pulse to be irregular. The nurse knows to follow up by auscultating the _____2_____ rate for _____3_____ minute(s).
    Answers:

Options for 1	Options for 2	Options for 3
Radial	Apical	One

Question 3: Select All that Apply/Analyze Cues

Health History	Nurses' Notes	Vital Signs	Laboratory Results

0430: Day 2 of admission to cardiac floor, General Hospital, 83-year-old

Daughter remains at the bedside. Patient A&O x1 with increase work of breathing, clutching her chest. Focused assessment of the thorax, lungs, and heart performed. Patient is lifted upright in a high fowler position with oxygen increased to 5 L nasal cannula. Symmetrical lung expansion, lungs with bilateral inspiratory crackles auscultated. No crepitus. S_1-S_2 normal, not accentuated or diminished, S_3 gallop present. No carotid bruit.

VS: T 101.0°F (38.3°C)/HR 110 bpm, irregular/RR 36 bpm/BP 101/70 mm Hg/Spo$_2$ 90% on 5 L nasal cannula

Provider notified of patient status. New orders received for STAT portable chest x-ray, EKG, troponin, BNP, and arterial blood gas. Call respiratory to place patient on heated high flow oxygen. Transfer patient to Intensive Care Unit.

What **significant changes** in the patient's status from day 1 admission notes to day 2 admission notes will the nurse include in their report? (**Select all that apply.**)

1. Clutching her chest
2. A & O X1
3. Increased work of breathing, RR 36 bpm
4. Oxygen increased to 5 L nasal cannula, Spo$_2$ 90%
5. Bilateral inspiratory crackles auscultated
6. S3 gallop present
7. T 101.0°F (38.3°C)
8. HR 110 bpm, irregular, BP 101/70 mm Hg
9. Symmetrical lung expansion
10. COVID positive

Answers: 1, 3, 4, 5, 6, 7

Question 4: Multiple Response Grouping/Recognize Cues/Analyze Cues

Choose the finding(s) and abnormal finding(s) that correspond with each body system.

A. Body System	B. Normal Assessment Findings	C. Abnormal Assessment Finding
Thorax and lungs	☐ BP 105/70 ☐ Confusion ☒ Symmetrical lung expansion ☐ Clutching of chest ☒ No crepitus	☒ Bilateral inspiratory crackles ☒ Spo$_2$ 90% on 5 L nasal cannula ☐ HR in the 120 s, irregular ☐ S3 gallop ☐ T 101.0°F (38.3°C)
Heart	☒ BP 105/70 ☐ Bilateral inspiratory crackles ☐ Symmetrical lung expansion ☐ Clutching chest ☒ No carotid bruit	☐ Confusion ☐ RR 36 bpm ☒ HR 110 bpm, irregular ☒ S3 gallop ☐ BP 105/70

Question 5: Highlight in Text/Recognize Cues

Highlight the cues the nurse should make note to follow up on in the Nurses' Notes

Health History	Nurses' Notes	Vital Signs	Laboratory Results

0930: Day 8 Follow-up visit post discharge from hospital, Primary Care Office

Patient follow-up visit after a 7-day hospitalization for COVID pneumonia and new onset atrial fibrillation. Daughter is with patient. Daughter reports she has hired someone to help with her mother until the patient regains some of her strength. Using walker with gait belt.

Patient is alert and oriented to person and place, which daughter reports is her baseline. Denies any complaints of pain. Skin tear noted to right lower extremity. Lungs with fine crackles bilaterally. Heart S_1-S_2, not accentuated or diminished, regular rhythm, 74 bpm. Grade 2/6 Murmur heard at apex. 1+ pitting edema to bilateral lower extremities. Appetite slowly improving. Daughter denies recent fever. Denies any falls. Denies any issues with current medications.

Question 6: Drop Down Cloze/Analyze Cues

Complete the following sentence by choosing from the list of options.

The nurse knows a murmur heard at the apex suggests a problem with the <u>mitral valve</u>.

Bonus Questions to Level Up With Critical Thinking

1. Describe what pneumonia versus congestive heart failure would look like in a patient, i.e., pathophysiology of condition, subjective findings, assessment findings?
   Answer: See Table 19.9, Unit 3: Physical Examination, Jarvis.
2. The patient had baseline confusion from dementia history. What else can cause acute confusion or an increase in confusion from baseline?
   Answer: Hypoxia, infection and/or sepsis, acute brain bleed or infarction, medications and/or recreational drugs, psychosis, delirium, abnormal labs such as sodium or glucose.

NOTES

NOTES

NOTES

NOTES

NOTES

NOTES

NOTES

NOTES